Ten tips for permanent weight l

1) Recognise that this is something you are going to do for *yourself* – not for your partner, not for your family or friends, but for *you*.
2) Weigh and measure yourself using reliable techniques.
3) Discover the real reasons why you struggle with your weight and fix the problems at their source.
4) Wait until you feel comfortably and physically hungry before eating or drinking anything containing kilojoules.
5) Don't let yourself get ravenously hungry, and eat enough of the types and amounts of mostly nutritious foods that make you feel genuinely satisfied.
6) Aim to eat at least two serves of fruit and at least five serves of vegetables every day.
7) Don't strive for some impossible standard of perfection. I'll show you how to lose weight while enjoying your favourite foods and beverages.
8) If you're not already very active, find ways to be a bit more active than you are now. Even a modest increase in your activity levels will help you to lose weight.
9) Take a weight loss holiday. Sometimes you just need to take a break from trying to lose weight.
10) Live your life to the full right now, as if you'd already lost all the excess weight you want to lose.

Others have done it, including myself, and *so can you*.

Amanda.

Dr Amanda Sainsbury-Salis, PhD

About the author

Dr Amanda Sainsbury-Salis is an internationally renowned Australian weight loss scientist with a PhD from the University of Geneva, Switzerland. Her groundbreaking research into weight regulation has been published in a number of prestigious science journals, including *The Journal of Clinical Investigation*, *Diabetes*, *Genes and Development*, *Nature Medicine* and *Cell Metabolism*. Her work has also been featured on national and international radio, including ABC Radio National's *Health Report* with Dr Norman Swan. Dr Amanda leads a research team investigating how the brain controls body weight at the Garvan Institute of Medical Research in Sydney, Australia, and is an Associate Professor in the School of Medical Sciences at the University of New South Wales. She lectures to medical professionals around the world about the science of weight regulation. Dr Amanda has received numerous awards for her research, including the 2002 Young Investigator Award from the Australian and New Zealand Obesity Society and the 2004 NSW Young Tall Poppy Science Award from the Australian Institute of Policy and Science. In 2008 she was selected by the International Association for the Study of Obesity to be the Chairperson of the International Conference on Sex and Obesity in Bangkok, Thailand. Dr Amanda lives in Sydney with her husband and their two children.

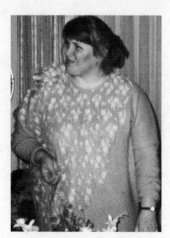

Dr Amanda before
losing weight

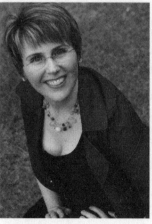

Dr Amanda today

Don't Go Hungry for Life

Dr Amanda Sainsbury-Salis, PhD

BANTAM

SYDNEY AUCKLAND TORONTO NEW YORK LONDON

A Bantam book
Published by Random House Australia Pty Ltd
Level 3, 100 Pacific Highway, North Sydney NSW 2060
www.randomhouse.com.au

First published by Bantam in 2011

Addresses for companies within the Random House Group can be found at www.randomhouse.com.au/offices

National Library of Australia
Cataloguing-in-Publication Entry

Sainsbury-Salis, Amanda
Don't go hungry for life

ISBN 978 1 74166 963 3 (pbk)

Reducing diets.
Weight loss.
Self-actualization (Psychology).

613.25

Cover photograph by Spanish Alex
Cover design by saso content & design pty ltd
Internal design and typesetting by Midland Typesetters, Australia
Printed in Australia by Griffin Press, an accredited ISO AS/NZS 14001:2004 Environmental Management System printer

10 9 8 7 6 5 4 3 2 1

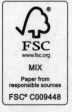

FSC
www.fsc.org
MIX
Paper from
responsible sources
FSC® C009448

The paper this book is printed on is certified against the Forest Stewardship Council® Standards. Griffin Press holds FSC chain of custody certification SGS-COC-005088. FSC promotes environmentally reponsible, socially beneficial and economically viable management of the world's forests

For all the people who kindly agreed to share their personal stories in this book so that others could learn from their experiences.

Contents

Getting started

Chapter 1

Escaping from Diet Dungeon

A man will be imprisoned in a room with a door that's unlocked and opens inwards, as long as it does not occur to him to pull rather than push.

Ludwig Wittgenstein, Austrian–British philosopher, 1889–1951

As a scientist specialising in weight loss research, and as someone who has lost 28 kilos and kept them off for what is now more than 13 years, I have written this book with one mission in mind: to help you escape from Diet Dungeon and to set you on the path to successful, sustainable weight management. Come with me on this new journey, and I'll show you exactly what to do and guide you every step of the way.

Diet Dungeon is a place I once knew well. Since you are reading this book, you've more than likely done time there yourself, or are still doing time. It's not literally a prison, of course – you checked yourself in, after all, 'for your own good' – but it feels like one. It's that dark, dreary place full of restrictions where your thoughts keep coming back to rules about what you can and cannot eat, and where your relationship with food is dominated by feelings of guilt. That dark place where on the first day of every week, month, year or decade you start the Diet To End All Diets, only to crash and burn before you reach your desired destination. That dark place where you loathe seeing photos or reflections of yourself, where you can't be the person you want to be, or give your full attention to the people close to you, because you're too busy hating the way you look or counting the kilojoule, fat, carbohydrate and protein content of every single thing you eat. That dark place to which you feel your genes, or your plain bad luck, have consigned you, and from which you feel there is no escape if you are to exert some degree of control over your weight.

In this book I explain the weight loss principles that will enable you to walk free of Diet Dungeon forever and lose weight for life in a healthier and more sustainable way. These principles are based on knowledge gained from my 20 years of medical research into successful weight management. Together, my research team and I have published more than 60 reports in leading international science journals, including *The Journal of Clinical Investigation*, *Diabetes*, *Nature Medicine* and *Cell Metabolism*, and we have attracted some $6 million in government and industry grants in order to further our research into successful weight loss. In this book, I'll show you how to lose weight and keep it off in a way that may feel foreign to you, a way that you may even think seems too simple to be effective, but one that really works – just like opening an unlocked door that opens inwards by pulling rather than pushing.

We now know from scientific research that our bodies are programmed to attain and maintain an ideal healthy weight. When you follow your body's signals about what, when and how much to eat, choosing from reasonably healthy foods, and combine this with some form of regular physical activity, you automatically lose excess weight until you reach the optimum weight for your body. Simply, and without having to count kilojoules, fats or carbs, or estimate portion sizes, or sacrifice your lifestyle and eat separate foods to your family, friends and colleagues. While you do need to be attentive to your food choices in order to lose weight in this way, you don't need to eat like the Dux of the Diet Club. You can eat normal foods every day and still lose weight: toasted wraps filled with roasted vegetables and chicken and dressed with pesto, or hummus made with adequate quantities of tahini, olive oil and full-fat yogurt (not the low-fat varieties that can seem so airy and bland), or a proper roast dinner with starchy vegetables such as peas, pumpkin, potatoes and parsnips. And if you enjoy an occasional choc bomb when you go to the movies, a pub lunch with your friends on Fridays, or a scone with jam and cream with tea at your favourite café, you can still enjoy these treasured treats from time to time as you lose weight. Many people simply can't believe that eating in such a normal way could result in lasting weight loss, but having seen the scientific evidence that it works from my research into body weight regulation, having used the information myself to escape from Diet Dungeon and subsequently lose 28 kilos – which I have kept off for what is now more than 13 years – and having seen many other people do the same, I know that it *does* work.

Why I wrote this sequel to *The Don't Go Hungry Diet*

I've seen many people struggle with their weight, usually because they were trying to lose weight by the conventional approach, which is at odds with how our bodies are designed to work. No wonder it seems such a struggle.

THE CONVENTIONAL APPROACH TO LOSING WEIGHT

Eat less, move more, and *keep going until you reach your ideal weight.*

However you go about it, to lose weight you need to consume fewer kilojoules than you burn. What most people don't realise, however, is that *continuous adherence* to conventional weight loss methods triggers strong physiological reactions that make it exceedingly difficult for anyone to continue losing weight and that also promote rapid rebound weight regain.

The overwhelming majority of diets are based on this conventional approach to weight loss, and in *The Don't Go Hungry Diet* I explained why they don't work in the long term. In that book, I explained what happens to your physiology when you try to lose weight, and why it's so much more effective to work with your body by eating as much as you need to eat when you feel physically hungry than to work against your body by trying to stick to rigid kilojoule allowances until you reach your ideal weight. Since then, I have given live workshops explaining these principles to thousands of people all around Australia, and I have been delighted to receive hundreds of emails from readers and workshop participants telling me of their experiences. Many wrote about the *Aha!* moments they had experienced when reading my book and putting its principles into action in their daily life. They wrote of newfound freedom, of finally being able to lose weight without constantly being obsessed about what, when and how much to eat. Some lost weight slowly, about half a kilo or one kilo a month, and others lost weight more rapidly, up to 2 kilos a week, depending on their circumstances. Regardless of their rate of weight loss or how much weight they lost, all of these people told me how delighted they were to be able to lose weight without feeling deprived or hungry. I felt that I was achieving my mission in life to have been able to help them.

Other people wrote and told me how much they loved my book or workshop and how excited they were at the prospect of trying this approach for themselves, but first they wanted to know if someone in their particular situation would be able to follow the program and if it would work for them. I spent many hours on my computer at night answering emails and helping people over those initial hurdles so that they could start losing weight by connecting with their body. I also initiated a regular newsletter to help people with the practicalities of losing weight by connecting with their body. (If you'd like to register for my newsletter, details of my website can be found at the back of this book.) Many wrote back some time later and told me that they had started losing weight, and that was always gratifying.

And then there was another kind of email, and it's mainly in response to these emails that I wrote this book. These emails were from people telling me that despite trying to follow the principles of *The Don't Go Hungry Diet* for a couple of weeks or a month, they hadn't lost any weight or had even gained a kilo or two. I know how awful it feels when your weight doesn't do what you want it to do, and so I'd write back as soon as I could to help these people start losing weight. Often it was a question of tweaking just one or two things, and after a couple of emails or a phone call they'd be off and running on their weight loss adventure. Other people wanted more intensive help, and so they enlisted my support in the form of coaching, via email, over the phone or face-to-face. I helped adults – mostly women – in all different circumstances in all different corners of Australia and New Zealand, and even as far distant as the US, Canada and the UK. In the process of helping such a wide variety of people, it became crystal clear to me that despite their differences in age, past dieting experiences and geography, all were making just one, two or at most three out of ten common mistakes, and these mistakes were preventing them from losing weight permanently. In other words, they were doing most things right, but then unknowingly sabotaging their efforts by falling down in one to three areas. Most of these people were being held back by ways of thinking instilled in them over years of conventional dieting, which goes against our natural physiology. Once I helped them to identify where they were going wrong, they were able to start losing weight in an effective and sustainable way. The difference that this self-awareness made to these people's lives was so gratifying to watch that I wanted more people to be able to enjoy the same benefits. That's why I decided to write this book, and I'm delighted that you're reading it now.

In this book, drawing on recent scientific studies as well as the real-life success stories of people I've helped to lose weight for life, I'm going to walk you through 10 diagnostic tests that will enable you to pinpoint the one or more mistakes that are keeping you from getting the results you desire. You will then know exactly which issues *you* need to focus on in order to attain and maintain your optimum weight – and live for the rest of your life in peace and harmony with food and your body. (If this book is your introduction to the Don't Go Hungry Diet, doing these diagnostic tests will alert you to the common mistakes you need to avoid if you are to lose weight effectively and sustainably.) In the process, I'm also going to explain the specific *sequence* in which you need to address these common weight loss mistakes in order to start losing weight as efficiently as possible. I know as well as anyone that it's impossible to be a saint all the time. It's not always possible to eat in the way you would theoretically prefer to eat, and it's not always possible to exercise as much as you would theoretically like to exercise. Sometimes life just gets in the way. But that's OK, as long as you tackle these lifestyle changes in order of priority as explained in this book. Doing so will enable you to continue losing weight, or at least maintain your lower weight and not go backwards, during such challenging periods. And then, when the time is right for you to lose more weight, the diagnostics and information in this book will show you exactly what *you* need to do to reach the optimum weight for your body.

Being in Diet Dungeon is unrelated to how much you know about dieting

Being in Diet Dungeon is totally unrelated to how much you know about food and nutrition, diets and dieting. In fact, some of the people I've helped to escape from Diet Dungeon and lose weight by taking a different approach have been nutritionists, weight loss practitioners or slimming club lecturers. Most of the people I've helped have spent at least five years, and usually more than 20 years, in on-again-off-again dieting. They have read dozens of books about food and nutrition, and many of them know the kilojoule, fat, carbohydrate and protein content of just about every single food they've ever eaten. As one of my clients, Kimberly, said, 'I've always had this terrible habit of counting calories. My husband made me burn my calorie counter when we met, but unfortunately it's all in my head!'

In my own Diet Dungeon days, I knew practically everything there was to know about healthy eating and how to lose weight.

I knew that in order to start losing weight I had to burn more kilojoules than I ate, and that I could achieve that either by eating fewer kilojoules or by burning more kilojoules through increased physical activity, and preferably both. I knew that I was better off losing weight by eating meals that were nutritionally balanced rather than on fad diets that cut out whole food groups, and I knew how to put together nutritionally balanced, reduced-kilojoule meals. I knew that in order to lose weight I had to cut out chips, chocolate, cake and other fun foods, and that, to help keep my hunger under control, I had to fill myself up with low-kilojoule foods and vegetables from the 'free list'. However, the fact that I was carrying 93 kilos on my 1.6 metre frame showed clearly that my knowledge wasn't doing me much good. By the time I was in the first year of my science degree at the University of Western Australia, I had so much 'back fat' spilling out from the top of my bra strap and under my arms that I could no longer put my arms down straight by my sides. I had chins on my chins and stretch marks on my stretch marks. Whenever I went to the beach with my girlfriends, they would strip down to their tiny swimsuits and splash about in the Indian Ocean, and I would swelter on the beach in the giant, tent-like clothes I'd made for myself. I marvelled at how they managed to get the support they needed from the spaghetti-thin straps of their dainty swimsuits, whereas I needed to wear military-style bras with triple hooks at the back and 22 millimetre-wide shoulder straps. Worst of all, every breath I took was laboured because I was in a permanent state of generalised anxiety, imagining that I was physically suffocating under all that fat.

I hadn't always been that knowledgeable about diets and dieting. Nor had I always been that fat.

I dieted myself fat

It all started six years earlier. New to high school and feeling awkward, I thought if I could just lose 3 kilos and get down to 50 kilos, I would feel better about myself. And so I began a no-carbohydrate diet, imagining how great I would feel in a tiny bikini and how everyone – especially the boy I liked most – would sit up and notice me. But the pleasure of imagining these scenarios soon paled in comparison to the pain of sticking to the diet. Within less than two weeks I'd blown it. I not only ate all the normal foods I wasn't supposed to eat on the diet, I began to eat in a way I'd never eaten before. Sneaking to the corner shops to buy lollies and ice-cream, then hiding in shame while I ate them.

Back at 53 kilos, I braced myself and tried again. But although this time I followed a 'sensible diet' that was nutritionally balanced, after about 10 days I began to yearn for more than its restricted portions. I tried to resist my escalating hunger, but after less than three weeks I was back at the corner shop buying junk and scoffing it in secret. This time my post-diet pig-out was grander than the last. By the time I got the courage to try another diet, I was a kilo heavier than my previous starting weight.

Panic set in. And so began the vicious cycle that held me hostage for six miserable years. Each dieting attempt was more elaborate and expensive than the last, and each time I was filled with even greater hope of reaching my ideal weight. And the higher my expectations rose, the greater the impact when I inevitably fell off the wagon. My post-diet pig-outs became increasingly grandiose and my weight rose steadily. The boy I liked most certainly noticed me. 'I remember when we were in year eight you were the best-looking girl in the whole year,' he told me during a deep and meaningful conversation when we were in year 12, by which time I weighed over 80 kilos. 'What happened to the beautiful, slim Mandy we all knew before?' I buried the excruciating pain of his comment with more food. I would eat chocolate bars until I felt sick and then go to bed to sleep off my discomfort and guilt. I remember eating a whole family-size pizza in hiding, feeling desperately alone.

In the midst of this turmoil, there was one thing that brought me peace: reading anything and everything I could find about food and nutrition, diets and dieting. I read every magazine and newspaper article on the subject, I read diet books, and I read textbook chapters on nutrition and digestion. One of my favourite sources of information was a particular slimming magazine from

England. I'd read it religiously every month, poring over every single article, every new product announcement, looking for clues to help me escape from Diet Dungeon. But most of all, I used to read the success stories. I'd hang off every word written about those beaming successful people and long to be one of them. I tore out all the success stories from that magazine every month for two years and filed them carefully in a secret folder, hoping their inspiration would rub off on me. But I never did find the inspiration I needed in that magazine. Instead, I found something else.

One day, while scouring the latest issue for clues, I was shocked to read the following letter in the Q&A section of the magazine. I still keep that letter to this day. It was obviously a letter from my mother. In retrospect, my mother was clearly beside herself with worry and hoped her letter would trigger an improvement of some kind. But I felt deeply humiliated and even more desperate about my predicament.

What can be done about my daughter Amanda – 60 kilos at 15, 70 kilos at 16, 80 kilos at 17, now 89 kilos and still putting on weight? I always kept an eye on her intake; but once she started work, she spent her wages on chocolate, etc. In desperation, I lost 19 kilos myself – but this was no incentive to her.

It's not that I wasn't trying to lose weight, nor that I didn't want to. The trouble was, nothing worked for me. Every six months I'd join a new diet club. In the beginning I'd follow the program to the letter, do some exercise and lose a bit of weight. After a few weeks, however, I'd inevitably stop losing weight even though I was continuing to do all the right things. I would not only hit that dreaded plateau, I'd also start to get really hungry. So I'd struggle on, but inexorably I'd start cheating and then give up, pig out and gain back all the weight I'd lost, plus more. Too embarrassed to show my face at the diet club again, I'd abandon ship, only to join a new club – where no one knew what a failure I was – in another part of town six months later.

One of the diet clubs I joined was led by a fantastic lecturer, a mature woman with a gravelly voice and a wicked sense of humour. And she had been fat, like me. I adored hearing her lectures so much that I swallowed my shame to rejoin her club several times. I wanted so much to stay in her club that I once devised a crazy plan to help me do so. Before my first weigh-in, I strapped a scuba-diving belt around my waist, complete with eight half-kilo weights threaded along it. Every week at the club I wore that heavy belt under my shirt. That way, whenever the going got tough, as I knew it would, I had eight half-kilo shots of ammunition up my sleeve. At the first sign of a plateau, I went to the club the following week minus a couple of those shots. Even though I obviously wasn't any slimmer, the scales registered a one-kilo loss. That gave me the courage I needed to continue with the program the following week. But the week after that I ate more than my program allowance, and so I probably wouldn't have lost any weight. Off came another two of the weights, and the club scales registered another encouraging loss. But, as you can imagine, I soon used up all my chances. While my lead weights allowed me to stay shame-free in my favourite lecturer's diet club for longer than I'd stayed in any club before, they only delayed the inevitable. Cheating merged into overeating, overeating into pigging out, and pigging out into all-out bingeing.

SIX SIGNS YOU ARE DIETING YOURSELF FAT
1. Before you start a diet, you pig out on loads of rich foods: you figure you may never eat them again.
2. When you're on a diet, you think constantly about what you're going to eat next, and how much and when.
3. You tend to wear the same clothes every day because you only have one or two outfits that fit.
4. Every time you give up on a diet, you eat loads of rich foods in a blind, senseless way, with little or no pleasure.
5. You are heavier now than when you started dieting.

6. If you ever forget about dieting for a few months, your weight doesn't escalate wildly out of control but either stays the same or goes down a little.

Six years after starting that first diet, I'd gone from 53 kilos to an unwieldy 93 kilos. For all my efforts, expense and anxiety, all I'd gained in six years of dieting was 40 kilos and a binge-eating disorder. I had dieted myself fat. It was shortly after that that I decided to make my career in medical research so that I could finally understand why I couldn't lose weight and, more importantly, what I could do to get back to a healthy size. I won a Swiss Government Scholarship and set off overseas to do my PhD at the University of Geneva.

What I learned from my medical research changed my life. I was finally able to walk free of Diet Dungeon, lose my excess weight and settle at a healthy 65 kilos, which I've maintained ever since (except during pregnancy). I came back to Australia to set up my own research laboratory focusing on weight management at a medical research institute in Sydney, and with my team I've been engaged in cutting-edge research ever since. In the next chapter I'm going to show you what I learned, and give you an overview of how you can use this knowledge to walk free of Diet Dungeon and lose your own excess weight once and for all.

Chapter 2

The science of weight loss

I tore myself away from the safe comfort of certainties through my love for the truth; and truth rewarded me.
Simone de Beauvoir, French author and philosopher,
1908–1986

If you long to free yourself from the tyranny of constant weight worries or diet obsessions (or both), you'll find everything you need to know in this book. It's a practical, step-by-step guide to doing exactly that. You will most likely find you need to do things a little differently from what you've done in the past. For instance, if you usually try to strip your fat intake back to the quick when you want to lose weight, I'll encourage you to incorporate more natural fats into your diet, as much as you feel like eating. If you usually eat five or six small meals or snacks per day while you're trying to lose weight (you've heard it will 'keep your metabolic rate high'), I'll encourage you to question whether you are actually comfortably and physically hungry before each of those meals and snacks, and if not, to ditch some of them and do something else besides eat. If you think it's normal to sometimes grapple with hunger while you're trying to lose weight, and to have to resist the physical urge to eat more than the paltry number of kilojoules your diet allows, I'll encourage you to eat more, as much of the types and amounts of mostly nutritious foods that make you feel genuinely satisfied. Doing these things may feel strange to you in the beginning. You may wonder how you could possibly lose weight and keep it off by eating in this way – and it's true that following the practical steps in this book can feel impossibly risky and difficult at times. That's why, in this chapter, I'm going to give you a brief overview of the science of weight loss, a summary of the scientific principles I explained in *The Don't Go Hungry Diet*. Once you understand the medical research that explains *why* listening to your body and eating accordingly helps you to attain and maintain the weight or size you're biologically meant to be, you'll find it so much easier to do the simple things you need to do to escape from Diet Dungeon once and for all and get on with enjoying your life.

The Famine Reaction

In my six years of failed dieting attempts, I always thought there was something wrong with me, because I could never lose more than a few kilos on a diet before piling it all back on again. When I started my PhD and began investigating how the brain controls body weight, I realised that there wasn't anything wrong with me at all; I was just a normal person having a Famine Reaction.

The Famine Reaction is a survival mechanism that protects you from wasting away in times of scarcity. It's what makes you feel hungry and slows your metabolic rate when you're trying to lose weight.[1] When I was doing research at the University of Geneva, I learned how to switch off my Famine Reaction so that I could lose weight without constantly fighting with my body, and I've now taught many others to lose weight in this easier way. But before we go into how to do this, you need to understand the Famine Reaction. The better you understand this beast and how it works, the easier it is to tame it.

The Famine Reaction is controlled by a part of your brain called the hypothalamus. Part of your hypothalamus's job is to keep everything in your body constantly optimal: body temperature, blood sugar, blood oxygen, blood pressure and so forth. Your hypothalamus also strives to keep the amount of fat you store on your body at a constant and optimal level. We still don't fully understand why, but once you've been carrying extra fat for a certain amount of time, your hypothalamus can come to accept that having that much fat is optimal for your body, and it strives to constantly maintain that level of body fat. In other words, the amount of body fat you have on you most of the time can become what we call your Set Point, and your body strives to maintain your Set Point level of body fat. Your Set Point is simply the amount of fat that your body perceives to be right for you at any particular time.

HOW TO ESTIMATE YOUR CURRENT SET POINT

- What's your 'normal' weight, when you're not dieting? For example, if you usually hover around 78 kilos, then your Set Point is probably around 78 kilos.
- What weight do you tend to revert to when you stop trying to lose weight? For instance, if every time you stop dieting you end up back around 78 kilos, then your Set Point is probably about 78 kilos.

Don't be concerned if your Set Point is higher than your ideal weight. You'll see later that your Set Point is not set in stone. Rather, it's a 'settling point' that can be reduced with the right strategies until you reach your ultimate Set Point, or optimum biological weight, the weight below which you cannot go without making it likely that you'll immediately regain weight.

Let's imagine that one Monday morning you wake up and start a new weight loss attempt. In the beginning, everything goes fine and you start losing weight. You're eating well, you're doing some form of regular physical activity, and you feel great. But after a while your hypothalamus gets wind of the fact that you're losing fat, and that can mean only one thing: that you're eating fewer kilojoules than you're burning off. In other words: *not enough food*. If you're carrying more fat than your current Set Point, your body doesn't care a hoot if you're not eating enough to maintain your fat stores. In fact, as you'll see later in this chapter, your body will actually *encourage* you to eat less so that you can get back to your Set Point. But if you continue losing weight and start getting too far below your current Set Point, this relative lack of food will trigger changes in the balance of natural chemicals in your hypothalamus, bringing on the Famine Reaction.

> **YOUR FAMINE REACTION IS ACTIVATED BY TWO THINGS:**
> 1. Consuming fewer kilojoules and fewer nutrients than your body needs to maintain its fat stores.
>   and/or
> 2. Having less fat than your Set Point.

How to recognise a Famine Reaction

A Famine Reaction is a sign that your weight is too far below your current Set Point for your body's comfort. The most common and obvious sign that you're having a Famine Reaction is that you start feeling hungrier than usual.[1-3] When you start a weight loss program, you might not feel very hungry at all. But once you get down to a weight that's too far below your current Set Point and you're having a Famine Reaction, you can eat your whole day's diet ration and *still* feel hungry . . . and it's only 10.30 in the morning. That's your Famine Reaction, pushing you to want to eat more and thereby helping to protect you from losing any more fat.

A second common symptom of a Famine Reaction is lethargy.[1,4] We all know that to lose weight and keep it off, regular physical activity is essential. Keeping active can be a challenge at the best of times, but when you're having a Famine Reaction you can feel like you're dragging your whole body through mud just to get through the bare necessities of life. That's your Famine Reaction, slowing you down so you don't waste precious energy and lose any more fat.

A third sign that you're having a Famine Reaction is when – barring other obvious causes – you feel really cold and shivery, even in the middle of summer. The reason for this is that the Famine Reaction can reduce your metabolic rate by as much as 4000 kilojoules (or 900 calories) per day.[1,4-7] That's a lot of kilojoules. Many diets require you to reduce your intake by about 4000 kilojoules per day, and in the beginning, of course, you lose weight. But then your clever Famine Reaction just goes and drops your metabolic rate by the same amount. The result is that your weight loss can come to a complete standstill even if you're still sticking rigorously to your diet and exercise plan.

These three major effects of the Famine Reaction (hunger, lethargy and reduced metabolic rate) are incredibly powerful. They explain why, if you've ever lost weight in the past, it's more than likely that you hit a plateau and then gained back some or all of the weight shockingly quickly.

It was when I was doing my PhD at the University of Geneva and reading the scientific literature in the field of weight regulation that I came across the missing link in my vast knowledge of diets and dieting. This was the missing link that ultimately set me free from Diet Dungeon.

I learned that you could deactivate the Famine Reaction by something very simple, very pleasant, and completely without side effects. And can you imagine what that very simple, pleasant and safe thing might be?

The Famine Reaction can be deactivated by eating

That's right, *eating* can deactivate the Famine Reaction.[7-18] It may sound obvious that if you're having a Famine Reaction you can switch it off by eating food. But in my six years of failed dieting attempts, I never once heard any mention of that concept. Whenever I hit a plateau, I was always advised to just keep going, or to eat less or exercise more, and told that if I felt hungry I should just quell my hunger pangs by drinking more water or eating vegetables from the 'free list'. Aargh! The free list! Have you ever noticed that when you're really hungry, no amount of vegetables from the free list is ever going to satisfy you?

As a weight loss scientist, I now know that these conventional plateau-busting strategies either don't alleviate the Famine Reaction[11, 19] or actually make it worse.[20-21] The harder you work to push against your Famine Reaction, the stronger it can get. If you use willpower and brute force to stick to your diet no matter what, the Famine Reaction can turn your body into a super-efficient fat-storing machine. The result is that when you give up on your weight loss program, you end up gaining all the weight back again, and more.

How to eat your way out of a Famine Reaction

Knowing about the Famine Reaction, and how to tame it, radically changed my approach to weight loss. Instead of using willpower and brute force, as I'd tried to do in all my past weight loss attempts, I worked *with* my body, not against it. As I lost weight and hit the nagging hunger of a Famine Reaction, instead of trying to deny my hunger, I fed it.

To give you a feel for the types and amounts of food you need to eat in order to deactivate a Famine Reaction as you lose weight, think back to a time when you broke your diet and ate in a 'diet-wrecking' way. When you experienced that diet-induced nagging hunger, what is it that you ate at that time in order to satisfy your appetite? Or, if you didn't break your diet too badly at that time, but you wanted to, what are the foods that would have stopped your hunger dead in its tracks?

When I ask this question of participants in my workshops, they often say things like 'A big slab of caramel mud cake' or 'fish and chips'. Maybe you answered with something similarly kilojoule-loaded. If so, you're certainly in tune with your body's instincts. To deactivate the Famine Reaction, research shows that you need to consume sufficient kilojoules.[11,19] You'll certainly get sufficient kilojoules from a slab of caramel mud cake or a feast of fish and chips. A diet jelly or carrot and celery sticks just won't do the job. But you also need something else besides kilojoules to deactivate the Famine Reaction, and that's *nutrients*.[22-27] Not nutrients from a bottle, but nutrients from food, the only place where they occur in the optimum concentration, the optimum combination with other nutrients and the optimum chemical conformation to benefit your body.

So if your favourite diet-breaker is chicken schnitzel, chips, chocolate or your colleague's home-baked jam drops, can you think of something that would give you the same degree of satisfaction but also offers greater nutritional value? For instance, instead of having fish and chips, would you feel just as satisfied to have a meal of fish, grilled with butter instead of deep-fried, a small handful of chips rather than a pile, and a salad with avocado and real olive oil dressing, finished off with a full-fat flavoured yogurt or a scoop of ice-cream if you still have room for dessert? If you ate as much of these mostly nutritious foods as you comfortably wanted, would that leave you feeling just as satisfied as a mound of fish and chips? Not only has it got way more famine-busting nutrients, it's more likely to leave you feeling elegantly satisfied rather than bloated like a boa constrictor. What if the only things that would quash your hunger and cravings were a blueberry and white chocolate scone and a mugaccino? Would you feel happy to enjoy it as part of a balanced day's eating that included a wide variety of wholesome and nutritious foods, not forgetting two or more serves of fruit and at least two meals that included generous amounts of vegetables?

Whatever it is that genuinely satisfies your hunger and also provides overall nutrition, that's exactly the kind of thing you need to eat in order to keep your Famine Reaction under control as you lose weight. By eating the types and amounts of *mostly* nutritious foods that make you feel genuinely satisfied, you convince your hypothalamus that there's plenty of food around. You probably won't lose much weight, if any, during this famine-busting time, but after a while your body will accept your lower weight as its new Set Point, your Famine Reaction will subside, and your appetite and metabolic rate will return to normal. If you're listening carefully to your body's hunger signals and eating accordingly, this drop in appetite will naturally lead you to eat less and enable you to lose some more weight.

After you've lost some more weight, several things will happen. You'll start getting too far below your new Set Point, your body will consequently have another Famine Reaction, and you'll therefore start feeling hungrier than usual – and that will be your cue to eat more in order to satisfy your hunger. Maybe you'll need to eat a little bit more than usual, such as a yogurt and a piece of fruit or a couple of crackers with peanut butter, or maybe you'll need to eat quite a bit more than usual, such as an additional meal. But if you listen to your hunger and eat accordingly, you'll deactivate that Famine Reaction and before long you'll start losing weight again.

Successful weight loss is not about trying to steamroller your way over your survival instincts by using your willpower to stick to predetermined diet rations no matter what. It's about listening to your body, doing what it tells you to do, and trusting that it will take you to the weight you're biologically meant to be. This will most often mean that you lose excess weight in gradual increments, with interim periods where your metabolism recharges itself and you patiently allow your body to adjust to progressively lower weights. When you lose weight in this stepwise manner, it will only be a question of time before you lose all the weight you want to lose, and all without ever going hungry.

HOW TO STOP YOUR FAMINE REACTION FROM THWARTING YOUR WEIGHT LOSS PROGRESS

Losing weight by any means – be it by diet, by exercise, or by diet and exercise combined – ultimately activates your Famine Reaction, a survival mechanism that protects you from wasting away. New research shows that you can calm your Famine Reaction and therefore lose weight more effectively by eating whenever you feel physically hungry, and stopping when you've honestly had enough.

The Fat Brake

Besides the Famine Reaction and how to tame it, my research taught me a second revolutionary concept that changed my life. Just as your body has a Famine Reaction that protects you from getting too far *below* your Set Point, it also has a Fat Brake that protects you from getting too far *above* your Set Point. [28, 29] The Fat Brake is your body's automatic weight maintenance system. It helps you to keep the weight off without having to think about it all the time. It's thanks to my Fat Brake that I've been able to keep those 28 kilos off for more than 13 years (and counting). Once you understand your Fat Brake – how it works, and how to make it work for you – you can say goodbye forever to depressing weight gain.

Like the Famine Reaction, the Fat Brake is controlled by your hypothalamus. The Fat Brake essentially works in the opposite way to the Famine Reaction. Let's imagine that you've lost some or all of the weight you want to lose. Once your body has come to accept your lower weight as its new Set Point, it strives to protect you from getting too far above that Set Point. Now let's imagine that you go on holidays or you stop being as active as you usually are for some reason, you eat more than you need, and you gain a bit of weight. This kilojoule excess sets off a series of changes in the balance of natural chemicals in your hypothalamus, thereby activating your Fat Brake.

TWO THINGS ACTIVATE YOUR FAT BRAKE
1. You're at your Set Point weight and you consume more kilojoules than your body needs to maintain its fat stores.
    and/or
2. You gain weight and your fat stores exceed your Set Point.

How to recognise your Fat Brake in action

There are various ways to recognise your Fat Brake in action. A major sign that your Fat Brake has been activated is reduced appetite. [30] Not only does the Fat Brake cut your appetite, it also reduces your tendency to want rich, fatty foods. Have you ever been on holidays, for example, and eaten more than you needed for a day or so and then noticed that you just didn't feel as hungry as usual when you got back into your regular routine? It was probably your Fat Brake, cutting your appetite in an attempt to help you get back down to your Set Point.

A second sign of your Fat Brake in action can be when you feel an urge to fidget and move about after periods of over-indulgence. In this case your body is trying to burn off excess kilojoules. When research volunteers are asked to overeat by 4200 kilojoules (1000 calories) a day but are requested not to do any exercise, they end up fidgeting and pacing uncontrol-lably, burning off up to 2900 additional kilojoules (700 calories) per day.[31] I once read an interview with Australian actress Toni Collette about what it was like to pack on 20 kilos in order to play roles such as Muriel in the film *Muriel's Wedding*. She said that the hardest thing about it was that she had to refrain from doing any exercise in order to gain enough weight in time for filming. No wonder she found this unpleasant. With her Fat Brake pushing her to move about, she must have felt really cooped up during the fattening process. So, if you ever get that restless feeling and you just can't keep still, take a moment to check whether you've recently eaten more than you needed. If so, it may well be your Fat Brake in action, helping you to burn off any excesses and so prevent you from gaining too much weight.

A third sign of your Fat Brake in action is that it can make you feel excessively warm. Have you ever noticed you felt hot after a particularly heavy meal? Either immediately afterwards, as you sit at the dining table with beads of sweat running down your face, or later, when you wake up in the middle of the night and throw off your bed covers in a lather of sweat, even in the middle of winter. The reason you feel so hot after overindulging is that your Fat Brake revs up your metabolic rate in another attempt to burn off excess kilojoules.[6, 28, 32] Unlike the heat you feel when it's hot outside, the heat from your Fat Brake burns you up from the inside out.

Can you see that with these three effects of your Fat Brake (re-duced appetite, increased propensity to move about and increased metabolic rate), if you simply listen to your hunger signals and eat accordingly, your Fat Brake helps you get back to your Set Point without too much effort? A lot of people mistakenly believe that if they eat something 'fattening', then they're going to balloon, so they may as well just give up and pig out on truckloads of fattening foods. But when you understand your Fat Brake and how it works, you know that occasional overindulgences at parties or on holidays don't make you gain weight overall, as long as you honour your hunger signals *most of the time*. The trick is to make a habit of eating *only* when you feel physically hungry, and to stop eating before you feel overfull. If you're not hungry, do your waistline a favour and do something else besides eat.

HOW TO MAKE YOUR FAT BRAKE WORK FOR YOU
To keep weight off in the easiest possible way, you need to make a habit of eating *only* when you feel physically hungry and stopping when you've honestly had enough. When you do this, your Fat Brake can work at its best, enabling you to maintain your weight automatically without having to think about it all the time.

Putting these insights into action in the real world
You've seen that to lose weight effectively, you need to eat enough to keep your Famine Reaction quiet. On the other hand, it's important not to eat too much; otherwise, your Fat Brake won't be able to do its job of keeping weight off. While this may sound like a delicate balance, all it boils down to is one simple thing: eating according to your physical needs. What this means is to simply:

A. Eat when you feel physically hungry (and only when you feel physically hungry).
B. Eat what you really feel like eating (within reason, and as long as you also eat fruit and vegetables every day, as I'll discuss in Step 2).
C. Eat until you feel truly satisfied.

When you eat according to your physical needs, choosing from a wide variety of mainly nutritious foods and including plenty of vegetables and fruit, and when you combine this with some form of regular physical activity, your Famine Reaction remains quiet as you lose weight, and your Fat Brake can work at its best. The result is that you'll find it much easier to lose weight and keep it off.

The adventure of a lifetime

In some ways the weight loss adventure you are embarking on will be easier than any weight loss experience you have had in the past. You won't need to turn your life upside down or eat separate foods to your family, friends and colleagues in order to start losing weight. If you currently equate losing weight with feeling naggingly hungry and lethargic, you'll no longer need to struggle with those sensations in order to lose weight, because you won't be provoking your Famine Reaction. If you currently do unreasonable amounts of gruelling exercise every day in order to lose weight and keep it off, you won't have to do that either, because you'll no longer be consuming more than your physical needs by eating meals and snacks when you're not hungry. If you currently equate weight loss with long lists of foods to avoid, you'll no longer need to deny yourself any wholesome nutritious food that you may fancy, nor will you have to do without a little of your favourite treats from time to time, in order to lose weight.

While this method of weight loss is incredibly simple, and flexible enough to accommodate almost any lifestyle, that doesn't necessarily mean it's easy. So in other ways the weight loss adventure you are embarking on will be harder than other weight loss experiences you have had in the past. You'll need to assess your situation honestly in order to find the key things you need to focus on specifically in order to manage your weight by this method. This will mean keeping a *written* record of how hungry and satisfied you feel before and after everything you eat and drink for at least two weeks, which is the only way to ensure that you're reading your body's hunger signals correctly. You'll need to walk bravely through walls of fear as you wonder whether this is really going to work for you. And, needless to say, fruit and veggies will be on the menu every single day, and physical activity will need to become a regular fixture in your life. Not easy feats, but I'm here to hold your hand and guide you step by step as you embark on this new adventure. Drawing on my own experience and the experiences of the many others who have kindly shared their stories in this book – all backed by medical research – I'll give you tried and tested methods of determining exactly what is impeding your progress and what strategies you need to implement to set you on the road to success. Once you've done the hard yards of discovering the specific things you need to do to lose weight by connecting with your body, and once you've been doing them consistently for a few weeks, you'll be rewarded by pulling on those favourite jeans that are currently too tight, only to discover that they now do up easily and fit you comfortably. And that jacket in your wardrobe, the one you always leave open because the buttons strain when you do it up? You'll find it will glide effortlessly over your body and do up like a dream. And once you've identified the particular strategies you need to implement to manage your weight, they'll be yours to keep forever.

Over to you

Here's something you can do immediately to put the ideas in this chapter into action.

Think back on your past experiences of losing weight. Can you pinpoint any instances where the Famine Reaction tripped you up? Can you see any past diet failures that you blamed yourself for but that in retrospect were caused by trying to fight the Famine Reaction with conventional weight loss strategies? If so, what did the Famine Reaction *feel* like to you? Did you notice anything unusual about how hot or cold you felt, your energy levels, your appetite and your desires for food – especially fun foods – at that time?

Similarly, can you think of any times when you felt your Fat Brake in action after a period of overeating? For instance, did you ever feel off your food, restless or unusually warm for no apparent reason after a run of heavy eating? Have you ever been surprised at how little weight you've gained or how quickly you've lost it again after a short period of overindulgence? Have you ever wondered why you don't weigh more than you do, despite the fact that you may go for long periods of time without paying much attention to what you're eating? These are sure signs that your Fat Brake is doing a fine job of protecting you from gaining weight.

The more conscious encounters you have with your Famine Reaction and your Fat Brake, the more confident you'll become about working with your body, not against it, in order to lose all the weight you need to lose and maintain your ideal weight for life.

Later in this section I'm going to show you how to apply these scientific principles in order to lose weight, starting from the very first practical steps you need to take to get the ball rolling. First, though, let's take a look at how much weight you actually need to lose.

Chapter 3

How much weight do you need to lose?

I have tried to do what is true and not ideal.
Henri de Toulouse-Lautrec, French painter, printmaker,
draughtsman and illustrator, 1864–1901

Once you've made the decision to lose weight, it's helpful to know what weight or size you are aiming for. But in a world where the prevailing idea of the 'ideal' male or female body is vastly different from what is biologically feasible for most people, how can you know if your target is realistic for you or if you are chasing an impossible dream? In this chapter I'm going to explain the acid test that will reveal *exactly* what weight you're biologically meant to be. But first I'm going to explain how you can get a useful ballpark estimate of your ideal weight and size based on crude measures of body mass index (BMI) and waist and hip circumference. This information is based on estimates drawn from medical research as to which values of BMI and waist or hip circumference are healthy for most people. I'll then show you how to narrow down your search and pinpoint the optimum weight for you.

Get a ballpark estimate of your ideal weight and size

Body mass index
One way to get a broad estimate of your ideal healthy weight is to calculate your body mass index (BMI). Your BMI is simply your weight in kilograms divided by your height in metres, squared

(kg/m^2). The easiest way to calculate your BMI is to enter your weight in kilos into a calculator and divide it by your height in metres. Press the equals button, and then divide the answer by your height in metres again. For instance, if you weigh 92 kilos and you are 1.65 metres tall, your BMI is 33.79 kg/m^2. (92 divided by 1.65 = 55.76; 55.76 divided by 1.65 = 33.79 kg/m^2)

According to the World Heath Organization's current classifications for Caucasians, as shown in the following table,[33] if your BMI is between 18.5 kg/m^2 and 24.9 kg/m^2, your weight is in the 'normal' range for your height. For someone with a BMI of 33.79 kg/m^2, their weight would be in the 'obese' weight range for their height.

Classification of overweight and obesity by BMI and relative risk of metabolic complications

	BMI (kg/m^2)	Risk of type 2 diabetes, hypertension and cardiovascular disease
Underweight	< 18.5	Low (but risk of other clinical problems possibly increased)
Normal	18.5–24.9	Average
Overweight (Pre-obese)	25.0–29.9	Increased
Obese Class I	30–34.9	Moderate
Obese Class II	35.0–39.9	Severe
Obese Class III	40.0+	Very severe

Current research suggests that having a BMI of 25 kg/m^2 or above puts you at significantly higher risk of hypertension, metabolic diseases such as type 2 diabetes, and cardiovascular disease. The greater your BMI, the greater your risk, as shown in the table.

Here's an easy way to estimate a range of body weights that would be considered 'normal' for your height.

- Your estimated minimum normal weight = your height in metres × your height in metres × 18.5
- Your estimated maximum normal weight = your height in metres × your height in metres × 24.9

So, for example, if like me you are 1.60 metres tall, the minimum and maximum weight you could be while still falling within the World Health Organization's definition of normal weight for Caucasians would be 47.4 kilos to 63.7 kilos respectively. As you can see, 'normal' covers a wide range.

Every time I punch these numbers into my calculator, I'm acutely aware of the fact that at my usual weight of 65 kilos I'm 1.3 kilos overweight according to the World Health Organization! It's important to know that BMI is not the only determinant of your ideal weight or metabolic health, and that BMI is not a validated predictor of disease risk in children, in adults who have not finished growing, in adults who are naturally very lean or very muscular, in people from certain racial or ethnic groups, or in adults over the age of 65. This is illustrated by the fact that many Olympic athletes have a BMI that places them in the overweight or obese category as defined by the World Health Organization, although metabolically they are extremely fit. On the other hand, some people with a BMI in the normal range store excess fat around the midriff, and this places them at significantly higher risk of metabolic diseases.

PROCEED WITH CAUTION IF YOU ARE OVER 65

For most of her adult life, Trishy had maintained her weight at around 70 kilos. At her height of 1.7 metres, her BMI was a healthy 24.2 kg/m^2. Having studied nutrition and worked as a high school home economics teacher, she continually 'practised what she preached' by eating nutritious foods and being active. However, since her late fifties Trishy had gradually accumulated some extra padding for no apparent reason, and now, at the age of 69, she weighed 77 kilos and had a BMI of 26.6 kg/m^2. As most of the extra weight had settled uncomfortably around her midriff, and as her BMI was now in the overweight range according to the World Health Organization's tables for Caucasians under the age of 65, Trishy was anxious to lose the extra weight for the sake of both her health and her appearance. However, there is emerging evidence that Trishy would be better off accepting this slightly higher weight than trying to slim down to the weight she was when she was younger.

In people over the age of 65, weight loss has been linked to numerous adverse outcomes that are observed regardless of whether the weight loss occurs intentionally through diet and exercise or unintentionally through illness or accidents.[34, 35] Such adverse outcomes include exacerbation of nutritional deficiencies, loss of muscle mass and bone density, reduced physical functioning, reduced quality of life and increased mortality. In fact, a BMI below 24 kg/m^2 in older people is related to an increased risk of disease and death.[36] There are emerging health benefits of carrying a bit of extra weight in older age, such as a lower risk of fractures due to a higher bone mass and more cushioning in case of falls.[35] Also, a little extra weight in older age gives you valuable reserves in case of weight loss due to illness or medications that blunt your appetite.

If you're over 65 years of age, many specialists recommend that you should only consider losing weight if your body mass index is over about 27–29 kg/m^2 *and* your weight is interfering with physical functions, or you have risk factors for heart disease such as hypertension or high blood lipids.[35] And if – after discussing the pros and cons of weight loss with your doctor – you decide that you do need to lose weight, it's absolutely essential to increase your levels of physical activity as much as you comfortably can as you slim down (preferably including some regular strength training). If you don't, up the a third of the weight you lose will be precious muscle that is critical to your physical abilities and independence in the decades to come.

Waist circumference

When it comes to being healthy, it's not so much how much you weigh but how much fat you have on your body and where you store it that counts. Carrying too much fat around the midriff, especially in the visceral space around organs such as the intestines, liver and pancreas (belly fat), is linked with a significantly higher risk of preventable lifestyle diseases such as diabetes, heart disease and certain cancers. Research shows that most Caucasian and Asian women with a waist circumference of 80 centimetres or over and most Caucasian men with a waist circumference of 94 centimetres or above are at significantly greater risk of developing preventable lifestyle diseases and metabolic complications, regardless of how tall they are (www.measureup.gov.au). For women and men with waist

---

HOW TO MEASURE YOUR WAIST CIRCUMFERENCE

The easiest scientifically validated way to estimate whether you have too much belly fat is to simply measure your waist circumference, the distance around your waist. To measure your waist circumference precisely and accurately, take a tape measure and run it around the narrowest part of your torso (as seen from the front) between the top of your hipbone and the bottom of your rib cage. If there's no obvious narrowing between these two landmarks, measure your waist circumference at the mid-point between landmarks. Make sure the tape measure is flat against your skin, but don't pull the tape so tight that it digs into your skin. Relax your abdomen – neither sucking it in nor letting it all hang out – exhale, and take your measurement. Take several measurements until you consistently hit the same, smallest number each time you take a reading.

If you've ever measured your waist circumference, you know how easy it is to pull the tape that teensy bit more to get a better result. The best way I've found to standardise the amount of tug you give the tape is to use a spring-loaded retractable tape measure. You hook it around your waist, press the button a few times, and zip! The tape measure snaps into place around your waist.

circumferences greater than or equal to 88 and 102 centimetres, respectively, the risk of metabolic complications is even higher.

Waist-to-hip ratio

Early last year I went for a coffee with my friend Barbara from work. Barbara brought along a young colleague, Zena, who had just started work at our institute that week. Upon hearing that I was doing research into weight loss, Zena asked me what she could do to lose weight. From what I could see of Zena as we stood in the coffee queue, I couldn't imagine why she would want to lose weight. She was dressed in a long black skirt and a canary yellow tank top that showed off her slim physique, willowy arms and perfect muscle tone. 'Why do you ask?' I enquired. 'I know I don't look fat,' Zena said. 'I'm even a bit skinny in my upper body. It's just that my bum and hips are way too big for me.'

Over coffee, I talked with Zena about new research suggesting that having a 'big bum' is actually a plus for your health, not something that healthy-weight women should be trying to get rid of. When investigators at the Garvan Institute of Medical Research in Sydney took fat from the inguinal ('hip and thigh') region from donor mice and transplanted it into the intra-abdominal (belly) region of recipient mice, the recipient mice were protected against fat gain and the development of insulin resistance and glucose intolerance, both hallmark features of type 2 diabetes.[37] Something about fat from the lower regions of the body seemed to have protective effects against weight gain and disease. In keeping with this, in a review I recently co-authored for the international journal *Obesity Reviews*, several epidemiological studies suggest that having a high waist-to-hip ratio (that is, your waist circumference divided by your hip circumference) is a better predictor of death from cardiovascular disease than having a large waist, regardless of your waist circumference or how much belly fat you have.[38] In brief, if you're a sufficiently pear-shaped, your risk of dying from metabolic disorders such as cardiovascular disease may be less than that of people who are more apple-shaped, even if you're larger overall.

ARE YOU AN APPLE OR A PEAR?

To calculate your waist-to-hip ratio, divide your waist circumference as determined above by your hip circumference. When measuring your hip circumference, look at yourself side-on in the mirror and measure your hip circumference at the point where your bottom sticks out the most.

Waist-to-hip ratio is not widely used in public health initiatives, partly because it's more fiddly to measure than waist circumference and also because more research is required to determine what the cut-off points should be (that is, the waist-to-hip ratio above which your risk of metabolic diseases is increased). Over the years, however, a waist-to-hip ratio of around 0.7 for women has been considered ideal in terms of attractiveness. For instance, Marilyn Monroe, Audrey Hepburn, Twiggy, Sophia Loren and even the Venus de Milo had a waist-to-hip ratio close to 0.7, even though they were all very different in terms of overall size. In terms of metabolic health, research suggests that if your waist-to-hip ratio is less than 0.8 for women and less than 0.9 for men, you're doing well.[39] With my own waist-to-hip ratio of 0.73 (74 cm divided by 101 cm), I'm feeling pretty good about my prospects for long-term metabolic health, even though I'm more Venus de Milo than Audrey Hepburn.

THERE'S NOTHING LIKE A REGULAR CHECK-UP

BMI and waist and hip circumferences are helpful tools for estimating and comparing the overall metabolic health of populations, but are not accurate tools for determining the health of individuals. To get an accurate assessment of your own metabolic health and risk of disease, see your doctor for a full check-up.

Fine-tuning your weight and size targets

Your body mass index (BMI) and body measurements can give you a ballpark estimate of your ideal weight and size. However, your actual best weight may wind up being a good few kilos above or below these cut points of 'normal' values. For instance, many people who successfully lose weight and keep it off never actually reach these 'normal' values of BMI or waist circumference, but that doesn't stop them from being the happiest they've ever been. On the other hand, I know a lot of women with a BMI that places them comfortably in the normal weight range for their height and whose waist circumference falls well below 80 centimetres, but who'd gladly lose 5, 10 or even 15 kilos. Here's how to fine-tune your weight and size target to a value that's physically feasible for you.

Look at your weight history

One way to know if the weight or size you're aiming for is realistic is to take stock of how much of your adult life you've spent at that weight or size. For instance, if all throughout your twenties, thirties and early forties your weight hovered around 62 kilos but in the decade since turning 45 you've gained 10 kilos, then 62 to 63 kilos is probably a realistic target for you. If, on the other hand, the only time in your adult life you weighed 62 kilos was when you went on a highly restrictive diet where you white-knuckled your way past multiple Famine Reactions and spent three months at that weight before promptly piling it all back on again, then 62 kilos is not likely to be a realistic target for you, even if you have a whole wardrobe of clothes that only fit you when you weigh 62 kilos.

What if you've never weighed less than you do now as an adult? Or what if the only time you weighed less than you do now was decades ago when you were a teenager or a very young adult? How do you know what's the right weight for you? As I mentioned above, my own healthy weight range according to the World Health Organization is 47.4 kilos to 63.7 kilos. For the past decade I've weighed 65 kilos, plus or minus a kilo (except during pregnancy). The last time my weight was stable at anything less than this was when I was 13, just before I started the yoyo diet cycle that saw me skyrocket from 53 to 93 kilos.

Although I was fully grown at that time and looked healthy as a 53 kilo teenager, would 53 kilos be a suitable weight for me now? It's for questions such as these that other people's opinions can be very helpful.

Listen to clues from other people

As you lose weight, you'll probably be thrilled to receive regular compliments on your appearance. Having personally gone through the transformation of losing 28 kilos, here's my tongue-in-cheek translation of what those compliments mean.

If people are telling you 'You're looking great', it means 'You look much better than you did before, and you will look even better if you keep doing what you're doing'.

If people are telling you 'You look great', it means 'You look great'.

If you keep losing weight and people stop commenting on your appearance, it means that you're starting to lose so much weight that you no longer look great.

If people start asking 'How are you?' with concerned looks on their faces, it means you look less radiant than you did before and they're wondering if your weight loss is due to some terrible disease you haven't told them about.

While you'd never want to live your life by what other people say about you, it's helpful to keep an ear out for what people are saying. The weight that is healthiest for you is often the weight at which you look most healthy to most people, and the weight where you receive the most compliments on your appearance. On a few occasions in the past 10 years my weight has gone below 64 kilos. While I'm always thrilled when this happens, I've also noticed that it reliably brings on those concerned questions from several people. Something tells me that if ever I tried to get below my current weight, I'd soon look like a skinned rabbit.

The opinions of important people in your life about how you look can help you to recognise when you reach the weight that's best for you. However, there's one acid test of what weight you're biologically meant to be.

Let your body be the ultimate judge of your own healthy ideal weight

The ultimate test of what weight you're meant to be is your own body.

I'm not talking about you and your opinions about how your body looks, which can be distorted. (Research shows that some people who are overweight or obese estimate their weight to be in the healthy range. On the other hand, there are many lean, healthy women who look fantastic but who think they need to lose weight.[40]) What I'm talking about here is you, your body and how it *feels* to be in your skin.

As you approach the weight that's right for your body, losing weight will become increasingly difficult. Your weight loss will slow down, and you may find that losing even just half a kilo in a month will set off a Famine Reaction that will make you need to snack all day to keep your hunger under control. When you reach this point, if you want to lose more weight, then you'll need to be *super-vigilant* about listening to your body and eating accordingly, choosing highly nutritious foods and being active. I'll show you exactly how to do this in Chapter 5. By doing so you will ensure that you eat enough to stop your Famine Reaction from sabotaging your efforts but not so much that you can't lose more weight. After a while, when you reach the ideal weight for your body, you will stop losing weight. You may lose a few hundred grams now and again, but doing so will stimulate your appetite to the point that you inevitably gain it back again. When you reach this point, you've reached your optimum biological weight.

Some people discover that their optimum biological weight is lower than they expected. Throughout this book you're going to read many stories of people who were surprised and delighted to be able to lose more weight, and to keep it off with greater ease and grace, by listening to their body than they'd been able to achieve with any of the strategies they'd tried in years of previous dieting. This illustrates how working *with* your body in order to lose weight is so much more effective than working against it.

Other people discover that their optimum biological weight is higher than they may have wanted. Every time I see magazine articles about people who've lost a significant amount of weight, their newly slimmed-down bodies are almost always larger than those of people who have never had a weight problem in their life. Even the rich or famous, who presumably have time, money and sometimes cheering squads of publicists to help them lose excess weight and reach their ideal biological weight, rarely get so slim that they pose in a bikini for magazines or on television. This suggests to me that their optimum biological weight is heavier than the current standard for a bikini shoot. The bottom line is that if you've been overweight or obese at any time in your life, your optimum biological weight may be somewhat higher than what is promoted as the current ideal in our society.

Whether your weight loss comes to a standstill at a weight that's higher or lower than what you might have expected or desired, the weight and size that you end up settling at when you eat mainly wholesome foods, live an active lifestyle and consistently listen to your body – and I mean *really* listen by writing down your hunger and satiety signals as described in Chapter 5 – is your optimum biological weight. For me personally, it seems that my weight will never go under 64 kilos, no matter what the World Health Organization may say about how much I should weigh. Even when I up my exercise and am super-vigilant about eating wholesome foods and eating only when hungry, I lose a few centimetres here and there but my weight always stays close to 65 kilos. Sometimes I've wished that my weight could be otherwise. When I came back to Australia over 13 years ago to start a new life, I decided that part of that life would entail being slimmer. Knowing that listening to my body wouldn't get me any lighter than 64 kilos, I joined a diet club for the first time in over six years and followed their restricted-kilojoule diet. I remember coming home from the lab in the evening feeling totally ravenous and eating two big bowls of diet jelly in order to quash my hunger pangs until I could prepare my carefully counted diet dinner. A few days after I found myself in the throes of an irrepressible Famine Reaction, bingeing uncontrollably on a family-sized packet of chips and eating anything else I could find in my flatmate's fridge and cupboards. I hadn't binged like that, and felt so disgusted with myself, in over six years. It took me back to those wasted years in Diet Dungeon where I was constantly dieting and bingeing. That was a deciding moment in my life: the moment when I decided once and for all to love my body just the way it is, curves and all.

Binge eating is not the only thing you risk by trying to steam-roller over your Famine Reaction to get below your body's optimum biological weight. The Famine Reaction induces and exacerbates the hormonal changes that occur with menopause and ageing, such as a drop in the levels of sex hormones[8, 41, 42] and insulin-like growth factor–1[8, 42] circulating in the bloodstream as well as an increase in the circulating concentrations of the stress hormone cortisol.[2, 42, 43] All of these hormonal changes are known to result in a greater propensity to store fat around the midriff and loss of muscle and bone, as well as detrimental effects on libido and fertility.[38, 44–49] Please don't do this to yourself. If you're struggling to attain or maintain a particular weight but find that in order to do so you're often hungry, often on edge, often feeling cold, often on the verge of a binge or often feeling out of control around food (classic signs of the Famine Reaction), you may like to reassess your view of yourself and your ideas of your ideal healthy weight. By accepting being a little bigger than the goal you may have set for yourself, you stand to gain so much more out of life.

Over to you
Here's something you can do immediately to put the ideas in this chapter into action.

As a first step towards determining your ideal healthy size and weight, it's helpful to take stock of how you measure up against research into metabolic health. If your body mass index (BMI) is over 25 kg/m^2 and you're less than 65 years of age, then aiming for a BMI of 24.9 kg/m^2 or less is a prudent move. Additionally, if your waist circumference is 80 centimetres or more for Caucasian or Asian women or 94 centimetres or larger for Caucasian men, then stripping weight until your waist falls under these cut-off points is one of the best things you can do for your long-term health and longevity. Every kilo you lose will result in a loss of approximately 1 centimetre from your waist.

These simple measurements of weight, height and waist circumference can give you ballpark figures to aim for as you lose weight. However, your actual best weight may wind up being a good few kilos above or below these cut-off points for 'normal' values, and you won't know for sure when you've reached your body's optimum biological weight until you actually get there. Additionally, it's difficult to know in advance exactly how long it's going to take you to get there. In some months you may lose record amounts of weight or waist, and in others you may lose less for various reasons (Famine Reactions, busy periods that eat up the time you need to fully care for yourself, and so on). One thing's for certain, however: if you keep listening to your body and following its lead, it will take you to the weight you're biologically meant to be.

With this journey of uncertain duration ahead of you, why not make yourself comfortable and enjoy the ride? What can you do right now to enjoy your life to the full as your body sets off on the path to its optimum biological weight for life?

Whatever it is, just get out there and start doing it.

Chapter 4

How to track your weight loss reliably

We must walk consciously only part way toward our goal, and then leap in the dark to our success.
Henry David Thoreau, American author and philosopher, 1817–1862

As you set out on your weight loss adventure, it's important to ensure that you're weighing or measuring yourself in a way that helps rather than hinders your progress. In the course of helping people to lose weight by connecting with their body, I've come across many whose relationship with their bathroom scales was making it impossible for them to lose weight effectively. To find out if your weighing or measuring techniques are sabotaging your progress, take this quick quiz. You don't need a pen; just keep reading.

Quiz: Are you weighing or measuring techniques sabotaging your progress?

1. **My relationship to my bathroom scales can best be described as follows:**
A. I rely on them to show me what I weigh. Whether I weigh myself once, or whether I weigh myself three times in a row, the result is always the same, plus or minus 100 grams.
B. What bathroom scales? I donated that useless piece of equipment to the charity shop years ago.

C. I find mine very dodgy. They sometimes get stuck at certain weights, and when I weigh myself again they show a different number. But it's all relative; if I'm losing weight, even my dodgy scales can detect it.

2. When it comes to measuring my waist circumference:

A. I can do it.

B. I just can't do it; the number never reflects my progress. Sometimes I've measured my waist circumference and it looks as if it's increased, even though I've lost weight on the scales. But I have a pair of trousers that tell me exactly how well I'm doing. When I'm doing well, my benchmarking trousers get looser. When I'm doing badly, my benchmarking trousers get tighter. They never lie.

C. What waist? I haven't looked for it in years. All my clothes are loose and stretchy; they help me to forget about my girth.

3. When I start a new weight loss plan:

A. I weigh myself first thing in the morning on a reliable scale and take my waist measurement. I wear well-fitted clothes so I'll know how I'm going.

B. I can't bear to weigh myself, but I measure my waist circumference or try on my benchmarking trousers so I know my starting point.

C. I can't bear to weigh myself: seeing that number might scare the pants off me. I pull on my loose stretchies and start the day. I may decide to weigh myself or at least try on my benchmarking trousers in a few weeks' or months' time, once I feel certain I've lost some weight.

4. I weigh myself:

A. Once or twice a month.

B. Every day. When I see a positive number, it encourages me to keep doing what I need to do to keep my weight the way

I like it. When I see a not so positive number, it motivates me to try harder so I can see the numbers I love.

C. Every morning and sometimes every night as well.

5. When I weigh myself and see a pleasing number:

A. It encourages me to keep doing all the things that have helped me to achieve it.

B. It has no effect on how I live.

C. It makes me slack off and sit back on my laurels.

6. When I weigh myself and see a not so pleasing number:

A. It encourages me to get back on track immediately.

B. It has no effect on how I live.

C. It makes me give up and go have a party in my mouth.

7. When I see my weight on the scale, it has the following effect on my mood:

A. I feel pleased when I see a positive number and disappointed when I see a less positive number, and that motivates me to keep doing the things that work for me.

B. It has no effect on my moods whatsoever. How could it? The scale is a piece of metal.

C. When I see a good number I feel elated. When I see a bad number it's worse than a bad hair day. The weight I see on the scales not only affects the way I feel, it also affects the way I interact with people.

8. There's a change in my daily routine (for example, due to holidays or work commitments) and I wind up eating more than I normally would for several days in a row. Curiously, although I fully expect to gain weight, my weight stays the same day in and day out, or it may even have gone down a little. I keep eating in this way because I've seen I can get away with it. Then one day I weigh in to discover that I've gained a kilo overnight

for no apparent reason. I wish I could blame it on dodgy scales, but I can't. I wonder why life is so unfair. My reaction to this scenario is:

A. This doesn't apply to me because I don't weigh myself every day.

B. This has happened to me once or twice before.

C. I've experienced this disheartening scenario many times.

Scoring

If you answered C to any of these questions, it's possible that you're inadvertently hindering your escape from Diet Dungeon with ineffective weighing or measuring techniques. I wrote this chapter specifically for you. But even if you answered A or B to all of the questions above, the insights in this chapter could still make it so much easier for you to manage your weight. That's what happened to Jessie, a vibrant, energetic woman who came to a workshop I gave in Sydney five years ago. In fact, these insights not only made it easier for Jessie to manage her weight, they liberated her from a ball and chain she had been carrying for more than 35 years.

Jessie took a leap of faith, and look what happened

If Jessie had done the quiz at the start of this chapter on the day she first came to my workshop, a sunny winter's day in August, she would have probably answered B to question 4. Ever since she was 17 years old, Jessie had weighed herself almost every single day. Being just one month short of her fiftieth birthday when I first met her, she had quite a few weigh-ins under her belt. Daily weighing was part of Jessie's strategy for keeping her weight under control, and she was continually trying to push it down towards her ideal of just under 8 stone (50 kilos), the weight she felt her best at. (Jessie recorded her weight in stones rather than kilos.) Invariably, however, Jessie's weight hovered at around 53 kilos or above, and once she even went as high as 64.4 kilos, a weight that sat heavily on her petite, 1.57 metre frame.

As Jessie would soon discover, weighing herself every day was not helping her as much as she thought it was. On the contrary, it was actually hampering her progress like a ball and chain.

Jessie didn't make this life-changing discovery immediately after that workshop. It wasn't until two and a half years later that something clicked in her mind and a marvellous change was set in motion. It was all triggered when she came and heard me speak once again at the launch of my first book, *The Don't Go Hungry Diet*, and then read the book. Four months after the book launch, I saw Jessie again at another workshop.

As the workshop got under way and the participants and I started to become better acquainted with each other, Jessie beamed from ear to ear and announced that she had something to show everyone. She dug into her bag, and I was intrigued to see what might possibly emerge. Finally, Jessie resurfaced with a thick, heavy, navy blue A4-sized diary. 'At home, I have many other diaries like this one,' she explained excitedly. Jessie opened the front cover of her diary, revealing a two-page overview of the year. In the little rectangle for each day was a neatly written entry.

'This is me *before* Dr Amanda's book launch,' explained Jessie as she proceeded to read out some of her daily entries. 'Eight stone five pounds, eight stone five pounds, eight stone four pounds, eight stone three, eight stone four, eight stone four, eight stone five, eight stone five . . .

'And this is me *after* Dr Amanda's book launch,' announced Jessie jubilantly, pointing to March in the two-page overview of her year. Whereas up until late March Jessie's yearly overview was crammed with daily weigh-in results, starting a few days after my book launch she had left the rectangles blank. Jessie had taken a leap of faith and had decided to weigh herself just once a month. In the past, various health care professionals had suggested she stop weighing herself every day, but she said she didn't trust them enough to put it into practice. After the book launch, however, she decided to take the plunge. 'When I finally weighed myself again after one month of putting into practice the things I learned from Amanda, I was *three pounds lighter*!' she told us.

After so many years of daily weighing, Jessie was astonished with the effects of letting go and allowing her body to control her weight for her. What's more, Jessie has continued to weigh herself just once a month, and her weight hovers reliably at around 50 kilos, even through life's adventures such as breaking her ankle and not being able to be as active as she would like for a few months, and leaving her family, friends, home, work and comfort in Sydney to go and live in Montreal with her husband. A year-and-a half after taking that leap of faith, Jessie sent me an update via email. I'm delighted to report that she's *still* enjoying the benefits of weighing in once a month and being at the weight she feels best.

> *I flew back to Australia last Saturday in preparation for my eldest son's wedding at the end of the month, and I went to the wedding boutique yesterday to get my whole outfit approved and fine-tuned. When I took my jeans off and put the outfit on, the woman in the boutique saw my body and she said, 'Look at you. You are perfect. How do you do it?' and so on. Honestly, Amanda, for a wedding dress connoisseur to say that, I was over the moon, especially as she knew I am in my mid-fifties and no spring chicken. I had just weighed myself and I'm a whisker under 49 kilos – pretty damn good given that I eat fabulous meals full of a variety of goodies.*

While this loss of a few kilos on Jessie's small frame feels wonderful to her, the effects on her mental wellbeing are more far-reaching. After years of rigid mental control over her weight, she's no longer afraid of gaining weight.

> *Letting go of this one behaviour [weighing herself every day] has been the key to tuning into my body. Knowing and trusting you was my safety net to do this. Not only*

that, it makes our mealtimes at home less stressful – not so precise, not so rigid – because I'm not following what a 'diet' says to do.

The other major benefit of letting go of this one behaviour is that it has allowed me to get on with living – a phrase that you have said again and again – because I'm no longer preoccupied and taking up valuable brain space with thinking about food and eating, namely:

I can't eat this or that because . . . ; I want to weigh less in the morning so I'll eat less tonight; what will my husband say if I don't eat; I don't want to go out because I may overeat or eat something I prefer not to; I have to be strong and rigid about what goes into my mouth . . .

These are just an example of the myriad thoughts that used to run through my brain that are now over!!!

For decades, Jessie had used her daily weigh-in as a tool to keep her weight under control. However, it wasn't until she let go and decided to weigh herself just once a month that she realised that her daily ritual was standing in her way. Throughout her life, Jessie had walked consciously towards her goal of keeping her weight under control. Luck played little part in her slim physique. She was always careful about what she ate; she conscientiously avoided the foods that weighed her down; and she always chose the most nutritious options she could find. But as Thoreau puts it in the quote at the start of this chapter, walking consciously to your goal can only take you part way there. To finally achieve success, you must leap in the dark. When Jessie leaped into the dark by not weighing herself every day, she not only reached her goal weight, she also achieved something she could scarcely have imagined in her previous life: she was now able to live in peace and harmony with food and her body.

If you currently weigh yourself every day or every week, you might like to consider whether weighing in less often will give you a better result. This doesn't mean that you shouldn't weigh yourself at all. As you'll read later, weighing yourself regularly can be an excellent tool for permanently controlling excess weight. However, there's a point at which 'regular' stops being helpful and becomes a ball and chain. The only way to find out if your daily or weekly weigh-in is helping or hindering your progress is to take a leap in the dark, weigh yourself once or twice a month, and see if this gives you a better result. If you normally weigh yourself every day or every week, you may be dead scared of gaining weight if you don't keep doing this. But remember that the information in this book is your safety net. And as with all leaps of faith, scary as they can seem, you may surprise yourself by achieving *even more* than you imagined.

Less can be more, but none is not necessarily better

While Jessie got a better weight loss result, plus an unexpected bonus, by letting go of daily weighing, this doesn't mean that you shouldn't weigh yourself at all. In 1994, Professor James Hill from the University of Colorado and Professor Rena Wing from Brown Medical School in Providence, Rhode Island, New York, set up a registry of people who have lost weight and kept it off. Currently there are more than 5000 people listed in the National Weight Control Registry, and every one of them has lost over 13.6 kilos and kept it off for more than a year. By studying the behaviour of people who are successful at keeping weight off (who the researchers call 'Big-time Losers'), we can obviously gain valuable insights into what might work for people who are still struggling with their weight. In a recent study published in the journal *Obesity*,[50] 79 per cent of Big-time Losers from the National Weight Control Registry reported that they weighed themselves at least once a week. The researchers hypothesised that regular self-weighing may help people to maintain their weight loss by alerting them to weight gains and allowing them to make the necessary behavioural changes to prevent further weight gain. No surprises there; and, of course, by weighing yourself regularly you can see whether your current weight loss strategies are working or whether you need to adjust your approach.

Whenever someone asks me to help them in their weight loss journey, I first of all ask them to do the following: weigh themselves first thing in the morning on a reliable scale, and preferably also measure their waist circumference; follow the simple instructions outlined in Chapter 5 for about 14 days; and then weigh in again on the same scale and measure their waist circumference again on the morning of their scheduled appointment. If the person doesn't possess a set of bathroom scales, I suggest they use the scales at their local pharmacy, shopping centre, gym or doctor's surgery, wearing similar clothes each time. And if the person is totally averse to weighing himself or herself – a situation I completely understand given the love–hate relationship I've had with my own bathroom scales – I ask them to measure their waist circumference instead. I make it very clear to my clients how important it is that they follow these instructions. By knowing how much your weight and waist circumference have changed in your first weeks on the program, you know how much you need to tweak your approach, if at all, in order to get the results you want. If you don't know how much your weight has changed, or at least your waist circumference, you have no idea what's working for you and what isn't, and losing weight will be harder than it needs to be.

Precision powered Yvonne

Taking precise statistics helped Yvonne, a 37-year-old woman from Melbourne, learn that losing weight doesn't have to involve the huge sacrifice she had known it to involve in the past. Six months after the birth of her third child, Yvonne was ready to tackle her excess weight once and for all. She had already lost 8 kilos since her daughter was born, but at 74.5 kilos and 1.7 metres tall, she knew there was a leaner Yvonne yearning to break free from her size 16 clothes. Long before children, in what felt like another life, Yvonne knew her naturally willowy figure looked great in the smartly tailored clothes she wore to work as a lawyer in a busy Melbourne practice. But since becoming a mum, she had never been able to get her weight under 70 kilos for longer than a few weeks, after which it would bounce back up to around 75 kilos. In order to conquer the dreaded plateau and rebound weight gain, Yvonne enlisted my support via email coaching.

In getting Yvonne started on the adventure that changed her relationship with food and her body, I asked her, as I do all my clients, to get some good starting statistics (that is, weight and waist circumference). Apart from her recurring problem of hitting a plateau and rebounding, the greatest weight loss challenge Yvonne currently faced was her need to unwind after she had put the children to bed by having some adult conversation with her husband and a little treat such as a few squares of chocolate or a glass of wine, or preferably both. From past weight loss attempts, Yvonne viewed this as a big 'no-no'. Knowing that Yvonne was thinking she'd have to give up her regular sanity treat, a sacrifice that's never sustainable in the long run, I suggested she try some simple strategies that would enable her to enjoy her little pleasures while still losing weight and keeping it off. You'll read more about these types of strategies in Chapters 15, 17 and 19. Two weeks after our initial correspondence, I was delighted to receive Yvonne's first fortnightly update.

From: Yvonne
Sent: Wednesday 21ˢᵗ April 2:21 PM
To: Dr Amanda Sainsbury-Salis
Subject: Yvonne's Email Coaching: First Steps

Hi Amanda,
Please find attached my scanned success diary for the past two weeks. And what a success it's been – I have dropped from 74.5 kilos to 71.5 kilos and 105 cm to 99 cm (at the widest part of my waist)!!! To be fair I think the Pilates is also helping with the waist measurement. The result is quite a miracle given that I had family visiting the first weekend and we ate and drank up a storm! Last weekend my husband and I had dinner out at a great restaurant for our anniversary and also had a dinner party

*at a friend's place the following night! I tried to prepare
my appetite for the events and concentrated on eating only
what I really wanted, e.g. sharing a cheese platter for dessert
rather than ordering a big dessert for myself! Evidently it
worked! Really looking forward to seeing what you have
to say about the diary. I am interested to see what happens
next . . . I find the 70 kilo mark a big one to break through,
and would love to be able to conquer this over the next
two to four weeks. Thanks again Amanda!*

> *Regards,*
> *Yvonne*

Seeing how her weight and waist circumference were responding
to her efforts, Yvonne and I knew that she was on the right track.
Although she was eating some things that would have broken all
the rules on the weight loss programs she had tried in the past,
we both knew it didn't matter, because it was working for her.
She didn't need to give up occasional treats, because they weren't
preventing her from losing weight. By continuing to weigh and
measure herself regularly (Yvonne has found that once every two
weeks works best for her), she now knows *exactly* what she needs
to do to keep her weight moving efficiently downwards. Six months
after starting her weight loss adventure, Yvonne lost 8 kilos, to
reach 66.5 kilos. When she recently went clothes shopping with her
17-year-old niece, Yvonne was chuffed to come home with several
new outfits that fitted her perfectly and made her feel magnificent.
Here's what Yvonne said about losing weight in this way:

From: Yvonne
Sent: Friday 4ᵗʰ June 8:43 AM
To: Dr Amanda Sainsbury-Salis
Subject: Yvonne's Email Coaching: P.S.

Hi Amanda,
*I thought I should also thank you for some of the little
ways you have improved my quality of life:*

1. *Never again having to order a 'skinny' latte – YUK!*
2. *Losing weight without everyone noticing me counting my food – I always found it somehow humiliating.*
3. *Not having to trade things off in my head – like OK I'll have this beer but then I have to go for a big walk tomorrow and I can't have wine with dinner. Not being someone for whom self-denial naturally flows I hated this!*
4. *Best of all, not feeling – 'Great I'm now 70 kilos!' And then a moment later – panic, 'how am I going to stop my weight from creeping up!' and realising that I have absolutely no idea!*
5. *Another BIG plus is to be able to model really healthy eating behaviour for my kids. For them to see a mum who is in control of her weight, neither starving herself nor thinking constantly about food and able to enjoy food with the family, is just fantastic.*
    Thanks again Amanda!
    Yvonne

Don't miss a golden opportunity to learn the secrets of *your* success

It may sound obvious that when you start a weight loss program you need to take reliable starting statistics – either your weight or your waist circumference, and preferably both – but I'm constantly amazed at the number of people who don't. If you don't take reliable starting statistics you miss a golden opportunity to discover whether your weight loss strategy is actually working. Additionally, one of the factors that have been shown to predict a person's overall success on a weight loss program is successful results in the beginning, possibly because of the positive reinforcement this gives. So why not take advantage of this? When Belinda, 60, called to make an appointment to help regain the lissom dancer's physique she had known up until 10 years ago, I asked her to take her starting weight and waist circumference first thing in the morning; to try to eat according to her physical hunger, using the specific instructions that you'll read in Chapter 5; and then to weigh and measure herself again first thing on the morning of our scheduled appointment. Ten days later, Belinda met with me in Sydney as planned. After the usual exchange of pleasantries, I asked Belinda how she had got on. 'I'm not sure,' she answered. 'My scales at home are pretty untrustworthy. I thought I'd wait until I got here and take my starting weight on your scales.'

You know that sinking feeling you get when you close a door behind you and realise you've left your keys inside? That's exactly how I felt upon hearing Belinda's response. I feared that our meeting might not be as beneficial for Belinda as it could have been. But wait. Maybe there's a chance we could sneak back in through the window. 'Did you notice any change in your waist measurement in the 10 days since we spoke on the phone?' I asked hopefully. 'No,' answered Belinda. 'With a belly as big as mine, I'm never sure if I'm measuring it correctly.' Unfortunately, the window was locked. 'How about your clothes,' I continued. 'Have you noticed a change in the way they feel in the past 10 days?' Belinda said Yes, her jeans did feel as though they'd been getting a bit looser around the middle.

Thank heavens for Belinda's jeans! They gave us an inkling that she was on the right track . . . but we couldn't be certain. Maybe her jeans had just stretched from running around after her grandkids during the school holidays. Belinda then mentioned that she had succumbed to one of her favourite delights during the week, fish and chips with salad. It was hard to eat super healthily when the grandkids were around, especially when they went out to eat and she wanted to join in the fun. I reminded Belinda that other mature women have lost weight while enjoying occasional pub lunches and the like, and given that she eats veggies and fruit every day, there was probably no reason why she couldn't continue to join in the fun every now and again as she had been doing in the past 10 days. *Probably*. I wish I could have jettisoned that word from my conversation with Belinda, but in the absence of concrete evidence from the scales or a tape measure, we couldn't be certain whether what Belinda was currently doing was working for her. If only we knew how much her weight and/or waist circumference had changed in the past 10 days, we wouldn't have had to pussyfoot around with 'probablies'; we would have known exactly whether her current approach was working or whether she needed to do some fine-tuning. It's clearly impossible to fine-tune when you don't have a draft to start with.

I didn't see Belinda again after that day, so I can't tell you how she got on in her weight loss adventure. However, I felt disappointed for her sake that she had missed out on an opportunity to see concrete and motivating evidence of success at an early stage of her weight loss efforts. It was after this experience that I started going to greater lengths, making at least two follow-up phone calls, to ensure that my clients weigh and measure themselves when they start their Don't Go Hungry Weight Loss Adventure and then again before coming to see me. And, as you can see, I've devoted this whole chapter to the importance of weighing and measuring. I don't want *you* to miss this golden opportunity for a motivating start to your Don't Go Hungry Weight Loss Adventure, either.

Back up your data with waist measurements

When 54-year-old Millicent started losing weight by listening to her body, she was pleased to register a loss of approximately half a kilo at each of her fortnightly weigh-ins. She was losing weight more slowly than she had while following restrictive diet regimens in the past, but she was happy with her results because they didn't come at the price of being constantly hungry. Then one day Millicent went interstate to host a trade display at a week-long conference. She was on her feet all day, every day, and she did lots of walking around the huge convention centre. She was so busy that she scarcely had time to eat. When she did eat, she was careful to eat according to her hunger, because she knew her next weigh-in was just around the corner. She felt certain that she'd see a great result this time. So when she came back to

Sydney and saw that she hadn't lost any weight in the past fortnight, she was so disappointed that she lost her momentum and
regained 2 of the 2.7 kilos she had lost in the previous 12 weeks.
Had she also taken a precise measure of her waist circumference
every two weeks, she would have had a second chance of receiving the positive reinforcement she needed to stay motivated.

It's quite common to lose centimetres from your waist even
if you don't lose weight on the scales, especially if you're more
active than usual, as Millicent was.[51] If you're substantially
more active than usual, you may even gain weight, even though
you're obviously shaping up, mainly because the increased activity
makes your muscles hold onto more water as I'll explain below.
Jocelyn, 56, is a case in point. Jocelyn bought a new little black
dress before Christmas. It was a size 12 and fitted her perfectly.
When she went to put it on again in early January, however, she
discovered that it was now too tight. Shocked into action, Jocelyn
started cycling again for 10 to 15 minutes three or four mornings
a week, as she had been doing before the party season began, and
she also took up swimming one to three days a week for 20 to
30 minutes per session. Within three weeks of implementing this
change in her exercise routine, Jocelyn actually *gained* 2.8 kilos
on the scales, even though she lost over 3 centimetres from her
waist and her little black dress was now loose on her.

You always hear that 'muscle weighs more than fat' as the
explanation for weight gain despite centimetre loss with increased
activity, and this is certainly part of the explanation in some
cases. However, if you're consuming fewer kilojoules than you
need to maintain your body's fat stores and you're therefore
shedding fat, it's very difficult to gain muscle mass; the body
doesn't easily make muscle when there aren't enough kilojoules
available for maintenance. Part of the reason why increased
physical activity can lead to weight gain despite fat and centimetre loss is that exercise causes your muscles to hold more
water than they otherwise would. Exercise makes your muscles
become more responsive to the actions of the hormone insulin,
and the result is that they become more efficient at capturing

glucose (a simple sugar) from your bloodstream and either using it as an immediate source of energy or converting it to a branched structure called glycogen,[52] which is a stored form of glucose that your muscles can use in future bursts of activity. Although a burst of physical activity initially causes your muscles to eat up their stores of glycogen, the heightened effects of insulin mean that after exercise your muscles can accumulate greater stores of glycogen than they did before. Your body can store about half a kilo of glycogen in total. The more muscle mass you have and the more active you are, the more glycogen you can store. The important thing to note about glycogen is that it's a bit like a sponge in that it holds roughly three times its weight in water. So if you increase your level of physical activity and therefore increase the amount of glycogen stored in your muscles, it's quite possible to gain a kilo or so from water weight alone. This change occurs much faster than your body can make new muscle cells and increase your muscle mass. It explains why, if you've ever weighed yourself on the morning before and after an unusually active day, you may well have noticed an increase in your weight, even if you ate particularly carefully during your active day. It's for this reason that I recommend you weigh *and* measure yourself precisely during your weight loss adventure, because then you get two bites at the cherry of positive reinforcement that will motivate you onwards. If weighing doesn't agree with you and you prefer not to deal with weights at all, at least measure your waist circumference regularly so that you can track your progress.

HERE ARE A FEW NUMBERS TO CHEER YOU UP

Have you ever felt discouraged and given up because your weight loss was slower than you would have liked or you felt so far from your target? The next time you doubt your progress and feel inclined to pack it all in, take a moment to remind yourself of exactly how much weight you've lost since your highest (in the case of women, non-pregnant) weight ever. This is another good reason to take your starting statistics! When I was losing those 28 kilos, I used to constantly remind myself of how far I had come since my top weight of 93 kilos. If ever I had a 'fat day', where I felt particularly large, I'd cheer myself up with thoughts such as 'well at least I'm 6.2 kilos lighter than my top weight'.

One way to help you appreciate just how far you've come is to make a collection of packaged foods from your pantry that weighs the same as the total amount of weight you've lost since you were at your top weight. You can use things such as one-litre cartons of UHT milk (they weigh about 1 kilo), one-kilo packets of flour or sugar, and 500 gram packets of lentils or pasta. If you put all that food into grocery bags and carry it around for a few minutes, you'll realise that you've actually lost a sizeable amount of weight. Aren't you glad you don't have to carry it around all the time like you used to?

Here's another number that you may find heartening, as have many of the participants in my workshops. In the dozens of obesity research conferences that I've participated in over the years, and in the many research reports I've read, I've seen the results of numerous clinical weight loss trials. When weight loss is achieved by lifestyle means (that is, by changing diet and/or physical activity levels, including trials where healthy food is eaten ad libitum as outlined in this book rather than restricted to a set number of kilojoules), the average weight loss is about 12 kilos a year. This means that if you were to volunteer to participate in a long-term weight loss trial at a leading research institute, supervised by a multidisciplinary teams of doctors, scientists, dietitians and psychologists, you could expect to lose an average of 1 kilo a month over a year. So, if you're headed towards a weight loss of around 12 kilos a year, you're doing just as well as, if not better than, people in long-term clinical weight loss trials that are conducted in research facilities and supervised by teams of experts.

Another way to cheer yourself up about your progress is to project how much weight you'll have lost 6 months and 12 months from now if you just keep going as you are. Since you put your mind to losing weight in recent weeks or months, how much weight have you lost, and over how many weeks did you lose it? First, calculate your average weekly weight loss by dividing the amount of weight you've lost by the number of weeks over which you achieved that loss. Then multiply that number by 26 to project how much weight you'll have lost six months from now if you keep going at this rate, or multiply it by 52 to project how much weight you'll have lost 12 months from now if you just keep going.

For instance, let's imagine that two years ago you hit your highest-ever weight of 86 kilos, but since that time – after all the highs and lows – your weight has settled at 79 kilos. In the past 12 weeks you've been focused on getting your weight down another notch and you've dropped a further 2.5 kilos, to 76.5 kilos. You still want to lose another 16.5 kilos and you loathe being this heavy. The estimated amount of weight you will have lost in six and 12 months from now is as follows:

Average weekly weight loss = 2.5 kilos ÷ 12 weeks = 0.208 kilos per week
Projected weight loss after six months = 0.208 kilos per week × 26 = 5.4 kilos
Projected weight loss after 12 months = 0.208 kilos per week × 52 = 10.8 kilos

Even if your projected 6-monthly or 12-monthly weight loss is less than you would have liked, take a moment to imagine yourself a year from now. Wouldn't you prefer to be the projected number of kilos lighter than you are now, even if it's not quite as much as you hoped? Or would you be happy to weigh the same as you do now or even to be heavier than you are now? Six or 12 months may feel like a long time over which to lose weight, but the time will pass *anyway*, whether you choose to keep going or throw in the towel. Which outcome would you prefer?

Get facts not frights

Not only does knowing how your weight and waist measurement are changing during your adventure tell you whether your weight loss strategy is working for you and encourage you to keep going, it can also save you from thinking you have to take drastic measures to achieve your goal. Five years ago I gave a workshop in Sydney's inner west. One of the participants at that workshop was Lauren, 53 at the time, a beautiful woman with 40-odd years' experience of failed dieting attempts under her belt. I ran into Lauren briefly a few weeks after the workshop, and I was pleased to learn that she was putting the principles I'd outlined into action and was feeling the benefits of a more peaceful relationship with food. She had also noticed that her white jeans were getting looser. Two months later, however, Lauren called me in a panic. She had been to see her doctor for a check-up and had been strongly advised to consider gastric surgery as soon as possible in order to reduce her escalating risk of heart disease. Lauren had a referral to talk with a gastric surgeon and was booked in for an information seminar at the hospital the following week, a seminar she desperately didn't want to attend.

'Didn't you tell your doctor you'd been losing weight yourself?' I asked Lauren. 'But I haven't lost any weight! I've *gained* weight,' she blurted out. At her check-up, Lauren's doctor had weighed her. Since the last time she had weighed in at her doctor's surgery 18 months earlier, Lauren had gained several kilos and was now 134 kilos. Given her height of 1.61 metres, plus high blood pressure, insulin resistance and elevated blood lipids, losing weight was becoming a medical emergency in her case. 'What about those white jeans of yours? Weren't they getting looser when I last saw you?' I asked. Lauren said Yes, her white benchmarking jeans were continuing to get looser, but how did that stack up against the overall weight she had gained in the past 18 months? Would her current rate of weight loss be fast enough to avoid the need for gastric surgery? And how much weight loss did a looser pair of white jeans equate to, anyway? She hadn't weighed herself when she started her Don't Go Hungry Weight Loss Adventure, so she didn't actually know how much weight she had lost.

Lauren was horrified at the thought of going under the knife. I'd be scared, too. The two main types of gastric surgery currently in use for weight loss are gastric banding, where a removable band is put around the stomach to restrict its size, and what is called Roux-en-Y gastric bypass surgery, where the digestive system is irreversibly cut and reconnected, so that food entering the stomach no longer makes contact with the lower parts of the stomach or most of the upper small intestine. Instead, food from the stomach is rerouted so that it enters directly into the end of the small intestine. For reasons that are not yet clear, both of these procedures result in dramatic weight loss. However, while gastric surgery – particularly the more invasive Roux-en-Y gastric bypass surgery, as opposed to gastric banding – is currently the single most effective strategy for permanent weight loss, the disturbing fact is that sometimes it doesn't work. One year after gastric banding or Roux-en-Y gastric bypass surgery, the average amount of excess weight lost is 40 to 60 per cent for gastric banding and 60 to 80 per cent for Roux-en-Y.[53, 54] Eight years after surgery, these average weight losses are found to persist.[53] Despite these impressive long-term statistics, approximately 5 to 10 per cent of people who have gastric banding or Roux-en-Y gastric bypass surgery lose less than 10 per cent of the weight they need to lose. Gastric surgeons classify these as 'non-successful' operations. Moreover, there is currently no fail-safe way of predicting who will have a successful outcome after gastric surgery and who will not. Having gastric surgery for weight loss is a bit like a lucky lottery. Admittedly, it's a lottery where there are far more winners than losers, but the price of the ticket is particularly high (major abdominal surgery and its associated risks, side effects and expense).

Realising that Lauren hadn't weighed herself when she started her Don't Go Hungry Weight Loss Adventure after my workshop (it's only since then that I've discovered the importance of explicitly asking people to take their starting statistics), I suggested that she start weighing herself so that she would be able to give some specific numbers to her doctor about her current rate of weight loss. I also suggested that we set up a time to talk over the phone every week for a few weeks until she felt confident of her ability to lose weight by connecting with her body.

This turned out to be a good decision. Lauren lost 12 kilos in eight months and shared her burgeoning success story in my first book, *The Don't Go Hungry Diet*. A couple of years ago, on a sunny winter's afternoon, I saw Lauren again. My husband and I were walking along the promenade at Manly Beach, showing some of Sydney's sights to one of my former colleagues from Geneva, who was visiting us on her way to a conference. As we chatted in the sea breeze and kept a watchful eye on our children, I was surprised when a woman came up to me and said, 'Hello Amanda', smiling as though she knew me. I smiled politely and said hello as I racked my brains, trying to remember who she was. Then, suddenly, I recognised her lovely, kind green eyes. It was Lauren! Given that she had lost 30 kilos since the workshop three years ago, it was no wonder I scarcely recognised her. She looked sensational in a chocolate-coloured leisure suit as she headed home to her husband after her daily walk along the beach. It has now been five years since she started losing weight by listening to her body, and I'm delighted to tell you that Lauren has kept those 30 kilos off to this day and is gradually losing more weight. At 99 kilos, 35 kilos less than her highest-ever recorded weight, and with normal blood pressure, normal blood lipids and no trace of the insulin resistance she had before, she definitely didn't need gastric surgery. 'You may be interested to know,' she told me in an email, 'that those white jeans became too baggy and were given a new life at St Vincent de Paul's!' Later in this book I'm going to show you some of the specific strategies that Lauren is using to keep her weight moving down and staying down.

How to weigh and measure yourself precisely

Now that you've seen some real-life examples of the benefits of weighing or measuring yourself precisely and not too often, let's look at the best way of doing it.

How to weigh yourself precisely

If you have a set of bathroom scales, can you believe the first thing they tell you? Or do you have to weigh yourself several times in a row before you're confident they're coughing up the truth? Even after you've taken five or six readings, do you still secretly wonder whether your scales are giving you an accurate result or whether the batteries are perhaps going flat? If so, I strongly recommend that you get rid of them and either buy yourself a reliable set or use the scales at the gym, your doctor's surgery or a local pharmacy. Losing weight and keeping it off isn't easy. It requires lifelong vigilance, although it does get easier with time. Don't make the journey unnecessarily difficult for yourself by using poor equipment.

Body fat monitors

When choosing a set of scales, the simpler the better. Here's why I say this. Nowadays you can buy personal scales that not only show your weight but also estimate your body composition. These scales use the principle of bioelectrical impedance to approximate how much fat, water and fat-free mass (such as muscle and vital organs) you have. When an electrical current moves through a substance, its speed and tenacity depend on the conductance of that particular substance. For instance, metals are excellent conductors of electricity, whereas dry wood and woollen blankets are not. When you stand on the metal electrodes of a scale that measures body composition, a minute and unnoticeable electrical current is shot up through your feet, into your legs and lower abdomen, and back down to the electrodes. When the current reaches microscopic pockets of water around your cells or a chunk of muscle or a piece of large intestine, for instance, it zips through, scarcely missing a beat. Water is an excellent conductor, and muscle and vital organs – being about 50 to 70 per cent water – also conduct electricity extremely efficiently. But when the current reaches a wad of fat, its course is significantly impeded. Because fat contains only about 15 per cent water, the remainder being lipids that conduct electricity poorly, the current wades through your hip, thigh, bum and tummy fat as though through a thick swamp. Based on the speed and strength with which the current reaches the finish line, the scales calculate the amount of fat, water and fat-free mass you have.

These kinds of scales are an excellent tool for getting a ballpark estimate of your lean and fat mass. They have been tested on large numbers of people in numerous scientific trials, and the estimates they provide stack up well against more accurate methods for estimating body composition, such as dual-energy X-ray absorptiometry.[55] (This is explained in the box below.) If there's a body composition analysing scale at your gym or doctor's surgery, for instance, it can be really motivating to hop on and get an idea of what proportion of your body weight is fat. It's important to note, however, that if your body mass index (BMI) is greater than 35 kg/m^2 (see Chapter 3 for details on how to calculate your BMI), research shows that these scales currently provide inaccurate measures of body composition.[55] Another major limitation of such scales is that the technology isn't yet good enough to track progressive changes in body fat and lean mass from month to month. The body composition data you get from bioelectrical impedance analysis are highly dependent on your hydration status (the level of fluid you have in your body) when you weigh yourself. You've undoubtedly already noticed that when you're retaining fluid, such as when you eat food that's particularly salty, your weight can go up even if you swear you haven't gained in girth. You also saw earlier in this chapter that increased exercise can increase the amount of water you carry in your muscles, often resulting in a measurable weight gain. Estimates of body fat using bioelectrical impedance are *even more* dependent on your hydration status than weight. Therefore, if there's a change in the amount of fluid in your body from one measurement to the next – keeping in mind that significant changes in body fluid happen all the time as a result of factors that are difficult to control, such as how long you've slept, your stress levels, illness, caffeine or alcohol consumption, variations in exercise intensity, prescription medications, the types and amounts of food you've been eating and the female menstrual cycle – your estimated body fat content will vary markedly *regardless* of whether your fat content has changed. Moreover, losing weight in itself changes your hydration status. So, if you ever jump on those scales and they say you've gained fat in the past month, don't let it freak you out; you may have actually lost fat. Similarly, if the scales indicate you've lost fat in the past month, don't let it make you complacent; you may not have lost fat. The best way to gauge your progress from fortnight to fortnight or month to month is to use simple but precise measures of your weight and/or waist circumference.

HOW TO MEASURE BODY COMPOSITION PRECISELY AND ACCURATELY

In weight loss research, a lot of ambiguity and controversy arises because changes in body composition are not always measured precisely and accurately. That's because sufficiently precise and accurate technologies for measuring body composition were not available until fairly recently. Even now that they are available, they are still relatively expensive and so it's often not feasible to employ them in clinical trials involving a large number of volunteers.

The gold standard technique for measuring body composition (that is, fat mass, bone mass and lean tissue mass) is the 4-compartment model. This is the optimum method for accurately determining changes in body composition during dynamic weight loss, and is the method that my collaborators and I prefer to use in research when we are assessing weight loss and changes in body composition resulting from various interventions. Below is a description of the procedures our research volunteers kindly agree to go through up to four times a year. It's a time-consuming and labour-intensive procedure. If we could get reliable data on the progressive changes in the body composition of these volunteers from quick and easy analysis of bioelectrical impedance (as used in body composition analysing scales), we would. Since we can't, and until improved forms of technology become available that will make it quicker, easier and cheaper to measure body composition, this is what we do.

The 4-compartment model calculates the percentage of body fat from separate measurements of total body density, total body water and bone mineral content. Here's how each of those items is measured.

Total body density is the mass, or weight, of your body divided by its volume (the amount of space it fills). This used to be measured by 'underwater weighing', where a volunteer submerges their whole body in a tank of water and the number of centimetres by which the water in the tank rises is used to calculate the volume of their body. This, in conjunction with their weight, is then used to calculate their total body density. Nowadays the volume of a person's body is measured by displacement of air rather than water, using air displacement plethysmography. Volunteers change into a Lycra swimsuit and rubber swim cap and sit in the measuring capsule for a few minutes until a consistent measure of their total body volume is reached.

Total body water is measured by a method called deuterium dilution. This involves drinking a dose of 0.05 grams of 'heavy water' (^2H_2O) per kilo of body weight. Heavy water weighs more than normal water because it contains deuterium (^2H) instead of hydrogen (H). Deuterium is chemically identical to hydrogen except that it has a neutron in its nucleus. Deuterium is found naturally throughout the environment at a concentration of approximately one in every 6700 normal hydrogen atoms. As such, heavy water is also found naturally throughout the environment and in our bodies, but not in the concentrated form used in this laboratory test. The heavy water mixes with the water in the body and is excreted in the urine in proportion to the total amount of water in the body. A urine sample is obtained both before and five to six hours after drinking the dose of heavy water, and the amount of heavy water in the two urine samples is then measured by isotope ratio mass spectrometry. The increase in the amount of ^2H_2O in the urine after drinking the dose of heavy water is used to calculate the total amount of water in the body.

Bone mineral content is determined by a whole-body dual-energy X-ray absorpiometry (DXA) scan. For this test the volunteer lies on a table for a few minutes while an X-ray emitting arm sweeps over their body. The intensity of the X-rays is low, less than one-twentieth of what you'd receive from an X-ray of a broken arm, but it's not appropriate for research volunteers to have a DXA scan more than four times a year. The degree to which the X-rays are blocked is used to calculate the total amount of mineral in bones.

These measurements of total body density, total body water and bone mineral content are then used to calculate the total mass of fat, lean tissue and bone in the body. As you can see, it's quite an effort to accurately and precisely track changes in body composition in people who are losing weight. That's why I don't trust the changes in body fat or lean body mass that are obtained with the currently available body fat analysing scales. I rely instead on weights and circumferences.

How to get optimum results from the scales

Whether you regularly weigh in on your own bathroom scales or whether you weigh yourself only outside the home, such as when you visit your doctor, here are some ways to ensure you get the precise data you need.

- If you are buying scales, look for accuracy and precision over additional whiz-bang features you don't need.
- Use the same set of scales from one weigh-in to the next. There's no point weighing in at the gym if you know you won't continue going there for longer than a few weeks.
- Be sure that the scales are on a hard, level surface such as a smooth bathroom floor. Even the best scales will give erratic results on carpet. If you use the scales on carpet, I recommend putting a thick non-slip wooden board underneath them.
- Weigh yourself on the same surface in the same place every time. If you move the scales around the room to find the spot that gives you the best result, weigh yourself in that spot every time.
- Weigh yourself in the same clothes, or without clothes, every time.
- Weigh yourself at the same time of day. Your weight changes significantly over the course of a day depending on such things as what and how much you eat and drink, how much you sweat and expire, and how often you go to the toilet. A good practice is to weigh yourself first thing in the morning after going to the toilet.

Using your clothes as a guide during your weight loss adventure

When you measure your waist circumference, you need to measure the narrowest part of your torso (as seen from the front), between the top of your hipbone and the bottom of your rib cage. If there is no obvious narrowing between these two landmarks, measure your waist circumference at the mid-point between the landmarks. (More details about how to measure your waist circumference precisely and accurately are given in Chapter 3.) But what if you physically *can't* measure your waist circumference? I know a man who calls himself Buddha. If you saw him you'd know why. Buddha's midriff is so perfectly round that there is no indent to act as a consistent track for the tape measure, and he can't find his hipbones or his lower ribs.

However, one thing that always settles into the same spot on his body is the belt holding his trousers up. Recently, 66-year-old Buddha started paying attention to his diet and doing hydrotherapy a couple of times a week. He knows for certain that he's on the right track, because in the past 11 months he has had to tighten his belt by 12 notches in order to keep his trousers from falling off.

When you use your clothes to gauge your weight loss progress, particularly if you don't weigh or measure yourself regularly, it's important to use *quantifiable measurements*. Examples include dress sizes, the number of notches by which you've been able to tighten your belt, the distance your waistband overlaps when you pull it firmly around your waist, and the number of fingers or hands you can fit under your waistband when it's done up. Losing weight for life is rarely a case of losing a kilo a week every week until you reach your goal. You're almost certain to face challenging times where you feel you're not making progress and are tempted to give up. That's when such measurements are invaluable. You may have one of those 'fat days' where you feel larger than you actually are, but when you see that you can still fit into your size 18s whereas before you could scarcely squeeze into size 20s, you'll have physical proof of how much progress you've made and this will help inspire you to keep going.

Feel your way in the dark

Regardless of how often you choose to evaluate your success with quantifiable data such as weights, waist measurements and belt notches, it's helpful to be constantly aware of your body and how it's responding to your lifestyle. For instance, when you wake up in the morning, take a moment to run your hands over your body. They'll tell you exactly how well you're going. I can tell instantly how well I'm managing my weight just by looking at my face in the mirror first thing in the morning. If I see a hint of puffiness, I know I need to take a bit more care. When Yvonne is losing weight, she gets a particular feeling she finds difficult to describe. When she stops losing weight, she stops having that feeling. She finds the feeling so pleasant that it encourages her to keep doing the things that bring it on, and in the past six months she has lost 8 kilos. When you're constantly aware of your body and how it's changing in response to your lifestyle, it encourages you to do the things you need to do to keep your weight doing what you want it to do.

How often is too often?

Is your mood for the day dictated by the numbers you see when you weigh or measure yourself in the morning? Does seeing your vital stats affect your actions in a way that sabotages your long-term progress or even your relationships? When you nod off to sleep at night, is your peace of mind affected by the numbers you hope to see in the morning? If so, you're probably weighing or measuring yourself too often and you'd do well to pare it back. Remember that sometimes you don't realise what a struggle something has been until you experience what it's like to live without it. If you're in any doubt as to whether you're weighing yourself too often, try doing it once a fortnight and see if this doesn't make you feel better. Like Jessie, you may find it feels a lot better.

When someone asks me to coach them in their weight loss journey, I recommend they start by weighing and measuring themselves once every two weeks. Two weeks is long enough for your weight or waist circumference to drop by a measurable amount if you're on track, but not so long that things get out of hand if you're not, and not so long that you risk losing your focus and slipping back into old ways. Two weeks without weighing will also give you a chance to get more in tune with your body's messages about what, when and how much to eat. The reason for this is that when you start your Don't Go Hungry Weight Loss Adventure you may be more inclined to listen to your scales than to your body in regard to how much to eat. The trouble with this is that if you're weighing yourself every day, you are sure to see some fluctuations in your weight that have nothing to do with your body fat content. You may be doing really well at eating according to your hunger signals and you may be losing fat, but one day you weigh in and see a half-kilo weight gain due to an increase in how much water your body is holding (you may have eaten particularly salty foods the day before or done more exercise than usual, for example), and this can lead you to mistakenly assume that your strategy isn't working. You may then be tempted to pay more attention to what the scales are telling you than to what your body is telling you, with the result that you either resist genuine hunger in an attempt to improve your results (invariably instigating a counterattack from your Famine Reaction) or give up altogether and binge to the point of feeling oversatisfied. Either way, you won't lose as much weight as you would have if you had simply continued to observe your body's hunger and satiety signals and ate in the way they told you to. On the other hand, you may weigh in and see that you've lost half a kilo or so – which may or may not be fat loss – and this can lull you into eating more than your body is telling you to eat simply because you think you can get away with it. It's for these reasons that, in the beginning, I *strongly* recommend weighing and measuring yourself once a fortnight. Some people prefer to switch to more frequent self-monitoring thereafter, and some people prefer to switch to a monthly weigh-in once they feel confident about managing their weight by connecting with their body. Wendy, for example, prefers to weigh herself officially just once a month, at the same time in her menstrual cycle, because she knows her weight changes by up to 2 kilos depending on what phase of the cycle she is in. Hannah prefers to weigh herself just once a month because at the rate she's going – losing just over one kilo a month on average – she wants to be sure she'll see a noticeable, encouraging loss on the scales every time she weighs in. Gabrielle prefers to weigh herself just once a month, because it helps her put her weight loss journey on the backburner of her life, where it can simmer away quietly as she concentrates on other matters.

Keep in mind that sometimes you may prefer to watch your statistics every day, and at other times you'll be happier and more successful if you do it just once or twice a month. Once you find the frequency that works best for you at any particular time, do what you need to do to stick to it, even if it means removing your bathroom scales from your house.

WHEN IN THE MENSTRUAL CYCLE ARE YOU AT YOUR LIGHTEST WEIGHT?

Scientific studies have shown small but significant fluctuations in body weight over the course of the menstrual cycle in women who are not losing or gaining weight overall.[56] The average weight change is small – to the tune of half a kilo – and in some women there is no weight fluctuation, whereas in others the fluctuation is as large as 1.5 kilos. Peak weights are recorded in the few days leading up to menstruation or in the first days of menstruation, and weight drops to its lowest point in the last few days of menstruation or just after menstruation. This low point persists until ovulation, which occurs about 14 days after and 14 days before the onset of menstruation in a 28-day cycle. Several days after ovulation, weight starts to climb again to its perimenstrual zenith. On average, therefore, premenopausal women are generally at their lightest weight in the week immediately after menstrual bleeding ceases.

If you experience noticeable bloating and swelling (for instance, in your belly and breasts) in the lead-up to your period, or if your weight fluctuates considerably over the course of your menstrual cycle, you'd do well to weigh yourself just once a month, in the few days after your period finishes. This was the main reason why monthly weighing worked best for me while I was losing weight. After the 'Big Bang', as I called it, that horrible bloated feeling would dissipate and I'd feel like me again. What a great time to weigh in.

Regardless of how often you choose to weigh and/or measure yourself, back up your measurements with daily reminders from your clothes and hands about how you're going. It's how tight your waistband feels that will be of most help to you when you're seated in a restaurant deciding whether to have a second serving of beef vindaloo with rice and a beer, or some salad and another glass of sparkling mineral water.

Over to you

Here's something you can do immediately to put the ideas in this chapter into action.

Having read this chapter, and in thinking back over your past weight loss attempts, have you ever been tripped up by a lack of precise weights or measurements? Alternatively, have you ever been tripped up by weighing or measuring yourself too often? If so, deciding now to weigh and measure yourself precisely and not too often can set you up with a much greater chance of success.

In the next chapter I'm going to show you exactly what practical steps you need to take to kick-start your Don't Go Hungry Weight Loss Adventure. Many people are surprised to lose weight or centimetres after just two weeks of following the simple steps you're about to learn, so make sure you have access to a reliable set of scales and a tape measure so that you can take your starting stats. Also, if you usually weigh yourself more often than once a week, try weighing yourself just once a fortnight for the next two weeks. I think you'll be surprised at what your body can do for you if you give it a little time.

Chapter 5

Kick-start your Don't Go Hungry Weight Loss Adventure

Start by doing what's necessary; then do what's possible; and suddenly you are doing the impossible.
Saint Francis of Assisi, Italian Catholic deacon and
founder of the Franciscans, c. 1181–1226

In this chapter I'm going to show you the practical things you need to do to lose weight and keep it off by connecting with your body. If you follow the straightforward instructions in this chapter to the letter, you will lose excess weight and keep it off. Simply and surely you will lose weight – without having to count kilojoules, fats or carbs, estimate portion sizes, or sacrifice your lifestyle and eat separate foods to everyone else. Your Fat Brake will be able to help you shift any excess weight, because you'll be eating the kinds of foods that help it to work at its best. When your Fat Brake tells you to eat less by cutting your appetite, the step-by-step methods in this chapter will enable you to follow its clever lead, thereby making it possible for you to eat the quantities you need to eat in order to lose weight and keep it off. And as you lose weight and your Famine Reaction starts pulling stunts to stop you from losing any more, these simple instructions will enable you to eat enough nutrient-rich food to appease the beast. You will then be able to tiptoe around it and peacefully continue losing weight until you reach the weight you're biologically meant to be.

When someone asks me to help them lose weight, the first thing I ask them to do is follow the specific instructions in this chapter for two weeks. The reason for this is that I want people to get results immediately, and I've tailored the information in this chapter to achieve just that. More often than not, people who follow this guide lose weight or centimetres within the first two weeks. Our bodies already know how to attain and maintain an ideal healthy weight, and this guide merely helps people to connect with their body and enable it to do what it's biologically programmed to do.

As you're about to see, this is an incredibly simple guide. This is because there are so few things you need to do in order to lose weight effectively and sustainably, and you won't need to turn your whole life upside down in order to do them. Additionally, this guide is simple in that it won't ever make you work against your body's natural instincts in order to lose weight or keep it off. Instead, it will teach you to work *with* your body to achieve what it's designed to do. Simple doesn't necessarily mean easy, however, and that's why I'm here to steer you systematically through this learning process until you realise with absolute certainty what I already know: that you *can* reach a healthier, happier weight for life, and that your body will show you how.

How fast can you expect to lose weight?

Most people lose 0.5 to 2 kilos in their first 14 days of following the instructions in this chapter, provided they follow them to the letter. Some people lose a little less than this and some lose more. Jane, 55, lost 0.3 kilos in her first fortnight on the program, and 12 months later she has lost 6 kilos and wants to lose another 3 kilos. Samira, 32, lost 4 kilos and 3 centimetres off her waist in her first two weeks of following this guide, and within four months she had already lost the 10 kilos she wanted to lose. (You'll read more about Samira's story in Chapter 9). People often tell me that although their weight loss would probably have been faster if they had followed a restrictive conventional diet in the first two weeks, they are happy to pay the price of slower weight loss if it means they can keep eating as liberally as they have. As Tabatha, 39, said, 'At first I was a bit disappointed to have only lost one kilo in these first 14 days, but then I looked back over everything I'd eaten in the past two weeks and how unlike dieting it had felt, and it's actually quite remarkable that I've lost anything at all.'

How quickly you lose weight while following this program depends mainly upon the following factors: how closely you follow the instructions in this chapter; how much weight you have to lose (if you've got 50 kilos to lose you'll lose weight faster than someone who has only 3 kilos to lose); your sex (men tend to lose weight faster then women); your age; and your genes. How fast you lose weight also depends upon what your Famine Reaction and your Fat Brake are up to. If you start following the instructions in this guide after a long period of overindulgence, for instance, you will probably weigh more than your current Set Point and your Fat Brake will therefore be activated. Consequently, you will lose weight much faster than if you had started using this guide immediately after losing a lot of weight on a very low-kilojoule liquid diet, in which case your Famine Reaction would slow your progress. But how fast you lose weight is not the most important factor in your weight loss adventure. The most important thing is finding a rate of weight loss that's fast enough to keep you motivated while at the same time allowing you to enjoy your food in a sustainable way. At the end of this chapter I'll show you exactly what you need to do to achieve that vital balance. The other thing that's more important than how fast you lose weight is how long it has been since you haven't been back to your highest weight. Research shows that the longer it has been since you were at that uncomfortable zenith in your weight, the less likely it is that you'll ever go back up there again.[57, 58]

So, if you're ready to see what your body can do for you, it's time to put those kilojoule counters, obsessive exercise routines and lists of forbidden foods in the rubbish bin where they belong, roll up your sleeves and follow me.

Overview of how to kick-start your Don't Go Hungry Weight Loss Adventure

Here's an overview of what you need to do to start losing weight now.

- Take your starting weight and/or your waist measurement and try on some clothes to get a feel for how they fit.
- Follow these three steps.

  Step 1: **The art of eating according to your physical needs**
  Use a Success Diary every day and aim for *all* 2s and 3s.

  Step 2: **The power and simplicity of nutrition for weight management**
  Enjoy at least two serves of fruit and at least five serves of vegetables every day.

  Step 3: **Move**
  Gradually increase the frequency, duration and intensity of your physical activity until you achieve the levels recommended for permanent weight loss.

  Don't worry if you don't manage to take all three steps simultaneously; just tackle them in the above order of priority. For instance, if taking only one of these steps feels feasible for you right now, focus on Step 1 initially. Then, if you need to choose between making time for exercise or making time to enjoy fruit and veggies every day, put your efforts at this stage into eating the fruit and veggies. This will ensure that you start losing weight as soon as possible.

- After 14 days, weigh yourself and/or measure your waist circumference and try on those benchmarking clothes again, and see how they feel on you now.

Now, let me whiz you through the essentials of each of these steps.

Weigh and measure yourself only twice in your first two weeks on the program: once as you begin, and once again 14 days later.

It's vital to know how your weight or waist circumference and size change in your first two weeks on the program, because this will show you how much you need to tweak your approach, if at all, and because seeing your early success will motivate you onwards. So as you start your Don't Go Hungry Weight Loss Adventure, it's essential to weigh yourself or measure your waist circumference, and preferably both. The best time to do this is after you go to the toilet first thing in the morning. In Chapter 4 you'll find details of how to weigh and measure yourself precisely. If you feel that seeing your actual weight or waist circumference will have an adverse effect on you, you may like to ask someone else (such as a friend or relative, a doctor or a gym instructor) to weigh and/or measure you and keep the numbers to themselves. All you'll need them to tell you is how much your weight and waist circumference have *changed* in these first two weeks on the program; your actual measurements are irrelevant for now. It's also helpful to try on some clothes and get a feel for how they fit you.

If you usually like to weigh or measure yourself every day or every week, there's nothing wrong with doing that if it really agrees with you, *but only after these critical first two weeks.* (Chapter 4 will help you decide whether the frequency with which you weigh or measure yourself is helping or hindering your progress.) For now, put the scales or tape measure out of sight and out of mind for 14 days so that you can focus on connecting with your body signals. The reason for this is that as you start the process of listening to your body, changes in your measurements can sound louder than your body signals, and this can make you respond to what the scales or the tape measure are saying rather than to what your body is saying. For instance, if you weigh yourself after two days and see that you've lost half a kilo, it can make you eat more than your body tells you to eat simply because you think you can get away with it, thereby slowing your progress.

Once 14 days have passed, it's time to take the scales and tape measure out of quarantine so you can re-assess your statistics.

Again, it's best to weigh and measure yourself after going to the toilet first thing in the morning. If you haven't tried on your benchmarking clothes in a while, try them on again and see how they feel now.

Step 1: The art of eating according to your physical needs

*Use a Success Diary every day and aim for **all** 2s and 3s.*

In order to achieve success with this program, it's *imperative* that you write down how hungry and satisfied you feel before and after every time you eat or drink anything containing kilojoules, using a Success Diary. A Success Diary is simply a food diary with extra columns in which to record your hunger and satiety, as shown on the following page. Using your Success Diary will teach you how to read your body signals correctly and therefore how to eat according to your physical needs.

I recommend that you use a Success Diary until you feel confident about losing weight by connecting with your body. While many people start losing weight within two weeks of using a Success Diary, becoming confident about reading your body's eating signals usually takes longer: up to three months. To get started, you need to prepare a Success Diary that you can use for the next 14 days or more. It doesn't matter what format your Success Diary takes, as long as it contains the elements shown in the example on the following page. If you prefer using pen and paper, you could download and print off free Success Diary pages from my website (details of my website are at the back of this book), photocopy the blank Success Diary from the following page, draw up pages like it in a notebook, or purchase some of my Success Diaries in purse-sized booklet format. If you prefer electronic formats, you could download a free Success Diary spreadsheet from my website to use on your computer, or draw up a spreadsheet to use on your mobile phone.

Your Success Diary

Notes:	Date:		
Time	Hunger	Foods eaten	Satiety	Other factors

Time	Today's physical activity – every bit counts

From *The Don't Go Hungry Diet* by Dr Amanda Sainsbury-Salis, PhD

You won't need to keep a Success Diary forever,
but if you want to lose weight by connecting with your
body, it's essential to keep a Success Diary for the
first 2 to 12 weeks. Once you feel confident about
losing weight in this way, you can cast your Success
Diary aside and fly!

How to use a Success Diary to lose weight

The *first and most important step* in losing weight by connecting
with your body signals is to eat only when you feel hungry and
to stop eating before you feel overfull. This may sound difficult
to do, but when you use your Success Diary you will find it easier
than you expect.

Every time you eat or drink anything that contains kilojoules,
be it a three-course meal, a mouthful of something on the run, a
caffé latte or an orange juice, write down in your Success Diary the
time, what you consumed, and how hungry and satisfied you felt
before and after, using the scale of −4 to +4 in the following table.

Hunger and satiety ratings

−4	−3	−2	−1	0
Ravenously Hungry	Very Hungry	Quite Hungry	A Little Bit Hungry	No Feeling
I could eat anything right now.	I'd like to eat something substantial now.	I'd like to eat something now, perhaps a snack or light meal.	I'd be comfortable to wait a while before eating.	I'm not hungry at all.

+ 1	+ 2	+ 3	+ 4
Unsatisfied	Just Satisfied	Elegantly Satisfied	Oversatisfied
I still feel a bit hungry and I'd gladly eat something else right now.	My body is relaxed and comfortable. If I ate any more I would still feel comfortable, but I don't need any more.	My body is relaxed and comfortable. If I ate any more I would begin to feel Over-satisfied.	I know in my heart of hearts that I've eaten more than my body wants, and I feel uncomfortable.

Keep your Success Diary in a handy place and jot down your progress through the day. Otherwise, write down as much as you can remember at the end of the day. If you forget to write in your Success Diary one day, just skip that day and move on to the next day.

Your mission is to:

A. eat when you feel physically hungry, and only when you feel physically hungry (that is, a Hunger Rating of –3 to –2);
B. eat what you really feel like eating; and
C. keep eating until you feel truly satisfied (that is, a Satiety Rating of +2 to +3).

 Aim to score *all* –2s and –3s in your Hunger column, and *all* +2s and +3s in your Satiety column.

As you use your Success Diary, watch carefully to see if you score any –1s or 0s in your Hunger column. If this happens, it means that you're eating or drinking when you're not yet comfortably and physically hungry, and you're therefore consuming more kilojoules than you need. If it happens, write down any contributing factors (such as boredom or anxiety) in the Other Factors column. Once you become aware of the circumstances that make you consume more than your physical needs, it will be easier for you to do something about them.

If you score a –1 or 0 in your Hunger column once every three or four days, it's not a problem. But if you see –1s or 0s in your Hunger column more often than that, this will probably prevent you from losing weight. To ensure that your efforts are rewarded with satisfying weight loss, adjust your approach to meals and snacks and aim to score *all* –2s and –3s in your Hunger column.

As you use your Success Diary, watch also to see if you score any +4s in your Satiety column. If this happens, it means that you're eating or drinking more than your physical needs. Again, write down any contributing factors in the Other Factors column so that you become aware of any circumstances that may make you consume more than you need.

It's normal to sometimes eat until you feel oversatisfied; naturally lean people do it, too. But if you notice +4s in your Satiety column more than once every three or four days, this will likely hinder your weight loss. If this happens, aim to finish all of your meals or snacks when you feel more comfortably satisfied, at a level of +2 to +3.

While it's important for weight loss that you don't eat *more* than you need, it's equally important that you don't eat *less* than you need, either. Through past dieting experiences you may have come to accept that feeling ravenously hungry (−4) before eating or unsatisfied (+1) after eating is simply the price you must pay in order to lose weight. Science proves that this is not so. If you frequently feel ravenously hungry before eating, or if you frequently feel unsatisfied after eating, you will activate your Famine Reaction. Your Famine Reaction will then slow your weight loss and contribute to rapid rebound weight regain. Don't do this to yourself. Aim for 2s and 3s before and after *every* meal and snack.

Don't try this without a Success Diary

I know from hard-won personal experience how ghastly it is to feel trapped in an uncomfortably large body. I also know from my own six years of yoyo dieting how utterly soul-destroying it is to start yet another new diet and fail. I don't want you to waste two weeks of your life on a diet that doesn't work. And trust me: trying to lose weight on the Don't Go Hungry Diet without using a Success Diary is not going to work. You won't lose any weight, and you may even gain weight. In my early days of helping people to lose weight in this way, I quickly learned that people who don't use a Success Diary in the beginning don't lose weight. In fact, every single person who has kindly agreed to share their success story in this book used some form of a Success Diary in which to record what they ate as well as their hunger and satiety levels for at least two weeks. Now when I make an appointment to help someone lose weight using the methods in this book, I don't confirm the appointment until I'm absolutely certain that he or she has used a Success Diary for about 14 days. Research into weight management clearly shows that it's only by writing down what you eat and drink that you can become sufficiently aware of your habits to be able to change them.[59] So, if you're ready to see your desire to lose weight realised in the form of actual weight loss on the scales and clothes that have become noticeably looser and more comfortable on you, there is no better time than right now to start using your Success Diary. The early victory it will help you achieve will motivate you onwards towards even greater triumphs over the coming weeks and months. Remember, you don't need to use a Success Diary forever, only until you feel confident about losing weight by connecting with your body.

Step 2: The power and simplicity of nutrition for weight management

Enjoy at least two serves of fruit and at least five serves of vegetables every day.

Once you've got your Success Diary under way and you're aiming for those 2s and 3s, it's time to take a look at your food choices. The wonderful thing about losing weight by connecting with your body is that you don't need to eat like a saint in order to do so. While people who've had success with this method of weight loss certainly don't have takeaway meals, chocolate-coated ice-creams or wine with their dinner every single day, they don't cut all the fun out of their diet, either. In fact, if there are certain treats you absolutely adore, and your world just wouldn't spin properly on its axis if you didn't have them from time to time, I *encourage* you to incorporate them into your diet occasion-ally; doing so will make this program sustainable for you in the long term. However, there is one thing you definitely *must* do if you want to lose weight in this liberating way, and that is to eat adequate quantities of vegetables and fruit every day. As with all foods, ensure that you eat your veggies and fruit only when you feel hungry, and stop eating before you feel oversatisfied.

In order to lose weight by connecting with your body, you need to eat at least two serves of fruit and at least five serves of vegetables every day. The greater the variety of fruit and vegetables you eat, the better. There is absolutely no need to weigh or measure any of the foods you eat on this program, because your body will show you exactly how much you need to eat to lose weight and keep it off. However, to be certain that you're eating at least two serves of fruit and at least five serves of vegetables every day, you do need to know what constitutes a serve.

One serve of fruit is 150 grams of fresh fruit or:
- one medium-sized piece of fruit, such as an apple
- two smaller-sized pieces of fruit, such as two apricots, two plums or four dried apricot halves
- one cup of canned or chopped fruit, such as fruit salad
- one-and-a-half tablespoons of dried fruit, such as sultanas or raisins (use sparingly)
- half a cup (125 millilitres) of 100 per cent fruit juice (to be drunk sparingly, if at all)

One serve of vegetables is 75 grams or:
- half a cup of cooked vegetables, such as steamed peas, beans or broccoli
- half a cup of cooked legumes, such as dried beans, peas or lentils
- one cup of salad vegetables
- one medium-sized potato

For example, one way to get the fruit and vegetables you need for weight loss (and good health) is to eat at least an apple and a banana, say, with your breakfast and morning tea (two serves of fruit), at least two cups of salad with your lunch (two serves of vegetables), at least one cup of cooked vegetables or legumes with your dinner (two more serves of vegetables), plus a serve of starchy vegetable such as a medium-sized potato or a small ear of corn (another serve of vegetables, making a total of at least five serves).

It doesn't matter so much how you get your veggies and fruit, just as long as you eat them every day. The only thing to note is that dried fruit, fruit and vegetable juices (including alcoholic drinks), and deep-fried vegetables such as potato chips are best consumed only occasionally or in small quantities.

If you like an occasional drink, enjoy it with caution
Because liquid kilojoules (especially alcohol) interfere with your body's hunger and satiety signals, any more than one to four standard alcoholic drinks per week will stop you from losing weight – even if you're doing everything else to the letter.

Fruit can be of any solid variety, whether fresh, frozen, tinned or stewed, even with a little sugar added if this makes you want to eat it. I've met a lot of people who say they don't like eating fruit but who would quite happily eat diced pears and peaches in juice from a tin, or forest berries from the freezer, thawed and stirred through yogurt with a pinch of sugar if desired. These are both fabulous ways to get more fruit into your diet. Then there's stewed apple, strawberries, mangoes, kiwifruit, cherries, water-melon . . . the list goes on.

Vegetables can also be of any solid variety, whether fresh, frozen, tinned, raw or cooked. Be sure to add the condiments that make vegetables appealing to you. For instance, maybe you're not keen on spinach, but if you sauté it with a bit of butter or cream and garlic, I'll bet you'll reach for it time and again. In my six years of failed dieting attempts, I used to eat salad only when I was trying to lose weight. I would force myself to eat it without so much as a drop of fat. But then I learned to be more liberal with to-die-for salad dressings, such as olive oil vinaigrette and creamy mustard sauces, and now just I adore salad. I'm sure you will, too, when you find the salad dressings that light up your taste buds.

The most important thing with vegetables and fruit is to find ways to make them so enjoyable and enticing that you want to eat a wide variety of them every day. It's easier to do this than you may think it is.

Step 3: Move

Gradually increase the frequency, duration and intensity of your physical activity until you achieve the levels recommended for permanent weight loss.

Once you've got your Success Diary up and running and you're managing to eat a wide variety and adequate quantities of vegetables and fruit every day, you can move on to the next step in your Don't Go Hungry Weight Loss Adventure: making sure you are getting enough physical activity for permanent weight loss. Science proves that regular physical activity not only speeds up weight loss but is also essential for preventing weight regain.[60-62]

Before changing your physical activity habits, check with your doctor or health care provider that it is safe for you to do so.

To address the physical activity factor, you obviously need to know your starting point. The easiest way to do this is to use a pedometer and clock up how many steps you usually take in a day. Once you've done this for a few days and have an average figure as a starting point, aim to increase your step counts in increments of about 1500 steps per day (or about 15 minutes of moderate-intensity activity, such as walking). For instance, if your average step count is around 2000 per day, aim to increase this to around 3500. Once you're comfortably doing around 3500 steps per day, aim to increase your average to around 5000 steps per day, and so on. You can achieve significant increases in your level of physical activity with modest changes, such as parking your car a bit further away than usual and walking a bit more, and using the stairs instead of the lift where possible. Incidental activities such as these have been proved to help people lose weight. Write down any physical activity you do (including your pedometer count) in your Success Diary every day; this will help you to be more active.

Once you're getting an average of around 8000 to 12,000 steps per day (approximately 60 to 90 minutes per day of moderate-intensity activity such as walking, with lesser durations for more intense activities such as swimming), there's no need to keep increasing your level of activity, because medical research shows that this level of activity is adequate to aid weight loss and prevent weight regain.[60–62] However, as you gradually increase your level of physical activity, aim to incorporate some activities that make you huff and puff (cardiovascular training) as well as activities that make you work against resistance (resistance or strength training). Such activities provide clinically proven health benefits, and new research also suggests that they provide additional benefits for weight management over and above the benefits of less intense forms of activity.[60, 61, 63]

If you're clocking up around 12,000 or more steps per day on average – including some intense activities several times a week – but you're frustrated that you're not losing weight, it's not because you aren't exercising enough but probably because you're simply taking in too many kilojoules. Rather than adding still more physical activity to your life in order to lose weight, you need to look at how and what you are eating. Revisit Step 1, take an honest look at your Success Diary, and you'll probably see that you're consuming some meals, snacks or kilojoule-containing drinks when you aren't hungry. Remember: any kilojoules consumed when you aren't physically hungry at a level of –3 to –2 are in excess of your needs and will block your weight loss progress. So aim for all 2s and 3s in your Success Diary. Also, revisit Step 2 and check that you're eating adequate amounts of a variety of vegetables and fruit every day and keeping liquid kilojoules, especially alcohol, to a minimum. If you're eating when you're not hungry, if you're eating until you feel oversatisfied, if you're not eating enough vegetables and fruit every day, or if you're having more than one to four standard alcoholic drinks per week, you can exercise until the cows come home but you won't lose any weight. So take the time you need to master Step 1 and Step 2 and your efforts will be rewarded handsomely.

Roadmap of your Don't Go Hungry Weight Loss Adventure

Here's a roadmap that will help you to successfully navigate your Don't Go Hungry Weight Loss Adventure, from the sometimes scary first two weeks of trusting your body, through the rough seas of real life and the challenges it presents, all the way to your optimum biological weight for life. Your roadmap is also summarised in the figure on the following page.

If you're happy with your progress

If after your first two weeks on the program you're happy with the rate at which you're losing weight, or your shrinking waistline, what you're doing is obviously working. Your ongoing success is really just a question of continuing to do what you're doing. You do, however, need to check that you can sustain your approach. Too many people fall spectacularly from grace before reaching their optimum biological weight because they take an overly restrictive approach to losing weight. This strategy almost always backfires. Beware of making the following mistakes, all of which can slow or even halt your progress. Once you've done the diagnostic tests in the chapters indicated, you'll find helpful advice on overcoming each of these common problems in the text following each test.

- **Habitually getting too hungry before eating.** Diagnostic N°1c in Chapter 11 will tell you whether or not you're doing this,

Roadmap of Your Don't Go Hungry Weight Loss Adventure

Start here

Weigh and/or measure yourself (preferably both) and try on some clothes (Chapter 4).

Step 1: **The art of eating according to your physical needs**
Use a Success Diary every day and aim for *all* 2s and 3s.

Step 2: **The power and simplicity of nutrition for weight management**
Enjoy at least 2 serves of fruit and at least 5 serves of vegetables every day.

Step 3: **Move.** Use a pedometer every day and see how many steps you're clocking up.
Aim to increase your step counts gradually in increments of ~1500 steps per day.

In 2 weeks' time

Weigh and/or measure yourself and try on your clothes again.

Losing weight and/or centimetres at a satisfying rate?

Losing centimetres but not weight at a satisfying rate?
If you've increased your level of physical activity in the past two weeks, you may have lost fat and gained lean body mass, and you may see this as a reduction in girth but not weight.

Not losing weight and/or centimetres at a satisfying rate?

Use the following Diagnostics to find what may be blocking your progress.

Diagnostic Nº1a (Chapter 7)
Are you eating only when hungry (i.e. no more than two -1s or 0s in your Hunger column per week)?
Diagnostic Nº1b (Chapter 9)
Are you stopping before you feel oversatisfied (i.e. no more than two +4s in your Satiety column per week)?
Diagnostic Nº2a (Chapter 14)
Are you eating at least 2 serves of fruit per day?
Diagnostic Nº2b (Chapter 14)
Are you eating at least 5 serves of vegetables per day?
Diagnostic Nº2c (Chapter 15)
What's your intake of fun foods and liquid kilojoules, notably alcohol? Cutting it back can help.
Diagnostic Nº2d (Chapter 16)
Are you getting enough variety in your diet (i.e. 30 or more different foods per week)?
Diagnostic Nº3 (Chapter 18)
Gradually increase your level of physical activity to around 60 to 90 minutes of moderate-intensity physical activity per day (about 8000 to 12,000 steps), including some vigorous activity and strength training several times per week.

Go through these diagnostics from top to bottom. It's likely that one to three of them pinpoint what is holding you back. If you tweak your approach and hit the target scores shown, you'll get a good 'bang for your buck' in terms of measurable weight loss for your efforts. Give priority to the diagnostics at the top of the list and then work your way down.

Whatever you're doing, it's working, so keep going! Check that your approach will give you *sustainable* weight loss.

Diagnostic Nº1c (Chapter 11)
Are you avoiding ravenous hunger (i.e. no more than two -4s in your Hunger column per week)?
Diagnostic Nº1d (Chapter 12)
Are you 'going all the way' when you eat (i.e. no more than two +1s in your Satiety column per week?)
Diagnostic Nº2d (Chapter 16)
Are you eating a wide variety of foods (i.e. 30 or more different foods every week)?
Diagnostic Nº2e (Chapter 17)
Is your diet too 'perfect' for your own good?
Diagnostic Nº3 (Chapter 18)
Gradually increase your level of physical activity to around 60 to 90 minutes of moderate-intensity physical activity per day (about 8000 to 12,000 steps), including some vigorous activity and strength training several times per week.

Keep using your Success Diary until you feel confident about losing weight by connecting with your body.

In 2 weeks' time

Weigh and/or measure yourself and try on your clothes again. Keep tweaking your approach until you start losing weight and/or centimetres at a satisfying pace.

Keep going until you either stop losing weight or decide you need a weight loss holiday (Chapter 19). If you want to lose more weight, go back to the start (when you feel ready) to kick-start your ongoing weight loss.

and in that chapter you'll find inspiration for avoiding this problem.

- **Not eating enough to satisfy yourself when you do eat.** Diagnostic N°1d in Chapter 12 will reveal if you're making this mistake, and in that chapter you'll find strategies for avoiding it in future.

- **Not eating a wide enough variety of foods.** Chapter 16 will explain why eating a wide variety of foods is essential to losing all the weight you need to lose and keeping it off. Diagnostic N°2d in that chapter will show you whether you need to become more adventurous in your food choices.

- **Having an unsustainably low level of fun in your diet.** Diagnostic N°2e in Chapter 17 will show you whether your diet is too 'perfect' for your own good, and that chapter will also show you how to lighten up and have some fun as you lose weight so that you can keep going until you reach the weight you're biologically meant to be.

- **Inadequate physical activity.** In order to continue losing all the weight you need to lose and keep it off, sooner or later you'll need to bite the bullet and check that you're getting enough physical activity for this purpose. Diagnostic N°3 in Chapter 18 will help you to determine how you're faring in this regard, and in that chapter you'll find practical tips to help you make physical activity a part of your life.

If you're not making progress

If you reach the end of your first two weeks on the program and you're *not* losing weight or centimetres at a satisfying rate, chances are you are making one or more of the seven common mistakes listed below. These, too, will slow or even halt your progress. No one I've ever helped was making all seven of these mistakes. In fact, none of my clients was making any more than three, and many have had to watch out for only one. If you've already started using a Success Diary, you'll find you need to make only a few adjustments to fine-tune your approach and start losing weight or centimetres at a motivating pace.

- **Habitually eating when you're not yet comfortably and physically hungry.** Diagnostic N°1a in Chapter 7 will reveal whether this is where you're slipping up, and in that chapter you'll also find tried and tested strategies for avoiding this insidious diet wrecker.

- **Habitually eating until you feel uncomfortably full.** Diagnostic N°1b in Chapter 9 will show you whether this is the reason why you're not making the progress you desire, and in that chapter you'll also find tips to help you get around this problem.

- **Not eating enough fruit.** Diagnostic N°2a in Chapter 14 will show you how to quickly assess whether you're getting enough fruit in your diet for permanent weight loss, and in that chapter you'll discover some easy ways to make friends with fruit.

- **Not eating enough vegetables.** Diagnostic N°2b in Chapter 14 will give you the acid test for knowing if you're eating enough vegetables to lose weight and keep it off, and in that chapter you'll find some easy ways to incorporate more vegetables into your diet without feeling like you're constantly ploughing through salads.

- **Are you having too much fun to lose weight?** While you certainly need some fun in your diet if you are to lose weight in a sustainable way, there comes a point where too much fun will stop your weight loss dead in its tracks. Diagnostic N°2c in Chapter 15 will show you whether you've passed that point, and that chapter will show you how to bring your intake of fun foods or beverages back to a workable level that doesn't leave you feeling deprived.

- **Not getting a wide enough variety of foods into your diet.** This easily remedied but common mistake can not only make your diet unsustainable but can also stop you from losing weight and make it difficult for you to keep it off. Chapter 16 will show you why, and Diagnostic N°2d in that chapter will show you whether this error is your downfall.

- **Inadequate physical activity.** Yes, it's that old friend, physical activity. Diagnostic N°3 and Chapter 18 will give you the scientifically based facts on just how much physical activity you need in order to lose weight and keep it off, and in that chapter you'll find proof that even modest increases over your starting level will bring you better results.

If, after doing the diagnostic tests summarised above, you find that you've been sabotaging your efforts by making any of these mistakes, taking steps to avoid them will pay off handsomely.

Getting your priorities in order

Lifestyle changes are never easy. Some people like to go 'cold turkey' and improve everything about their eating and exercise habits all at once. This approach often brings better results. In fact, research shows that being physically active can make it easier to eat according to your physical needs.[64] When Alexia started using a Success Diary, she found it extremely difficult to hear her body's hunger and satiety signals. It wasn't until she started being more physically active that the signals became clearer, she felt more motivated to eat fruit and vegetables, and she was able to start losing weight. Other people (myself included) prefer to change just one or two things about their lifestyle at a time, allowing new habits to become entrenched before taking on any more challenges. This line of attack can often feel more do-able and sustainable. If this applies to you and you want to focus on tweaking just one or two things about your approach at a time, start with factors that are higher up in the list on the previous page and work through the list in order. For example, if you discover that eating when you're not hungry, not eating enough fruit and insufficient exercise are blocking you from losing weight at a motivating pace, there is no point in increasing your exercise level to speed things along unless you are also taking care of your kilojoule intake by eating only when hungry and eating more fruit. It's almost impossible to offset excessive kilojoule intake with exercise, and as you'll see in Chapter 8, even cyclists in the Tour de France don't lose fat after one of the most gruelling sporting events in the world. On the other hand, many people are able to start losing weight by focusing first on eating according to their physical needs (Step 1) and making appropriate food choices (Step 2), and it's only once they feel comfortable doing these things that they choose to focus on increasing their level of physical activity (Step 3), which speeds up their weight loss and helps them to keep the weight off. Tackling Steps 1, 2 and 3 in this order of priority will help you to achieve a motivating rate of weight loss as soon as possible.

Getting down to your optimum biological weight

Once you're losing weight or centimetres at a satisfying pace, you can keep going if you wish until you've lost all the weight you want to lose. For most people, however, weight loss will stall *at least* once before then. For example, once you've lost a certain amount of weight, your Famine Reaction will wake up and start trying to slow your progress. This will probably make you hungrier than you were when you started your journey, and as you'll be following your body's natural urges instead of working against them, as you probably did in the past, this will lead you to eat more than you were eating when you started your journey. As a result, your weight loss will probably slow down or stop. Rest assured that if you continue eating mainly nutritious foods (including fruit and vegetables) in accordance with your physical needs and do some form of regular physical activity during this time, then sooner or later your Famine Reaction will realise that there's no need to pull stunts like that, the beast will retreat to its corner, your appetite will return to how it was before, you'll no longer need to eat as much in order to allay hunger or feel satisfied, and you'll continue losing weight.

Do you need a weight loss holiday?

Often weight loss stalls not because of the Famine Reaction and a physical need to eat more but because of psychological reasons such as losing focus or momentum. For example, it may some- times seem a lot easier to pop a chocolate-covered sultana or 30 in your mouth than to find other ways to relieve boredom or introduce some fun into your life. If this happens and you don't feel ready for the effort required to lose weight, you may like to consider taking a weight loss holiday.

A weight loss holiday is a period in which you focus on maintaining your weight instead of trying to push it down (Chapter 19). While you'll never struggle against hunger while you're losing weight by connecting with your body, it does take commitment and focus. You need to be very attentive to eating *only* when hungry and stopping before you feel oversatisfied; you need to make sure you're eating adequate amounts and an adequate variety of fruit and vegetables every day; you need to consciously keep treats to a workable minimum; and you prefer-ably also need to be physically active. On the other hand, weight maintenance is considerably easier. It's easier to do it without the discipline of using a Success Diary, and you can, for example, enjoy slightly more treats than you would if you were trying to lose weight. So if you navigate periods in your life where losing weight is just not feasible, such as the festive season, holidays or work crises that steal your exercise and veggie-chopping time, taking a weight loss holiday and focusing on weight maintenance instead of weight loss can give you the sanity break you need. You can stay on a weight loss holiday for as long as you like, because whether you're losing weight or maintaining your new lower weight, you're winning.

Getting your engines started again

If your weight has been stalled for a while, for whatever reason, but you're ready to get it down to the next level, the best place to re-start is at Steps 1 to 3. If you haven't been using your Success Diary for a while, there's nothing better than bringing it back for a couple of weeks, or at least a couple of days, to help you achieve the almost exclusive 2s and 3s you need to achieve in order to lose weight. Your Success Diary will also make you more mindful of eating the vegetables and fruit you need for your weight's and waist's sake, as well as of how physically active you are.

Weight maintenance

When you've lost all the weight you need to lose and you've reached your optimum biological weight, your weight loss will naturally cease. Then, no matter how vigilantly you follow the instructions in this chapter, your weight just won't go any lower. Of course, your weight will go down a bit if you don't eat as much as your physical needs dictate (for example, if you're too busy to eat enough for a few days), but because you were already at your body's optimum weight, this change will result in a feisty Famine Reaction and a hearty appetite that's impossible to deny, and very soon you'll be back at your optimum biological weight. It's for this reason that when you're maintaining your weight at your Set Point by listening to your body, you'll naturally eat a bit more than when you were losing weight. Every time you lose a few hundred grams (and this will happen naturally on account of daily variations in how much you eat and exercise), your Famine Reaction will make you so hungry that you gain it back again. On the other hand, if you keep following the instructions in this chapter, you won't gain excessive weight, either. Whenever you gain a little weight (and this will also happen naturally from time to time), your Fat Brake will help you to lose it again, as long as you continue listening to your body signals and eating accordingly, choosing nutritious foods and staying active. In other words, once you reach your optimum biological weight, your weight will not be maintained in a static way but will naturally fluctuate within a narrow range. Your body will automatically look after weight maintenance for you, and all you have to do is listen to your body and eat accordingly, as outlined in this chapter.

Over to you

Here's something you can do immediately to put the ideas in this chapter into action.

To lose weight by connecting with your body, there are only three steps you need to take: eat according to your physical needs; eat nutritious foods (including vegetables and fruit every day); and gradually work up to the level of physical activity that has been scientifically proved to help prevent weight regain. As you set sail on your Don't Go Hungry Weight Loss Adventure, the most important of these three steps is eating according to your body signals – using a Success Diary to show you the way.

The best time to continue reading the rest of this book is once you've started filling in your Success Diary. By using your Success Diary in the coming days or weeks as you read through the remaining chapters, all of the insights you're about to learn will make so much more sense. You'll read many real-life tales of people who've unwittingly made one or more all-too-common mistakes that either prevented them from losing weight sustainably or prevented them from losing weight at all. By doing the simple diagnostic tests throughout the remainder of this book (you only need to have recorded three days in your Success Diary to be able to start running my Diagnostics over them), you'll be able to spot whether you're at risk of the same fate as the people in these cautionary tales. But unlike them, instead of spending a whole fortnight, or a whole month or more, trying to lose weight without success, you can spot potential problems from afar, remedy the situation right away, and thereby help ensure that you lose a satisfying amount of weight, or waistline, from your very first fortnight onwards.

So, have you started your Success Diary yet?

Step 1: Master the art of eating according to your physical needs

Inmates of Diet Dungeon tend to be of two types: those who can't lose weight or keep it off because they are eating too much, and those who can't lose weight or keep it off because they are not eating enough, thereby activating the Famine Reaction and inadvertently hindering ongoing weight loss.

While you undoubtedly know by now that if you eat too much or too little you won't lose weight, do you know whether you are obstructing your own success by doing one of these things, and if so, which one? I've been astounded by the number of people who don't know when they're eating too much or too little for permanent weight loss. Sure, if you regularly eat until you feel as full as a boa constrictor, you know you are eating too much. But eating too much isn't always so obvious. I've met many people who were baffled by their inability to lose weight despite eating only healthy foods and doing loads of exercise but who were actually overeating. It was only when they realised this and cut back their intake that they were able to lose weight. On the other hand, I've known many people who have imposed impossible restrictions on the amount they eat, thinking that the reason they weren't losing weight was that they were still consuming too many kilojoules, but who were actually eating too little. It was only once they started eating *more* at certain times while they were trying to slim down that they were finally able to lose their excess weight.

In this step I'm going to walk you through four simple diagnostic tests that will definitively show you whether you are eating too much or too little for permanent weight loss. I'm then going to help you find your own specific solutions, drawing on strategies that other people have found worked for them. Just as accurate diagnosis of a medical problem makes it faster and easier to find the most effective treatment, accurate diagnosis of overeating or undereating will enable you to quickly apply the most appropriate and effective solutions for you. Instead of feeling like you're forever trying to lose weight but not getting anywhere, your efforts can be rewarded with efficient and sustainable weight loss.

These four simple diagnostic tests are incredibly effective. Everyone I have worked with who has done them has gained valuable insights into how they can lose weight more effectively. But be warned: they are not for the faint-hearted. Doing them will require that you reflect on your body signals for approximately three minutes a day for at least three days. Some people won't do this, perhaps because they want instant or external solutions to chronic problems. If you do take the time to do these four simple diagnostic tests, however, I promise you that they will show you exactly what you need to do in order to successfully manage your weight, now and for the rest of your life. That's because using these tests will help you to *eat according to your physical needs*. This is important because although your metabolic rate will naturally change at various times in your life and for various reasons, your physical hunger will also change to match your metabolic rate. This means that when you listen to your physical hunger signals and eat accordingly, you won't eat more than you need, you won't gain weight, and you'll steadily attain and maintain the weight you're meant to be. As you'll see from the success stories in this section, it *is* possible to lose weight and keep it off through circumstances that can significantly reduce your metabolic rate, such as menopause, low thyroid function, and periods of inactivity due to time constraints, illness or disability.

Overview

Step 1 is the most important part of this book. Here's an overview of the journey I'm going to take you on. First, I'm going to help you determine whether you're eating too much to lose weight and keep it off. By far the easiest and most common way to eat too much is to eat when you are not yet comfortably and physically hungry, but another way to eat too much is to keep eating until you feel oversatisfied. Second, I'm going to help you determine whether you may be eating too little to lose weight and keep it off. One way to eat too little for weight loss is to wait until you feel ravenously hungry before eating. By far the most common way to eat too little for weight loss, however – and a mistake I have seen time and again among my clients – is to stop eating before you feel comfortably satisfied. If you try to lose weight while repeatedly failing to 'go all the way' when you eat, you will find it unnecessarily difficult to lose weight.

In summary, if you are not seeing results for your efforts, it's most likely because you are making one of the four following mistakes: eating when you're not hungry; eating until you feel oversatisfied; becoming ravenous before eating; and/or failing to 'go all the way'. If you're ready to find out which of these four mistakes is thwarting your progress towards the leaner, healthier you, read on.

Chapter 6

Are you eating too much to lose weight and keep it off? Barushka's story

A crust eaten in peace is better than a banquet partaken in anxiety.

Aesop, slave and storyteller from ancient Greece,
c. 620–564 BC

In a world where the average girth of people in developed and developing nations is expanding, an excess of kilojoules – resulting from overeating or underactivity or both – is the culprit. If you're carrying excess weight, it's because at some point in your life and for whatever reason – be it emotional or environmental or both – you consumed more kilojoules than your body needed. The solution is to take in fewer kilojoules than you burn.

The beauty of connecting with your body in order to lose excess weight is that your body will show you exactly how to do it. All you need to do is listen to your hunger signals and eat accordingly. Because human bodies the world over share the same physiology, this method of weight management transcends all geographic, language and cultural barriers. For this reason, when I was writing my previous book, *The Don't Go Hungry Diet*, I felt like I was sending out a message in a bottle. I wondered where my message would land, and what difference it would make to the people who found it. A few years later, I had the great pleasure of finding out.

When 25-year-old Barushka found my message on the shores of her computer's internet connection, she had recently landed a job in a busy law firm in Prague, in the Czech Republic. Finding her new job stressful and demanding, and having been through a tough few months finishing her law degree, Barushka had fallen into a rhythm of overeating for comfort. 'I used to eat lots of greasy things, not that many sweets (except chocolate), more like open-faced sandwiches, stuffed baguettes, deli meats, mayo salads, you name it . . .' she later told me in an email. 'However, one time after I had "stuffed myself for comfort", I realised that comfort may well be the only thing I did not get from overeating! Also, realising that I was the largest woman in our department was no good.' With her weight reaching its highest point of 76 kilos for her 1.64 metre frame, Barushka could no longer fit into any of her clothes. That was her deciding moment, the moment she decided to stop using food for comfort and instead to find other ways to cope with her stress. 'I got back into my favourite hobby, needlework, read more books and enjoyed my wonderful marriage more fully.'

One of the books that Barushka read at this time was *The Don't Go Hungry Diet*. Something in it clicked for Barushka and helped her in her mission. 'When I realised that food was just food, I decided that the only characteristics the food is going to have for me from then on is whether it is healthy or not. Teamed with lots of sports and exercise, I just decided to eat when hungry, eat what I like, but stick with healthy things. Soon the cravings sorted themselves out,' she said. To help her stop using food as a form of stress relief, Barushka removed overwhelming temptations from her environment by no longer buying foods she used to overeat. 'As for chocolate, I buy chocolate that is not a whole bar but divided into smaller bites and I have only one or two of them when I feel like it.'

Within eight months of eating no more than her body told her to eat and of being more active, Barushka had lost 10 kilos. She says that the best thing about being 66 kilos is being able to wear nice clothes, having 'way way better moods', and the compliments. 'My husband keeps on telling me how amazing I am. I don't get many nice comments from female friends and colleagues (this does not happen much here), but just a bit of envy, which is rather amusing.'

One of the things I love about Barushka's story is that in conquering her weight she also grew in other areas of her life, by learning to cope with stress without overeating. 'My work is still very stressful, and I suppose it will always be, however, getting to know it better helped me to get appreciation and even promotion, which negates the stress for me a bit,' she said. 'It is a very pleasant feeling to know that I no longer have to eat a lot to numb my insecurity and other unpleasant feelings.'

Over to you

To finish this section, I'd like to share with you the three most important things that Baruskha feels have helped her to shed these 10 kilos.

Remembering these:
Food is just food.
Eat when you are hungry until you are not hungry.
The chocolate you don't eat just now will be there later;
it is not going to run away.

Chapter 7

Step 1a. The number one barrier to weight loss: eating when you're not hungry

Hunger is the best sauce in the world.
From the novel *Don Quixote* by Miguel de Cervantes
Saavedra, 1547–1616

When you eat more than you need, it's nearly always because you are eating when you're not hungry. It's one of those things that, like snoring, almost everybody does at some point in their life, although they don't usually know when they're doing it . . . or if they do know, they don't like to admit it. Eating is such a basic survival instinct that it can be done in a practically unconscious state. In studies that have measured exactly how much people eat compared to how much they *think* they eat, absolutely everybody – and I do mean everybody, including slim dietitians and people who are vigilant about what and how much they eat – think that they eat less than they actually do.[65] It's all too easy to quaff a few olives or chocolate truffles or nibble a cracker or three when they are in front of you without realising how many you've eaten or giving any thought to whether you were hungry before tucking in.

Eating when not hungry is the single most insidious diet wrecker I've ever known. Whenever I help people to escape from Diet Dungeon, they often start off by telling me that the reason they can't lose weight is that they eat too many of the 'wrong' foods, or that they overdo it in restaurants or at dinner parties a tad too often. In fact, when we look at the data, it usually becomes apparent that the real reason they are carrying excess weight is not those extra-large lunches or dinners outside the home two or three times a week, or that slice of carrot cake while out for coffee with friends on Sunday afternoons. It's not that these things *don't* have any effect on weight; it's just that their infrequency, plus the fact that people who want to lose weight are usually acutely aware of them, mean that the damage is contained. No, the real culprit in the case of corpulence is the constant daily onslaught of food or drink – *any* food or drink that contains kilojoules – consumed once or twice *a day* when you're not hungry. It's the fruit and cereal eaten every day at breakfast despite a total lack of physical hunger at that time (more about breakfast later). It's the milky cappuccino drunk every weekday morning at 10 o'clock come hell or high water, even though a wholesome breakfast two hours ago means there is not the slightest hint of peckishness at that time. It's the full-sized lunch at midday, because that's the time lunch always is, even though you're not yet feeling hungry. It's the nut bar that gives you a lift on the drive home from work, despite a little voice inside saying 'You don't *really* need this right now.' This kind of daily onslaught of subtle overconsumption is the worst thing you can do for your weight. It's the surest way to prevent weight loss, and the easiest way to promote kilo creep. That's because when you're not hungry, your body just doesn't need any kilojoules, and any kilojoules eaten or drunk at that time are in excess of your needs and will contribute to excess bulk on your body. This is such a fundamentally important and widely misunderstood concept that I'm going to stand up on my soapbox and say it again:

Any kilojoules that you consume when you're not yet comfortably and physically hungry – whether in the form of a bucket of chips, a chocolate bar, a healthy balanced meal with lots of vegetables, a small handful of nuts, a flat white coffee (even if it's made with skim milk), an orange juice or whatever – will contribute to excess bulk on your body.

Does this apply to you?

The question is not 'Do you eat when you're not hungry?', because I know for a fact that you do, at least sometimes. Everyone sometimes eats when they're not hungry, including myself. (That's why I use sure-fire strategies for making sure I don't do it too often, as you'll read later in this chapter.) The *real* question is 'How often do you do it?' Is it so infrequent that it doesn't affect your weight in the slightest? Or is it happening at a rate that's seriously setting you back in the weight loss stakes? If so – and you'll find out for sure with the simple diagnostic test below – the good news is that cutting back on how often you eat when you're not hungry will give you a bigger 'bang for your buck' (in terms of weight loss for your efforts) than you probably ever imagined possible, and you won't even need to banish restaurants, carrot cakes or other fun foods completely from your life in order to see the benefits.

> ### Dr Amanda's Diagnostic N°1a: Are you eating when you're not hungry?
> To do this simple diagnostic test, use your Success Diary for 3 to 14 days as described in Chapter 5. For best results, aim to use your Success Diary for 14 days. That's because you may feel a bit wobbly about using your Success Diary in the first week as you experiment with reading your body signals and eating accordingly, but in the second week you'll feel more confident and your average result over both

weeks will give you a good estimate of what you're currently capable of.

Bonus offer

If you feel reluctant about using a Success Diary, I'd like to make you a special bonus offer for doing so. Once you've completed 3 to 14 days of your Success Diary, you'll be able to use those same pages for not one, not two, not three but 10 – yes, 10 – diagnostic tests in the book! That is, you'll be able to use the same Success Diary to complete Diagnostics N°s 1a, 1b, 1c, 1d, 2a, 2b, 2c, 2d, 2e and 3. For the 'price' of thinking about your body signals for approximately three minutes a day for 3 to 14 days, you'll receive 10 insights into the things that may be impeding your progress along the path to permanent weight loss. Knowing your own problem areas will enable you to focus your efforts on the things that will make a positive difference to your weight, and it will also save you from wasting energy on things that don't make your weight go down and may even make it go up.

How to do it

Once you've used your Success Diary for several days, your next step is to work out how many times per week you are eating when you're not yet comfortably and physically hungry. In other words, how many times per week are you scoring a –1 or a 0 in your Hunger column. This is straight-forward.

If you've used your Success Diary for exactly 7 days, you simply count how many –1s and/or 0s there are in the Hunger column of your Success Diary over that period. If you've kept your Success Diary for more or less than 7 days, here's how to calculate how many –1s or 0s you're scoring in a week on average, or how many –1s or 0s you'd be scoring in a complete week if you kept going at the same rate.

• Count the number of days you've used your Success Diary for the whole day.

- Count how many –1s or 0s you scored in the Hunger column of your Success Diary on those days.
- Divide the total number of –1s or 0s you counted by the number of days on which you used your Success Diary for the whole day. This will give you the average number of –1s or 0s you're scoring per day.
- Multiply this number by 7 to get the number of –1s or 0s you score on average (or would score) per week.

For example, suppose that you've used your Success Diary for 11 days, but yesterday the dog got hold of eight pages and chewed them into a ball, so you've got three full days of your Success Diary. In those three days you count a total of three –1s and two 0s in your Hunger column (that is, five –1s or 0s). So the number of times per week you're eating when you're not yet comfortably and physically hungry, on average, is:

5 times ÷ 3 days = 1.67 times per day
1.67 times per day × 7 days = 11.69 times per week

That is, you're scoring a –1 or a 0 in your Success Diary approximately 12 times a week.

Interpreting your results
If you're eating when you're not yet comfortably and physically hungry (that is, scoring a –1 or a 0 in the Hunger column of your Success Diary) around twice a week or less, well done and keep it up! By not eating when you don't feel hungry, you're helping your body to gravitate towards your ideal weight for life. Read on for reinforcement as to why it's important for long-term weight management that you keep eating only when you feel comfortably and physically hungry.

If, on the other hand, you eat when you're not yet comfortably and physically hungry more than twice a week and you're not losing weight as fast as you'd like, reducing the number of −1s and 0s you score in your Success Diary to two or fewer times per week will help you get much better results. For your waistline, those −1s and 0s are like cockroaches in your home; the faster you eradicate them, the better. Read on for inspiration on how to conquer those −1s and 0s, taken from real-life examples of others who have done it and who are now reaping the benefits.

Sharon overcame the mystery of weight loss by becoming aware of −1s and 0s

Thirty-four-year-old Sharon was a classic example of someone whose weight loss was being thwarted by −1s and 0s without her realising it. Sharon came to see me during the break at one of my introductory workshops. After losing 10 kilos using a variety of methods, she found that her weight loss had come to a grinding halt. Determined to get over her plateau, Sharon enlisted the help of a personal trainer. However, despite having watched what she ate and drank and having thrashed it out in the gym six days a week for the past six months, Sharon had not only *not* lost any weight but had *gained* 2 kilos. Considering that her training regime had been quite a step up in intensity and duration compared to her previous level of physical activity, Sharon's weight gain would almost certainly have been due to an increase in muscle mass and muscle water content. Nonetheless, there's only so much brawn you can gain from exercise, and if Sharon had been consistently losing fat in the past six months she would have noticed it on the scales by now.

Sharon asked me whether there could be some biological reason why she couldn't lose weight despite such a determined effort. Among the women I've met who can't lose weight despite exercising intensely, eating well and listening to their hunger signals, a common reason for lack of weight loss is that they've reached their optimum biological weight, as discussed in Chapter 3. However, given that Sharon weighed 92.5 kilos and was 1.65 metres tall, it seemed unlikely that this was the reason why she wasn't losing weight. I wondered whether a strong Famine Reaction – spurred on by her previous weight loss of 10 kilos – might have been the culprit, but as Sharon had not lost any weight in the past six months, this also seemed an unlikely explanation. Any Famine Reaction she might have had would probably have subsided by now. I asked Sharon whether she had been to her doctor to see if there might be any medical reason for her lack of weight loss. There are a few medical conditions that can make it exceedingly difficult for you to lose weight, even if you are heavier than your optimum biological weight. Some examples are polycystic ovarian syndrome, Cushing's syndrome and the type of diabetes that is treated with insulin. However, Sharon had recently had a thorough check-up and had been given a clean bill of health. Her personal trainer had suggested that she stop eating out in restaurants in order to get her weight moving downwards. Initially this seemed like a real party pooper of an idea, but when I learned that Sharon ate at least eight meals per week in a café or restaurant, I agreed that cutting it back a bit could help. After all, it's easier to get an overdose of kilojoules in cafés and restaurants because the food tends to be more generously laced with fats and oils than if you had prepared it yourself, plus such meals are often light on veggies. Add to these factors the thought 'I've paid for it, so I'd better eat it all', and it's obvious that someone who eats out a lot can easily consume more kilojoules than they need. It soon emerged, however, that cutting back on meals outside the home was something that Sharon was not prepared to do. Being single, she considered eating out to be an essential part of her social life.

It was getting close to the time I needed to start the second part of the workshop and we weren't any closer to finding the reason for Sharon's predicament. Clearly, it was time to go back to basics. I suggested to Sharon that she use a Success Diary for a few days and email it to me so I that I could see what might be standing in the way of her weight loss. Sharon obliged, and when I received her Success Diary I was relieved to see that her lack of weight loss was not due to some undiagnosed, difficult-to-treat condition but simply to a common hiccup. Can you spot it in the following example page from her Success Diary?

Notes:			Date: Tuesday 23rd October	

Time	Hunger	Foods eaten	Satiety	Other factors
07.30	–2	a couple of spoonfuls of passionfruit yogurt 4 sesame seed crackers with 1 slice of cheese cup of tea	+2	
10.30	–1	glass of pear and apricot juice 2 sesame seed crackers 4 grapes 1 date	+2	Wanted energy before going to the gym
12.30	–2	vegetables and mozzarella cheese on Turkish toast 1 spice cookie with a cup of tea	+3	
	?	grazed throughout the afternoon on crackers, yogurt, grapes and dates	?	Felt agitated after a phone call from Dave
19.30	0	slice of sourdough bread with olive oil and dukka Caesar salad with grilled chicken half a chocolate pancake	+2	Dinner out with Paula and Dana
21.00	0	2 crackers with goat's cheese and jam 3 spice cookies large handful of sesame seed crackers tub of yogurt	+4	Was in a bad mood and was craving chocolate but didn't have any so ate this instead. At least I stopped eating before I felt totally bloated, as I would have done before.

Time	Today's physical activity – every bit counts
11.40	60-minute workout at gym
18.30	30-minute walk

Did you notice that delicious-sounding chocolate pancake and the spice cookies in Sharon's Success Diary? Well, it wasn't those kinds of things that were holding her back; I'll tell you why in just a moment. Rather, the reason Sharon wasn't losing weight was that her hunger level had been no greater than a –1 when she ate that chocolate pancake and those spice cookies, plus all the other foods she ate in the same sitting, not to mention that snack she had before setting out for the gym. Sure, it was mostly nutritious food that she was eating, but it was just too much for her.

I suggested to Sharon that she try waiting until she felt comfortably hungry – at a level of –2 to –3 – before eating or drinking anything containing a significant number of kilojoules. She was unsure whether this would work for her, knowing she had a tendency to flick from feeling satisfied and content to ravenous and crotchety with very little warning, but she decided to give it a try. At first, avoiding the –1s and 0s was tricky. She was sometimes caught unawares and left feeling uncomfortably hungry when she was still a long way from a wholesome feed. Moreover, she needed to learn other ways of dealing with frustrations and disappointments than by eating when she wasn't hungry. But learn she did, because within a couple of weeks, pages such as the following started appearing more frequently in her Success Diary. Can you spot the difference from Sharon's previous Success Diary page?

Notes:			Date: Thursday 8th November	
Time	Hunger	Foods eaten	Satiety	Other factors
09.45	–3	banana muffin with passion-fruit icing	+3	
		orange and mango juice		
		skim mocha		
14.50	–3	1.5 small slices of mushroom pizza	+3	
		side serve of broccoli, cauliflower and carrot with butter		
		large bowl of leaf spinach salad with thousand island dressing		
		1 square of dark chocolate		

| 19.30 | –2 | 1 vegetable spring roll | +2 |
| | | salmon in teriyaki sauce with a small side of rice | |

Time	Today's physical activity – every bit counts
08.00	half-hour pump class plus 10 minutes on the stationary bike
08.50	20-minute walk

As you can see, Sharon was still obviously eating out and enjoying some fun foods as she was doing before, but the difference was that she was *no longer eating when she wasn't hungry*. And as the other pages in her Success Diary showed, she was managing to do this most of the time. Another difference that was clearly apparent was that she was eating significantly less. This usually happens when you eat only when you feel physically hungry. I know that the idea of eating less can seem like a storm cloud at a picnic, but the silver lining is that doing so usually results in weight loss. Indeed, three months later, Sharon had lost 3 kilos, all while continuing to eat out regularly and enjoying several end-of-year parties. Not only was she delighted with her weight loss, Sharon was pleasantly surprised to discover that her hunger was more predictable than she had previously thought. She now rarely got caught out by ravenous hunger. Most importantly, Sharon gained confidence that she could not only lose weight but could do so without turning her lifestyle upside down. Last time I heard from Sharon she had lost a total of 20 kilos, 10 of which she had lost after starting her Success Diary, and she has kept that weight off now for more than a year and a half.

With that, may I be so bold as to jump out of the pages of this book and ask if you've used that Success Diary yet and tried out Diagnostic N°1a? If you were to do this one thing, I guarantee that, like Sharon, you'd make some surprising discoveries about yourself and your body. Remember to weigh and/or measure yourself before you start, because once you banish those –1s and 0s and achieve almost *all* –2s and –3s in your Hunger column, and almost *all* +2s and +3s in your Satiety column, you'll be in for a nice surprise when you weigh and measure yourself again in two weeks' time.

Will I ever be able to eat normally again?

People who start trying to eat only when they're hungry often fear that they'll never be able to eat 'normally' again. Last spring, while running an advanced weight loss workshop, I invited participants to do Diagnostic N°1a by going through their Success Diary and counting how many −1s and 0s they had 'n their Hunger column. One woman flicked through the pages of her Success Diary, poised her pen over the page and started circling unenthusiastically, then sighed, closed her Success Diary and put it back down in her lap. When I asked her if anything was wrong, she told me there was no point in counting how many −1s and 0s she had in her Success Diary because *every* meal or snack involved a −1 or a 0. I must have looked unconvinced − I go to great lengths before workshops to ensure that participants understand the importance of avoiding −1s and 0s − because she opened her Success Diary and showed it to me. Sure enough, I didn't see a single −2 or −3. 'If I waited until I was hungry before eating,' she explained, 'I'd never eat.' I could see how concerned she was about this, because she had been eating three regular meals and one or two snacks every day regardless of her hunger levels. I did my best to assure her that a lack of hunger is only ever a temporary situation and that hunger will always come back to you if you give it half a chance.

If you've got surplus weight to lose, it's highly likely that when you start using a Success Diary your Fat Brake will be chugging away, trying to help you get rid of the excess. Remember, your Fat Brake is activated when you have more fat than your body's current Set Point, and one of its effects is to cut your appetite. So if you're vigilant about waiting for comfortable pangs of hunger before consuming kilojoules, you may find that in the beginning you eat breakfast and then don't feel hungry enough to eat again until dinnertime, or even until breakfast the next day. While this may sound appalling to some people, it's actually a cause for celebration. It shows that you have a Fat Brake and that it's in good working order. As well as quashing your appetite, your Fat Brake has probably also upped your metabolic rate, and it may also be pushing you to move around more than you otherwise might and in so doing helping you to burn through layers of past overindulgences. These are the days when you need to either get stuck into activities that are so fulfilling that you don't feel deprived if you skip a few lunches or dinners, or to eat something very light at mealtimes, such as a rocket salad with a few slices of pear and thin shards of parmesan cheese. Be sure to weigh and/or measure yourself as you start using your Success Diary, because with the Fat Brake blowing in your sails like this, you'll probably slim down at a terrific rate of knots. It's time to enjoy the ride!

THERE ARE ONLY THREE SITUATIONS IN WHICH I'D RECOMMEND EATING IF YOU DON'T FEEL HUNGRY

1. Breakfast, because scientific evidence shows that eating breakfast helps people to make better food choices later in the day. More about that later in this chapter.
2. If you know in your heart of hearts that skipping a meal will leave you feeling deprived or unsettled and lead you to make poor food choices or to binge later on.
3. If you have fixed mealtimes and you know that not eating now will mean you get ravenously hungry before your next opportunity to eat, thereby making you more likely to make poor food choices or binge.

In any of these three circumstances, eat something light and nutritious that your body and soul equate with a good meal but that doesn't make you feel overfull.

As you shed fat over the ensuing days, weeks or months, sooner or later you'll no longer have more fat than your body's current Set Point. Since your Fat Brake is only activated when you have more fat than your Set Point, this will be its cue that it's no longer needed, and your friendly Fat Brake will switch off. You may notice that your weight loss slows down at this time, no longer aided by the invisible ally that was stimulating your metabolic rate. On the other hand, you'll most likely enjoy the return of your appetite. Whereas before you might not have felt hungry at breakfast time, you may now start getting so reliably hungry for breakfast that you no longer need an alarm clock to wake yourself up in the morning. And you may start being able to set the clock by your body signals, so unfailing will be the hunger that heralds the arrival of lunchtime and/or dinnertime. If you stick it out for long enough to see your Fat Brake switch off and your hunger return, you'll be glad you did. Have you ever noticed how much better food tastes when you feel nicely hungry before eating? Instead of one or two opportunities a day to enjoy food seasoned with the most delectable sauce in the world (hunger), you'll enjoy two, three or more occasions every day to take true pleasure in your tucker.

If you keep eating only when you feel hungry, there will come a time when you lose so much fat that you get *below* your body's current Set Point. And that's when the real fun starts, because your Famine Reaction will kick in and will make you hungrier. When this happens, you may find that in addition to your usual meals you now need a snack or two to keep from falling into the jaws of ravenous hunger (–4). And you may also find that in order to reach the point of feeling just satisfied or elegantly satisfied (a +2 or a +3 of satiety) you now need to eat larger servings than usual. If you're a Food Lover like me, this will be another cause for celebration, because it will give you even more opportunities to enjoy satisfying your appetite. In the beginning you may not be sure that it's a Famine Reaction you're experiencing, but with time you'll become more confident about spotting it when it pays you a visit. Beth, 65, lost 9 kilos over 10 months using the method outlined in this book, getting down to 68.5 kilos for her 1.6 metre frame, and her weight has now remained stable at 67.5 to 68.5 kilos for more than 10 months. She now has a good understanding of her Famine Reaction and the effects it can have on her appetite. Beth's first Famine Reaction came after 12 weeks, by which time she had lost 5.3 kilos. As you'll read in her account below, it took her a couple of days to realise what has happening.

For the first few days, I wasn't sure that I was having a Famine Reaction as it wasn't how I expected it would be. I started waking during the night feeling hungry but I wasn't sure if it was indigestion, as I felt acidy and belchy. During the day I wasn't getting ravenously hungry, but I was a −3 at lunchtime whereas normally I'm only a −2, and I needed to eat a bit more than usual to fill myself up to +2 to a +3. After a couple of similar days the gnawing in my stomach during the night and the fact that I needed to add an afternoon snack to my day's eating convinced me that this was a Famine Reaction. I decided to have a snack before bedtime (a cup of cocoa and some trail mix), and that stopped me from waking up at night feeling hungry. This lasted for a total of six days (including the first two days when I wasn't sure). I thought I might be on a plateau now, but I'm not as I've lost 0.3 kilos this fortnight, with the Famine Reaction taking up six days of it.

THE THREE YESES TEST

To do this one-minute test, first make sure that you're physically hungry and then choose something that's available to you that you think you'd like to eat. Then ask yourself these three questions.

1. Will this food feel good while I'm eating it?
2. Will this food feel good once it's in my stomach?
3. Will this food still feel good one or two hours after I eat it?

If you can *honestly* answer Yes to all of these questions about the food you think you'd like to eat, then that food is exactly what you need to eat. But if you answer No to any of the three questions, choose something else that's available to you that you think you'd like to eat and put that through the Three Yeses Test. If you keep applying this test to various foods you think you fancy eating, then within a minute or so you'll know exactly what you really feel like eating, whether it's fruit and yogurt, a toasted cheese sandwich, a chicken Caesar salad, or a cappuccino and a slice of sticky date pudding.

As you can see from Beth's account, the Famine Reaction brought her a bounty of extra opportunities to eat with a hearty appetite. In order to make the most of these golden opportunities, it's important to ask yourself what you really feel like eating and going for that. Eating what you really feel like eating will give you the maximum pleasure from your food. The Three Yeses Test on the previous page can help you determine what you're really craving.

When you're having a Famine Reaction, you may find that the Three Yeses Test leads you to richer foods more frequently than usual. In fact, sometimes this will be the *only* change you notice in your appetite with the Famine Reaction, as was the case for Stephanie.

From: Stephanie
Sent: Tuesday 24ᵗʰ November 09:39 AM
To: Dr Amanda Sainsbury-Salis
Subject: Tired and Lethargic

Dear Amanda,
  I am soooo dopey and lethargic and wanting sweet energy food at the moment. I am really struggling to do my walking but I am about to go today nonetheless. I gave into my cravings on Sunday night and ate quite a lot of fruitcake – but I just loved it and off I went to bed and slept so deeply.
  I'd appreciate your thoughts . . .
  Thanks,
  Stephanie

Knowing that Stephanie had already lost about a kilo and that she didn't have much weight to lose, I strongly suspected that she was experiencing a Famine Reaction. I didn't need to point this out, however, because less than an hour later she realised what was happening and emailed me again.

From: Stephanie
Sent: Tuesday 24th November 10:16 AM
To: Dr Amanda Sainsbury-Salis
Subject: Famine Reaction

Dear Amanda,
I just realised it is called a Famine Reaction!!!!
How can I be going through this when I have hardly lost any weight?
I am going back to my diary for a couple of weeks . . . see if I am doing it right.
Will report.
Cheers,
Stephanie

When you hit a Famine Reaction, enjoy it and eat what you really feel like eating, because it won't last. If you continue to eat the types and amounts of mostly nutritious foods that really satisfy your hunger and cravings, your Famine Reaction will abate as your body accepts your new lower weight as its new Set Point and your appetite will return to how it was before. But fear not, because as you continue losing weight your Famine Reaction will kick in with increasing frequency as it seeks to protect you from wasting away. And then, when you reach your ultimate Set Point, the optimum biological weight below which you cannot naturally go, your Famine Reaction will visit you more frequently. Now that I'm at my optimum biological weight of around 65 kilos, I have a Famine Reaction whenever I eat particularly lightly for a day or two, such as when I'm giving a workshop interstate and don't have as much time as usual to eat regular meals. The next day, my Famine Reaction is back with a vengeance and I'm greeted with joyous opportunities to enjoy more of my favourite foods, such as Turkish dried apricots, honey-roasted cashew nuts and raisin toast. Since I love eating, but since I only get genuine pleasure from eating when I'm physically hungry, my Famine Reaction is now one of my favourite houseguests.

To sum up, if you don't feel hungry more than once or twice a day when you start using your Success Diary, there's absolutely nothing to worry about. There *will* be times when you're virtually not hungry at all, such as after you've been eating more than you need. However, if you follow your body's lead and eat only as much as you need, you will lose weight and your hunger will kick in again. Hunger *always* comes back. It's a survival instinct, after all.

WHEN YOU'RE NOT HUNGRY BUT YOU STILL WANT TO HAVE A PARTY IN YOUR MOUTH: DIET SOFT DRINKS

Knowing that I'm a strong advocate of whole foods, people often ask my opinion on diet soft drinks, the antithesis of the word 'natural'. Indeed, diet soft drinks contain many chemicals, such as artificial sweeteners, some of which have been linked to adverse effects such as bladder cancer when given in large doses to experimental animals.[66] Additionally, the acid in carbonated fizzy drinks has been linked to tooth enamel erosion and may contribute to reduced bone mineral density,[67] and it seems wasteful to use up so much of the world's resources to produce a product with absolutely *zero* nutritional value, particularly in light of such issues as global warming.

Despite all of this, I confess it gives me such a thrill to release the cap and hear that exhilarating fizz! Diet soft drinks are my guilty pleasure. When I was losing excess weight, I relied on diet soft drinks a lot, up to one or two a day. They enabled me to have a party in my mouth at times when I really needed to have a party in my mouth but just wasn't hungry. As such, diet soft drinks helped me to consume kilojoules only when I was hungry, and they therefore helped me to shed those 28 kilos. I got quite addicted to them. I remember feeling most put out when I was a patient in the Gastroenterology unit at the Geneva University Hospital in Switzerland, having just had my gallstones removed, and the nurses sternly advised me against buying diet soft drinks from the hospital vending machine.

The thing is, although diet soft drinks contain chemicals that we're certainly better off without, especially in the wake of liver surgery, the available evidence for detrimental effects of diet soft drinks on human health is sketchy and weak. What *is* compelling, however, is the overwhelming evidence that carrying excess weight is bad for human health. From what is known from research to date, the benefits of keeping excess weight at bay far outweigh the possible detrimental effects of a few diet soft drinks. Therefore, if a diet soft drink helps you to deal with situations where you just don't feel hungry but you really want to consume something, my advice is go for it.

Of course, the ultimate solution to eating when you're not hungry is to get out of the habit of putting something in your mouth if you're not hungry. This concept was not my idea; I first heard it from a hypnotherapist who tried to help me to lose weight when I was a teenager. He was right, of course, and more than 20 years later I've made great progress. (I'm now down to about one diet soft drink a month instead of one or two a day.) So if you're just starting your journey of learning to eat according to your body signals and you get the urge to put something in your mouth but you're not hungry, don't be shy about using a low-kilojoule crutch such as a diet soft drink. Other low-kilojoule alternatives that are possibly more healthful include tea with a splash of milk, chamomile tea with a dash of honey, a diet cordial with ice cubes tinkling in it, sugar-free chewing gum or – best of all – just plain water.

Are you making the mistake of eating five to six small meals a day?

Have you ever heard the concept that if you want to lose weight you should eat 'little and often' – five to six small meals per day – in order to 'keep your metabolic rate up'? This kind of advice is frequently given out in good faith at health clubs and gyms, but it's not backed by strong scientific evidence. In fact, following this advice has led many people down the path of eating when they're not hungry, thereby preventing weight loss and contributing to weight gain. To understand why this is so, it's helpful to look at the science underpinning this advice.

The concept of 'eating little and often' if you want to lose weight arose from cross-sectional investigations of populations that showed that the people who eat more frequent meals tend to weigh less than those who eat less frequently. Subsequent research, however, showed that this relationship between meal frequency and body weight only holds true for men, not for women.[38] Given this, it's somewhat ironic that it's women who so often strive to follow the advice of eating little and often. Moreover, just because a relationship exists between feeding frequency and body weight, it doesn't tell us whether one factor is causing a change in the other factor, and if so, what the *direction* of causality is. It may be that frequent feeding helps people, or men at least, to keep their weight down. Or it may be that the men with a lower body weight have a higher metabolic rate, and this means that they actually need to eat more frequently in order to meet their energy requirements.

Seeking to determine which of these two scenarios is more likely, Dr Michelle Palmer and colleagues at the University of Newcastle asked 180 obese men and women to follow one of three kilojoule-reduced diets for six months, each diet having an equivalent kilojoule, carbohydrate, protein and fat content.[68] The first diet was divided into three meals a day, the second diet was divided into three meals and three snacks a day, and the third diet was divided into six small meals a day. Now if it's true that eating little and often helps people to lose weight, you'd expect that the people who ate six times a day would lose more weight over six months than those who ate three meals a day, right? It seems it's not true. At the end of six months there was no difference among the three groups with respect to how much weight they'd lost, how many centimetres they'd stripped from their waistlines, or how much body fat they'd shed. There was no difference between men and women reported in that study. As for the relationship between meal frequency and body weight that's been reported from population studies in men, it would seem, therefore, that a lower body weight is *not* the result of higher meal frequency. Rather, it may be that leaner men have a faster metabolic rate, which means that they need to eat more often, or it may be that there's *no* causality between body weight and meal frequency, and that both parameters are simply influenced by independent factors such as the type of work the men do. Not only does this much-given advice about eating little and often if you want to lose weight not stand up in the light of current research findings, it also does a disservice to many people, as you'll see below.

Raylene was duped by her meal plan

A classic example of the negative effects of trying to eat five to six small meals per day without listening to your body is Raylene, a 44-year-old woman who wrote to me a couple of winters ago. At 1.65 metres tall and 61 kilos, Raylene was certainly in the healthy weight range for her height. However, while her usual weight was 58 kilos, in the past seven months she had gained 3 kilos, which had settled uncomfortably around her middle and made her feel unhappy. Something in her email alerted me to the likely cause of her weight gain: 'I currently eat three small meals and three small snacks every day, and this is a high-protein diet plan that was written for me by my personal trainers last year as I wanted to lose some body fat,' she wrote. I quickly replied to Raylene to alert her to the mistake I suspected she might have been making.

From: Dr Amanda Sainsbury-Salis
Sent: Thursday 5th June 8:51 AM
To: Raylene
Subject: Meal plans and weight loss

Dear Raylene,

If you aren't sufficiently hungry when you eat those three meals and three snacks every day, then they will stop you from losing weight and may even make you gain weight. This is likely what is happening for you.

When you keep your Success Diary as described in my book, it's important to aim for ALL −2s and −3s in your Hunger column, and ALL +2s and +3s in your Satiety column.

Many people who eat five or six small meals a day notice that they aren't actually hungry when they eat some of them, and this is a major problem.

Anything that you eat when you aren't hungry is in excess of your needs, and is stored as excess bulk on your body that you don't want.

So go the 2s and 3s! Even if that sometimes means only eating two meals a day.

If you'd like to let me know how you get on, I'd love to hear your experiences.

Sincerely,
Amanda

Two weeks later, Raylene excitedly wrote back with her results. As you'll see in her email below, it's clear that eating six small meals or snacks per day was to blame for her weight gain. When she connected with her body signals, she realised that she only needed to eat three times a day. By cutting out unnecessary snacks, she was able to lose weight and drift back towards her usual, optimum weight.

From: Raylene
Sent: Friday 20ᵗʰ June 5:00 PM
To: Dr Amanda Sainsbury-Salis
Subject: Re: Meal plans and weight loss

Hi Amanda,

How are you?

Just thought I would update you after two weeks as I promised.

I am, if I can use the word, 'gob smacked' at my results. I have lost 1 kilo in two weeks and nearly 1 cm off my waist, which is fantastic. I haven't felt as though I was eating less than I had been before, far from it, to be honest.

I haven't felt ravenous once. I have been eating three times per day, I always feel elegantly satisfied afterwards, and I haven't felt the need to eat anything else. I have been having lunch at around 12.30 pm and then not needing anything until 6.30 pm.

It has been so easy to do. Before, trying to think of what I was going to eat five times per day and packing it all up to take to work was a drag, now it is nowhere near as hard. I am still eating nutritious foods, salads, grainy bread, veggie soup, fruit and vegetables, mainly, as well as beans and legumes, which I love, and a bit of tuna. On the plan that I was following before, I had to eat a lot of protein and was eating a lot of fish which I don't particularly like as I would rather get my protein from vegetable sources. However, because I work out three times per week with weights, I was always advised to eat a lot more protein. But even though I have been eating less protein, I still have energy to do all of my workouts and cardio, which is great.

It has been cold this week so I have been having a lot of soups and chickpea curry and ricey things like that to fill myself up. I have found it so enjoyable to eat the things that I hadn't been eating on my higher protein diet, as supposedly there is not enough protein from these sources.

It has been so pleasurable to eat what I want (nutritious and whole foods though) and enough of it to keep myself elegantly satisfied, it is so different to thinking, 'I must eat every three hours' to supposedly 'keep my metabolism' working properly.

I have used a food diary every day to record what and when I have been eating. I was doing that before, so using a food diary is second nature to me and not a problem, but it has been invaluable to see exactly what I am eating, how hungry I feel before and how it is easily filling me up. It has just been so nice to eat the kinds of foods I would like to eat and in enough quantities so I am not snacking on anything in between meals.

Sorry I have waffled on a bit, but wanted to tell you how valuable I have found reading your book and following your instructions. As you say, it is simple and the foods taste great!

If you want to use any of my words on your site I am more than happy for you to use them, and I will certainly be spreading the news to family and friends about your book.

Take care and thanks again,

Raylene

Within six months, Raylene lost the 3 kilos she had gained in the previous seven months of exacting meal plans, and she's now maintained her svelte 58 kilos for almost two years, including the time when she was diagnosed with an underactive thyroid gland, as you'll read in the next chapter. By eating wholesome foods and eating only when she was hungry, Raylene found her ultimate solution.

Professional development for personal trainers

One of the things I love to do is to help personal trainers and exercise physiologists to understand the science of weight management and feeding frequency, because then they can use the information to help their clients. It's for this reason that when I was recently invited to lecture to first-year Human Movement students at a local university, I relished the opportunity to share what I've learned. As part of my lecture, I explained the concept of the Fat Brake to the class. Remember, the Fat Brake is your natural weight maintenance system. It helps you to lose excess weight after short periods of overindulgence by cutting your appetite and revving up your metabolic rate. 'Therefore,' I said to the students, 'If someone is not physically hungry, there's no reason why they should consume anything at all – apart from breakfast or a very light meal that would prevent them from subsequently pigging out. By only eating when hungry – even if it sometimes means eating just two meals per day – the Fat Brake helps people to gradually attain and maintain their optimum healthy weight.' At this, one of the students asked the question I'd been waiting for: 'I work part-time in a gym as a personal trainer, and we tell our clients to eat five to six small meals per day; otherwise, their metabolic rate will drop and they won't be able to lose weight. How does this fit with what you're saying about the Fat Brake and only eating when hungry?'

Bingo!

Here was my golden opportunity to help set the record straight on a well-intentioned but wrong piece of advice that has spread far and wide. 'Please,' I answered emphatically, 'don't do that to your clients!' In addition to telling the students about the research on meal frequency and body weight mentioned above, I explained that if a person was feeling hungry enough to eat five, six or more meals or snacks per day, then it was important that they eat five, six or more meals or snacks per day – whatever it takes to allay genuine hunger. Doing so would indeed help to prevent the Famine Reaction from lowering their metabolic rate and making it harder for them to keep losing weight. However, if a person was going through a phase where they just weren't particularly hungry (for instance, if they'd just come back from holidays a kilo or so heavier than usual and their Fat Brake had blunted their appetite, or if they'd just spent the weekend eating like there's no tomorrow because they knew they'd be starting a new diet or joining the gym on Monday), then eating five to six small meals per day when they weren't hungry would slow or even block their weight loss. Worst of all, encouraging people to eat five to six small meals per day regardless of how hungry they feel only serves to alienate them from crucial body signals that could help them to regulate their weight naturally.

The verdict on meal frequency

There is nothing wrong with eating five, six or even ten or more times a day, as long as you feel hungry at a level of −2 to −3 before every meal or snack. If you want to achieve a motivating rate of weight loss, take a few moments to note how hungry you feel before ingesting kilojoules, be they from solids or liquids. If you're frequently consuming kilojoules when you're not yet comfortably hungry (that is, you're scoring more than two −1s or 0s in your Hunger column per week), it's time to either cut back on the amount you ingest at each sitting, so that you get nicely hungry in time for your next feed, or cut back on the number of meals or snacks you eat. While you probably tend to follow a similar pattern of snacks and/or meals every day, a pattern dictated by your preferences and your environment, it's important to let your hunger signals be your ultimate guide as to whether to eat. Only they can tell you exactly what's right for you at any particular time in your life.

Wake up to a hearty appetite

Another time when many people repeatedly eat when they're not hungry is breakfast. No, I'm not about to say that you shouldn't eat breakfast if you're not hungry, because there's so much scientific evidence that eating breakfast helps prevent overeating later in the day.[58] However, scientific studies also show that repeatedly eating when you're not physically hungry puts you at risk of weight gain.[69] So, if you don't feel hungry at a level of −2 or −3 at breakfast time, keeping in mind that the hunger you feel before breakfast may feel different from the hunger you feel at other times of the day, the best thing to do is to eat your breakfast anyway; otherwise, you're more likely to say Yes when someone offers you a free doughnut with your coffee. However, if you scored more than two −1s or 0s in your Hunger column per week in Diagnostic N°1a and the wayward −1s and 0s are occurring mostly at breakfast time, you may start to wonder why your 'love handles' won't budge even though you're 'doing all the right things'. To help keep your weight moving satisfyingly downwards, you need to train your body to get comfortably hungry in time for breakfast. That way you get the double-edged weight loss benefit of eating breakfast *and* of eating only when hungry.

How to boost your appetite for breakfast

One way to boost your appetite for breakfast is to eat it a little later in the morning. This strategy works well for people with flexible timetables, such as retirees and those who work from home. Zeynep frequently noticed that she wasn't hungry first thing in the morning, but by the time she had gone for a morning walk, showered, and done some tasks around the home, she was pleasantly hungry for breakfast. What do I call breakfast? Provided you eat within an hour or so of waking, before you start the main activities of your day, consider it breakfast.

Another way to boost your appetite for breakfast is to eat your dinner earlier in the evening. Have you ever felt like the lady in Frank Sinatra's song, the one who gets too hungry for dinner at eight? Every evening at eight, 46-year-old Roseanne would sit down to a quiet dinner with her husband after the children had gone to bed. The only trouble was that Roseanne usually wasn't hungry at this time because she had been snacking since late afternoon while she fed the children. Her evening meal would often spoil her appetite for breakfast the next day, too. All this made for a lot of −1s and 0s in her Success Diary and no weight loss at all in her first month of using the diary. When Roseanne decided to stop waiting for dinner at eight and instead started eating dinner at around 5.30 in the evening – when her children ate and when she was actually ready for a proper meal – things started to change. Once she was able to look forward to her dinner at an hour that suited her, Roseanne got more pleasure from her food and found it easier to avoid eating meals and snacks when she wasn't hungry. This change – along with the realisation that if she wanted to improve her health she just had to put herself first – was instrumental in Roseanne's success. The last time I heard from her she had lost a total of 24.2 kilos in the 20 months since hitting her highest weight ever, and she had lost 20.5 of these kilos in the 13 months since she learned to eat according to her hunger signals. And what about her relationship with her husband? Roseanne tells how she manages this balancing act.

> *While I started out eating dinner earlier with the kids, I've had to re-think doing it every night! Eating at 5.30 with the kids meant that I was missing out on the all-important 'us time' with my husband. He wants to wait until the kids are in bed to have dinner, so I've come up with a plan whereby I eat later with him two nights a week and have an apple and a piece of cheese while the kids are eating their dinner at 5.30. On the nights when I don't eat with my husband and eat with the kids, I make myself a lovely pot of tea and have some kind of treat food like a small piece of chocolate or some really delicious yogurt and I join him while he's having dinner. This is working well for us at the moment but I keep it constantly under review and try to balance my needs with those of the family . . . not easy!*

If you can't change the time at which you eat breakfast or dinner, another way to boost your appetite for your morning meal is to eat a little less in the afternoons and evenings until you start consistently waking up with a decent appetite for breakfast. For instance, if you usually have a snack before bed, try eating a smaller or lighter snack, or no snack at all. I often get hungry before bedtime, and I've learned that if I don't feed that hunger I'll have a fitful night's sleep. But I'm often surprised at just how *little* food it takes to see me peacefully through to morning. Sometimes, when I've thought I would have needed a few table-spoons of toasted muesli with milk to help me sleep, I've eaten a couple of tablespoons of tinned peaches instead and had a divine night's sleep. At other times I bravely do without the security of my night-time snack, drinking just a chamomile tea with honey instead, and I've slept perfectly soundly. My night-time 'hunger' is often more a fear that I'll get hungry during the night than actual hunger. By being true to my body and eating only what I need to see me through the night – no more and no less – I consistently wake up feeling hungry for breakfast. That always puts me in a great mood.

WHY AM I SO RAVENOUS THE MORNING AFTER A BIG FEED?
While eating less at night usually increases your appetite for breakfast, have you ever woken up ravenously hungry the morning after a big feast at a restaurant or dinner party? The reason for this is that excess food (particularly processed carbohydrates) stimulates a large increase in the amount of insulin in your circulation. This flood of insulin efficiently pushes food-derived fuels such as glucose out of your bloodstream and into your muscles, liver and fat. Here, some of it is immediately used for energy, but most of the excess is stored as glycogen or fat. The result is that your blood glucose levels can plummet and your hunger can soar overnight, even though you have overeaten. To ensure that your morning hunger is a sign that you are burning and not storing fat, be sure to eat foods that are as minimally processed as possible (brown rice instead of white bread, for example) with plenty of fruit and vegetables, eat only when you feel comfortably and physically hungry, and stop eating when you feel pleasantly satisfied.

Another way to boost your appetite for breakfast is to be scrupulously honest about how hungry you are before having afternoon snacks. Are you really hungry at a level of –2 to –3 when you tuck into that homemade apple and walnut muffin with your cup of tea? Or are you eating to fulfil some other need? I've met many people who enjoy an afternoon snack as a way of rewarding themselves for completing certain tasks or as a break before moving on to other tasks. There's nothing wrong with that, as long as you're comfortably and physically hungry at the time. But if you're not actually hungry when it's time to take a break, think about ways to give yourself a break that don't involve food. When I finish my day at the institute where I work, I face the sometimes overwhelming task of picking up my children from day care and school and taking them home on the crowded train. I never know what kind of mood they'll be in or how tricky it will be to keep them well behaved on the train. However, I've found that things go a lot more smoothly on the days when I take a 10-minute break before leaving work to make myself a cup of tea, close my office door, gaze out the window and daydream.

When cutting out unnecessary afternoon or evening snacks, the idea is not to leave yourself feeling hungry and deprived at those times, but rather to eat just enough to satisfy your physical needs and then to simply get on with doing the things that fulfil your other needs. When you do this, within a short space of time you'll start waking up with a hearty appetite for breakfast, you'll annihilate those breakfast –1s or 0s, and losing weight and keeping it off will be much easier.

How can you tell the difference between physical and emotional hunger?

People starting their Don't Go Hungry Adventure often ask me how to tell the difference between physical hunger and the desire to eat for non-physical reasons. Although distinguishing between physical and emotional hunger may seem difficult to you now, once you start using your Success Diary to track your hunger and satiety signals the difference will soon become crystal clear. Here are some of the ways that people have described their sensations of genuine physical hunger versus a desire to eat for non-physical reasons.

- *Physical hunger starts slowly and builds gradually, but emotional hunger descends immediately and asks for instant gratification . . . usually with tiramisu choc tops.* – Wendy
- *Physical hunger can be easily satisfied with food, but emotional hunger can't be satisfied no matter how much I eat.* – Anne Marie
- *When I'm physically hungry I know exactly what I want to eat, but when I'm not hungry I umm and ah and I don't know what I want.* – Georgia
- *I know it's an emotional desire to eat when I feel full but I still want to eat.* – April
- *I'm physically hungry when I can feel there's something missing in my body.* – Bruce

My favourite definition of the difference between physical and non-physical hunger comes from a woman named Cindy. I think she sums it up beautifully.

- *If I have to think deeply about whether I am hungry or not, then I am not hungry.* – Cindy

Top tips for not eating when you're not hungry

As you'll see in the next chapter, the 'secret' of attaining and maintaining a healthy weight throughout life, including those times when your energy requirements are reduced for whatever reason, is to get into the habit of eating only as much as you need. If you wait until you feel genuinely hungry (that is, at a level of –2 or –3) before eating or drinking kilojoules, you've practically guaranteed you'll be able to manage your weight no matter what life throws your way. Not consuming kilojoules when you're not hungry will sometimes mean saying No to your favourite snack with your morning or afternoon tea, or some-times doing without that milky caffé latte unless you're genuinely feeling peckish at the time (yes, even if it's a skim milk caffé latte), perhaps having tea with a dash of milk instead. Not eating when you're not hungry will also sometimes mean skipping an odd lunch or dinner if it doesn't upset you to do so, or eating a *very* light meal (such as a miso soup or a plate of steamed veggies with a tiny dash of butter) if you don't like to skip lunch or dinner but you're just not hungry at the time, or eating less at one sitting so you'll feel nicely hungry in time for your next meal or snack. And, of course, not eating when you're not hungry will also mean ignoring weight loss advice you may have been given about eating five to six times a day if you're not actually hungry five to six times a day. In brief, eating or drinking kilojoules only when you feel physically hungry usually means consuming less than you might otherwise like to consume.

I speak from experience when I say that although you'll never need to fight against genuine hunger in order to do this, it's far from easy. We're genetically programmed to want to eat kilojoule-dense foods when they're available to us – regardless of how hungry we may or may not feel – and in most developed countries today kilojoule-dense foods are available 24/7. Additionally, food fulfils so many needs besides the basic physical need for sustenance. Whenever I eat my favourite brand of Swiss chocolate truffle, an instant wave of comfort and security washes over me. This partic-ular taste and texture has soothed so many of my frustrations over the years, and it's wonderful to know that I can always rely on it. My favourite chocolate is multifunctional; it does so much more than provide comfort and security. Whenever I feel trapped in the routine of work and commuting, as most of us do from time to time, a shot of Swiss chocolate on the way home gives me an instant dose of fun and excitement. With food offering so much more than simple sustenance, here are some strategies that I've found help me to avoid consuming kilojoules when I'm not physi-cally hungry, despite the fact that I must have been a Labrador in a former life and could easily eat whenever food is in front of me.

Kryptonite foods and quarantine

First and foremost, it's important to keep food out of easy reach. Kilojoule-rich food is now so cheap and readily available in our environment that the default route is to eat tasty morsels all the time and become obese. As you'll read in Chapter 15, new research shows that constant exposure to and overconsumption of highly processed, fatty foods trigger similar changes in the brain to those that are seen in drug addiction, which in turn drive the development of compulsive overeating and excessive weight gain.[70] If you don't want to go down the default route, there is no other way than to take control of your immediate environment. As an example, I rarely keep ice-cream and Swiss chocolate truffles in my house, because – like Superman when he comes into contact with kryptonite – they make me weak and I scoff them regardless of whether I'm hungry. I do eat these kryptonite foods regularly, but only when I'm out and I buy a single serving. What are *your* kryptonite foods? And what difference does it make to you when they are not readily accessible in your home, office or car?

Another thing I do to control my environment is to keep favourite everyday foods out of easy reach. I'm a giant fan of hot cross buns and raisin toast, but I always keep them quarantined in my freezer. Knowing that I have to go through the awareness-raising process of zapping them in the microwave or toaster for a moment before eating them means that I rarely bother to do so unless I'm genuinely hungry. If it's not possible for you to keep certain foods in quarantine, another thing you can do is to make sure that your readily accessible foods are plain and uninteresting. At work I keep a permanent stash of food in my desk drawer in case I forget to bring my lunch or I don't have time to go out and buy it. Knowing my Labrador-like tendencies, however, my stash consists of only those foods that I currently find pretty boring – wholemeal crackers, nut paste, raw almonds, wasabi peas and dried chickpeas. I know that I won't bother eating them unless I'm genuinely hungry.

Another effective way to control your environment is to be proactive about your social life. Whenever my family and I agree to meet up with friends, I'm quick to suggest active meetings, such as going for a walk in the rainforest, going for a swim at a beach or pool, or going to Sydney's Luna Park . . . *anything but the dreaded picnic*! If I could banish picnics from my life forever, I would, because they always leave me feeling fat and uncomfortable. I eat while I prepare the picnic food so that I can see if it tastes OK; I eat when I unveil my picnic food at the picnic so that I can see if it still tastes OK; and I eat to taste all the food that everyone else has prepared, even though I'm almost never hungry at picnics. Sure, when I go on active excursions with my family I might eat in the great outdoors when we get to the waterfall hidden in the forest, or between rides on the slides at Luna Park, but what I eat on those occasions is something like a single kebab or some crackers with cheese and tomato and an ice-cream. Eating only when I'm hungry is so much easier in these circumstances because, unlike at picnics, I don't have food in my face the whole day.

WALK AWAY FROM FREE FOOD

My friend Michael has lost 15 kilos using the principles outlined in this book and has kept them off for over 18 months. One of the things that has helped him to eat only when hungry was to deliberately walk away from free food. If he's at a function and a table full of snacks appears with tea or coffee, for example, he walks to the other side of the room so that he's less tempted to eat high-kilojoule foods with little nutritional value (as free foods often are), especially when he's not hungry. Another thing that has helped Michael to avoid eating when he's not hungry is to say, 'It's probably delicious. I'll have it later.' None of these cognitive efforts to keep from eating when you're not hungry are easy, but when I see Michael today, bursting out of his skin with radiant health, vitality and good looks, it's obvious his efforts are paying off big-time.

Controlling your environment is one of the simplest and most effective ways to avoid consuming kilojoules when you're not hungry. Moreover, because you can organise your environment when you're not in the throes of a giant craving for excess food, it's actually easier to do than you might imagine. Are there any simple things *you* could do to make your environment more conducive to eating only when you're hungry?

Remember your reasons for wanting to lose weight or keep it off

A second way to avoid eating when you're not hungry is to keep reminding yourself of your reasons for wanting to lose weight or keep it off. As I write this, I'm staying at my mum's place in Perth with my children during the long summer school holidays while my husband tends to things he needs to do in Europe. To tell you the truth, I was nervous about taking such a long holiday alone with our children, because this situation is reminiscent of the one that saw me gain 40 kilos in six years as a teenager. I was babysitting full-time for friends' children over my long summer holidays and eating all day to relieve my boredom and loneliness. I was afraid of ballooning this summer as I'd done in the past. Therefore, I wrote myself a little paragraph to remind myself of why I want to stay lean and trim these holidays, as well as how I'm going to do it (by waiting until I'm nicely hungry before eating or drinking anything containing kilojoules and by getting a minimum of 8000 steps in incidental activity per day), and I read that paragraph every single day. In brief, my current reason for wanting to stay lean is that it makes me feel really happy in myself and helps me to wholeheartedly connect with the people I love, whereas being on the high side of 65 kilos makes me feel cranky and short-tempered – not a good look, especially for the school holidays. Also, when I go back to Sydney in the cooler days at the end of the summer, I want to slip back into my favourite jeans and feel the exhilaration of being able to do them up easily. This constant reminder of my reasons for wanting to stay in shape motivates me to be nicely hungry before hoeing into anything, and it also encourages me to go for an extra trip to the pool, park or beach with the kids. So far so good: it has now (as I write) been a week (that week being the week between Christmas and New Year's Eve) and my clothes still feel satisfyingly loose on me. This is such a great feeling that I'm now on a roll and am confident I can continue to do what I know I need to do.

So, what are *your* reasons for wanting to be lean? Would it help you to write them down as a constant reminder to yourself, especially when opportunities for unnecessary eating abound?

Set yourself challenges and get involved in activities

Another excellent way to avoid eating when you're not hungry is to get involved in activities that are so absorbing that you don't even think about eating unless your hunger alerts you to it. That's where having goals and setting yourself challenges can be a huge help. Your goals and the challenges you set yourself can be as modest or as ambitious as you like. The important thing is to make room in your life for activities that you find fulfilling rather than sitting back and eating for lack of having anything better to do. In my own case, my mission this summer, in addition to giving my children a proper long break from school and day care, is to write so much of this book that I feel confident about meeting my publisher's deadline in three-and-a-half months' time. My goal is fulfilling, because writing a book makes me feel that I'm using my knowledge and abilities to their best advantage and in a way that can benefit others. One of the things I love doing is to sit in a private corner of a clattery café for a few hours and write, or put the children to bed early and write some more, a soothing cup of tea by my side. My goal is also exciting, because while I'm not entirely sure that I can make it on time, I also know how euphoric I'll feel if I do. The result is that – in contrast to those fateful summer holidays when I was a bored, bingeing babysitter – I'm doing what I love and feeling fantastic. Why would I want to eat to the point of feeling fat and stodgy when I feel like this? Eating only when I'm hungry is the easiest thing in the world for me right now.

Over to you

Here's something you can do immediately to put the ideas in this chapter into action.

Everyone eats when they're not hungry, at least sometimes. There's nothing unusual about this. The surest way to know if you're doing it too often for successful weight loss, however, is to keep a Success Diary and use Diagnostic Nº1a, as outlined in this chapter. If you discover that you're too often consuming kilojoules when you're not yet comfortably and physically hungry, you can do something about it. It won't be easy, but if you have good reasons for wanting to lose weight, it will be a great deal easier than doing unreasonable amounts of exercise or eliminating all the treats from your diet and then wondering why you're not getting results.

One of the best strategies to help you learn to eat only when you're hungry is to get involved in activities that will absorb you and take your mind off food. Take some time out to think about your own interests and what would give you a sense of achievement and satisfaction. Whatever it is, just do it.

Chapter 8

'Menopause makes you fat' and other myths

Don't make excuses – make good.
Elbert Hubbard, American editor, publisher and writer,
1856–1915

One of the many benefits of learning how to connect with your body and eat accordingly is that doing this will see you through much of what life throws at you without undue damage to your waistline. This includes situations that are frequently associated with weight gain, such as periods of inactivity due to illness or other factors, going through menopause and being diagnosed with impaired thyroid function.

Weight management during periods of inactivity

Periods of reduced activity are a well-known danger zone when it comes to gaining weight. In my weight loss Q&A for a health magazine, I received a question from a woman who had gained 20 kilos since having back surgery and being unable to walk without crutches. Surgery is just one of countless situations that can reduce your level of physical activity and contribute to weight gain if you don't take care. Maybe you move house or change jobs, and the only way to get to work is to drive instead of walking to the bus as you used to do. Or maybe someone in your family needs more of your time and attention than usual, and the only way to keep your head above water is to skip your regular dance or exercise classes. That's what happened to Dana, who gained 7 kilos when her husband had a health scare and needed to spend a good part of a year in and out of hospital. Or maybe you have a major project on the boil at work or college, and the only way to meet your deadline is to keep your nose to the grindstone every waking hour. When your level of physical activity is reduced for whatever reason, it doesn't have to result in weight gain as long as you listen to your body and eat only when you feel comfortably and physically hungry. That's because your appetite is closely matched to your energy needs, and when your body's need for energy is reduced, so too is your appetite.

Sometimes, the more active you are, the hungrier you are

How physically active you are dictates how hungry you feel. You might have noticed that when you're more active than usual you also feel more physically hungry than usual. Research suggests that this is especially true for women.[38, 60] I recall a particularly active day I had last month. I had a day at home alone to get things done, and whereas this usually sees me glued to my computer all morning, on that day I ran several errands before midday, walking to the bank, the library, the post office and the supermarket, then wheeling an especially large trolley-load of food back to our apartment and unpacking it all. Soon after lunch I returned the trolley and then went for a swim at the local aquatic centre. I often do this when I have a day to myself, but on that day I was caught off-guard. I got so uncharacteristically ravenous that I couldn't finish the one kilometre I usually swim. I went home shaking with hunger and downed two handfuls of almonds, a snack box of sultanas, two cups of extra milky tea and a handful of dark chocolate cooking drops. This is about three times as much as I usually eat in the afternoon when I'm at home alone . . . but then I'm not usually as active as I was on that day. Two hours later I was hungry again and hoed into fish with salad and mashed potatoes with my husband and children at dinnertime. Despite regular situations such as this, where I move more and eat more than usual, my food intake exactly matches how much food I need to maintain my weight, and from one month to the next my weight stays stable at around 65 kilos.

Research suggests that the more active you are, the closer the match between how much energy your body burns and how much you spontaneously eat.[64] This was illustrated beautifully in a study of five men competing in the 22-day Tour de France in 1986.[71] The Tour is considered to be one of the world's most strenuous endurance endeavours, and that year the race covered some 4000 kilometres, including 30 mountain passages at altitudes of up to 2700 metres. During the race, the average amount of energy the athletes burned each day was a massive 25,400 kilojoules (6048 calories). That's three to four times as much as an average adult burns in a day. But the astounding thing is that although they were burning up massive amounts of energy, the cyclists maintained a steady level of body fat during the 22-day race. That's because they spontaneously consumed an average of 24,700 kilojoules (5881 calories) per day, *just 700 kilojoules (167 calories) less than they burned per day*. This is all the more remarkable given how much they needed to eat in order to achieve this hefty kilojoule intake, and the limited time they had in which to scoff it down.

To give you a taste of what it would be like to eat that much, let's imagine that the only food the cyclists eat is Nori hand rolls like the ones you get at takeaway sushi shops, and the only drinks they consume are sweetened sports drinks such as Gatorade. In fact they don't eat only sushi, but they do drink a lot of sports drinks to keep their fluid and carbohydrate intake up. So in this hypothetical example, our cyclists would wake up and eat six Nori rolls and drink a 600 millilitre bottle of Gatorade for breakfast. If you think back to the last time you had sushi, how many of those big Nori rolls did it take to fill yourself up? Maybe two or three, perhaps fewer if you had a sugary drink at the same time, and almost certainly less than six? After breakfast the cyclists jump on their bikes and pedal for a good deal of their waking day, downing in the process another six Nori rolls and eight bottles of Gatorade. When they dismount at the end of the day, they need to down another three Nori rolls and another bottle of Gatorade to tide them over until dinner shortly thereafter, which consists of a massive eight Nori rolls. But that's not all, because before bed they would need a bedtime snack to see them through to morning: not a couple of tablespoons of tinned peaches or even muesli, but a couple of Nori rolls. That's the equivalent of 25 Nori rolls and 10 large, 600 millilitre bottles of sports drink that they've consumed every day. The difference between how many kilojoules they burned and how many kilojoules they spontaneously ate and drank was equivalent to a single Nori roll, just 3 per cent of their total daily energy expenditure. This is an astoundingly close match. Such is the precision of the body systems that match hunger to physical needs.

HOW CAN I LOSE WEIGHT IF MOVING MORE MAKES ME WANT TO EAT MORE?

If exercise can increase your appetite, and if elite athletes don't lose significant amounts of fat when they ramp up their level of physical activity to extreme levels, you may wonder how you can possibly hope to shed fat if you do the hard yards of being more physically active. In fact, I've met some women who actively avoid exercise when they want to lose weight because they know it makes them hungrier. This is a mistake, because physical activity is an essential component of successful long-term weight loss (more about that in Chapter 18).

The reason why most elite athletes don't lose a significant amount of fat when they do extreme amounts of exercise is that they are already as lean as they can naturally be and their Famine Reaction is especially vigilant about preventing fat loss. Being at their optimum biological weight, any hint of a deficit between how much energy they get from food and drink and how much energy they burn is met with a strong Famine Reaction that brings on a hearty appetite, pushing them to eat up to four times as much as what most people would usually eat. On the other hand, if you're not yet at your optimum biological weight as outlined in Chapter 3, increasing your level of physical activity will result in a loss of fat and centimetres, provided that you're only eating as much as you need to satisfy your appetite. Moreover, you will lose this fat even if your appetite increases and you need to eat more than usual in order to satisfy your hunger. The reason for this is that whenever you're heavier than your optimum biological weight, your body knows that you can safely, and beneficially, lose fat with no danger of your wasting away. Your body will therefore take some of the energy it needs to fuel itself and your daily activities from the excess energy stored in its fat deposits, and it will push you to eat and drink only as many kilojoules as it needs to make up the difference, which may or may not involve an increase in how much you usually eat.

As you continue in your weight loss adventure, you will most likely hit one or more Famine Reactions and plateaus, where your weight loss slows down or stops even though you continue to eat only as much as you need in order to satisfy your hunger and you stay active. This is normal, and is the result of your body reprogramming your Set Point to progressively lower levels. If you keep going, you will reach your ultimate Set Point, or your ultimate biological weight, the weight below which you cannot go without feeling hungry and deprived. That's when you'll be like one of those cyclists taking part in the Tour de France, when even a massive increase in how much physical activity you do won't make a jot of difference to how much fat you have on your body, provided that you're listening to your hunger and following its lead.

One of the reasons why people who are clearly heavier than their optimum biological weight don't lose weight despite exercising more is that they eat more than they need after exercise.[64] People do this for several reasons. Some people use food as a reward for exercise; some just feel they should eat, believing that exercise increases hunger; and some believe that it's important to refuel their body immediately after exercise.[64] While refuelling as soon as possible after exercise is important for optimum performance in elite athletes,[72] if you have excess weight to lose and you aren't trying to break an Olympic record or win a world championship, this practice will only hinder your weight loss. If you're snacking on a packet of trail mix with your billy tea and you're not in the slightest bit hungry, the kilojoules are going to be stored as extra bulk on your body, even if you've just done an 8 kilometre bushwalk.

So the moral of the story is that if you increase how much activity you do and you want to enjoy the benefit of losing excess fat, you need to be scrupulously honest about how much you really need to eat. You may find that in order to satisfy your hunger through periods of greater activity you need to eat a little a bit more than you normally would, such as a small handful of trail mix or an extra piece of fruit, or significantly more than you normally would, such as an extra meal or more, depending on how much you usually eat and how active you are. On the other hand, you may also find that doing more exercise doesn't make you need to eat more than usual, as has been shown in numerous studies,[64] or that you may even need to eat less than usual in order to satisfy your hunger. In fact, some studies have shown that exercise can decrease appetite, possibly by increasing the concentrations of hormones in the bloodstream that make you feel satisfied ('satiety' or 'stop eating' hormones)[64] and by influencing the parts of the brain that control the Famine Reaction.[73] If you use a Success Diary, you'll ensure that your exercise efforts will be rewarded with efficient fat loss that will have you doing up your favourite jeans or that special jacket in pleasing time.

The less active you are, the less hungry you tend to be

While an increase in physical activity is often, but not always, associated with increased hunger, the reverse is also true: the less active you are, the weaker your biological drive to eat tends to be. However, there's one important difference. Although the signals that drive you to eat when you're more active than usual can be impossible to ignore, the signals that reduce your hunger when you're less active than usual are all too easy to discount. You may not be in the slightest bit peckish, but it's lunchtime so you eat anyway. Or you may have a small appetite at dinnertime, but because you always eat this much at your evening meal, you clean your plate and end up feeling oversatisfied. This kind of Clock Hunger and Habit Hunger – not to mention non-hungry eating related to boredom, anxiety and other emotions – contributes to the weight gain so many people experience in periods of reduced activity. But it doesn't have to be that way. If you listen to your appetite and wait until you're genuinely hungry before consuming kilojoules, you can still maintain your weight despite a temporary drop in physical activity. You may not lose any weight in that time, but at least you won't go backwards and reverse the progress you've made to date. The most telling example I've seen of this is a woman named Sally who was struck down by post-streptococcal glomerulonephritis at the age of 38.

It all started one year in autumn, when Sally, her husband and their three young daughters were sick with colds and sore throats. After Sally had nursed everyone back to health, her sore throat persisted. By the end of the week Sally came down with the shivers and the shakes, and six days later she was in the emergency department of her local hospital with acute renal failure and her liver in jeopardy of packing it in as well. Sally's sore throat had been caused by a strain of streptococcal bacterial infection, which had unfortunately affected her kidneys and liver. The liver and kidneys are vital organs needed for many functions, particularly for neutralising toxins and clearing them from the body. If they stop working, you're in deep trouble. As such, post-streptococcal glomerulonephritis can be a life-threatening condition. Sally was given a continuous intravenous infusion of the strongest available antibiotics in hospital for two weeks, followed by three months of oral antibiotics at home and several visits to the hospital to help limit the damage to her kidneys. Needless to say, the ordeal sapped Sally's energy levels.

> *My body was incredibly weak. I was ordered to rest and rest and nothing else but rest. I could not even carry my baby when I came home from hospital; my muscle weakness was incredible. For the four months from May to August I was not allowed to do any exercise. It was not until the end of September that I was permitted to do a five-minute walk every day, and then only if I felt refreshed when I returned from that walk.*

This was a massive drop in activity levels for Sally, who normally got a lot of incidental activity walking her daughters 5 kilometres to and from the eldest's school every weekday and running around after her pre-schooler and toddler all day, not to mention three to four sessions of cardio and weights in the gym in some weeks. Despite this massive drop in physical activity, Sally didn't gain any weight. In fact, she temporarily lost 4 kilos in her five months of near-total bed rest, probably owing to loss of muscle mass from disuse. So how did she manage to prevent weight gain throughout her ordeal? By eating only when she was hungry, of course!

'It was very tough, but I really did not want to gain weight again,' Sally told me in an email. Having reached her highest ever weight of 86 kilos after her second pregnancy, Sally had worked hard to whittle her 1.73 metre frame down to 78 kilos over several years, including the 2 kilos she lost on The Don't Go Hungry Diet in the six months before becoming ill. She knew that inactivity would make her start gaining the weight back again if she wasn't super-careful, having gained several kilos when she had switched from active work as a nurse to inactive work as a graphic designer eight years earlier. The last thing she wanted in her convalescence was to have to deal with weight regain as well. 'I was determined to be a healthy parent, not an overweight, unhealthy parent. Also, I wanted my clothes to feel comfortable.' To help her remain focused on her mission, Sally was mindful of her clothes size. 'For my birthday, my husband bought me some clothes which were a size 12. I am a size 14 and I squeezed into them and thought they looked surprisingly good! So having the firm-fitting clothes reminded me that I needed to stay in control if I was to continue wearing my lovely three-quarter length jeans and groovy fitted T-shirt,' she wrote.

In the beginning, eating only when she was physically hungry was easy, because Sally would sleep during the day instead of eating between meals. Later, as she needed less sleep, Sally distracted herself with various activities.

> My favourite distraction was getting my eldest daughter to read to me in bed and I to her. This was a magical time as I had missed my girls like crazy when I was in hospital and was so glad to be back with them again. I also used to put my girls' hair in lots of plaits which was great fun and better than sticking a biscuit in your mouth because the enjoyment lasted longer.

Other strategies Sally used to keep herself from eating when she wasn't hungry were to drink cups of tea and, in the later stages of her recovery, to start using make-up. 'I had a make-up party and a make-up artist showed my friends and me some make-up tips. It was a lot of fun and I have been cleansing and moisturising twice a day and finding the time in the morning to put some subtle make-up on. It is not only a good distraction, it also makes me feel good about myself,' she wrote. Besides controlling needless snacks between meals, Sally also controlled *what* she ate. 'I started eating what I actually wanted more often by asking for and later cooking the healthy foods I craved instead of just eating what I was given. And I used my fridge and cupboard as my friend and did not fill them with rubbish.'

Although being ill is never fun, Sally sees a bright side to her experience. First, she learned how to listen to her body, and second, she gained a sense of control over her weight.

> *To be honest I did not realise how to really listen to my body until after I was sick. Before I was sick I used to walk five kilometres every Monday to Friday and write down everything I ate, but I must have still been eating too much as I only lost a couple of kilos in six months. When I look back over my food diary from those six months, it's no wonder I hardly lost anything. I was just eating the same as I always did; takeaway bacon and egg muffin sandwiches, endless cappuccinos, dim sums and not enough fruit and vegetables, and my hunger and satisfaction ratings were a joke. Anyway, I feel great now that I really know what my body is asking for, and if ever I do overindulge I am aware of what I am doing and I make a conscious choice to do so, so I always feel in control.*

While there's no doubt that an overall active lifestyle is essential for preventing weight regain, if you do happen to go through temporary periods of reduced activity, don't despair, because listening to your body and eating wholesome foods in accordance with your reduced appetite will go a long way towards preventing weight regain until you can start being more active again. Sally is a great example of this principle in action, and I've seen many others who have similarly prevented weight gain – or at most gained a kilo or two – despite being unable to be as physically active as usual for weeks or months owing to surgery, illness, depression, or just being inescapably overwhelmed by other obligations at home or at work.

Move over menopause

Menopause – the end of menstruation – is a life stage that sees many women battling to keep excess weight at bay. If you're going through menopause, understanding what's happening can make all the difference.

Most of the effects of menopause are caused by the fact that the ovaries cease to produce oestrogen at this time. A decline in ovarian oestrogen production – and the symptoms of menopause – usually begin naturally in the mid-forties, and within about five years oestrogen production is so low that menstrual bleeding ceases altogether. On average, women have their last period at the age of 51. If you're around that age and you haven't had a period in the past 12 months, you'll know you've reached menopause. Menopause can also occur as a result of surgery or medical treatments that affect the ovaries, such as a hysterectomy in which the ovaries are removed as well as the uterus, or chemotherapy. Some of the effects of menopause can also be mimicked by medicines frequently used to help conquer breast cancer. When 42-year-old Rowena's oncologist announced that her breast cancer was under control – thanks to surgery, chemotherapy, radiation therapy and ongoing hormone therapy – she had every reason to celebrate life. However, one of the things that Rowena had to come to terms with was the fact that her cancer was the kind that is exacerbated by oestrogen, and keeping it at bay would therefore require long-term use of tamoxifen, a medication that blocks the effects of oestrogen. While drugs such as tamoxifen help prevent oestrogen from stimulating cancer re-growth, they also prevent other actions of oestrogen, and this is particularly noticeable in pre-menopausal women such as Rowena, who effectively went through menopause in her early forties. Lack of oestrogen action, combined with comfort eating from the stress of a life-threatening illness, saw Rowena go from a healthy size 12 to a size 20 in just two years. I'll come back to her story a bit later in this section.

One of the most noticeable and bothersome effects of menopause for many women is an increase in body fat, especially around the midriff. Before menopause, you may find that clothes that skim your hips and bum will easily fit your waist, but after menopause it can become harder to do up those fastenings around your middle. Increases in total body fat and belly fat at this time are caused by the lack of oestrogen, because giving replacement oestrogen to women who no longer produce ovarian oestrogen helps to prevent or reverse these effects.[38] While replacing oestrogen through hormone replacement therapy might sound like an ideal solution to this problem, it's not without side effects. For this reason, hormone replacement therapy is usually only given to women who suffer severe menopausal symptoms, or to women at risk of metabolic diseases such as diabetes and cardiovascular disease. In these women, the benefit of reducing total body fat, particularly fat around the midriff, and thereby reducing the risk of cardiovascular disease, is considered to far outweigh the possible adverse effects of hormone replacement therapy. Fortunately, there are other things you can do to help prevent or reverse menopause-induced fat gain, as you'll read below.

CARDIOVASCULAR DISEASE IS NO LONGER FOR MEN ONLY

Heart disease used to be considered primarily a man's disease, something from which women rarely suffered. New data show that this is not so.[38] For example, women with type 2 diabetes are *twice* as likely to die from coronary disease than are men with type 2 diabetes. In men with diabetes, mortality rates dropped in the 30 years from 1971 to 2000, but this was not the case for women. In fact, cardiovascular disease now kills more women than men in Europe (55 per cent versus 43 per cent). Despite these emerging realities, women with risk factors for cardiovascular disease, such as glucose intolerance, hypertension or elevated blood concentrations of lipids such as triglycerides, are less likely to be offered treatment than men are.

The message from these statistics is that it's just as important for women to have regular medical check-ups as it is for men. And if you're a woman and your doctor mentions anything about your blood pressure or blood lipids being on the high side, or if a glucose tolerance test shows you're not clearing glucose from your bloodstream as efficiently as you should, fixing the problem is just as urgent and important for you as it is for the man who is waiting to see your doctor after you. In many cases, losing some excess weight will do the trick, but in the meantime you may need help from medications that lower blood pressure or blood lipids. In menopausal women, hormone replacement therapy can also help. Talk with your doctor about the most appropriate treatment plan for you.

What can you do to prevent or reverse menopause-induced weight or waistline gain?

The best way to deal with the propensity to become more apple-shaped than pear-shaped after menopause is to focus on reducing the total amount of fat you have on your body, and this will result in fat loss from your midriff as well as from other areas.[74] To this end, it's helpful to understand the cause of menopause-induced fat gain. The only way you can gain fat is when the number of kilojoules you consume in foods and beverages exceeds the number of kilojoules your body expends in carrying out basal metabolic processes such as digestion and repair, the amount of heat your body produces, and the amount of physical activity you do. Research has shown that women, on average, do not consume any more kilojoules after going through menopause than they did before menopause.[75] This shows that weight gain around the time of menopause, on average, is unlikely to be caused by increased food intake. On the other hand, a recent study revealed a sharp, 50 per cent decrease in how much physical activity women did at the time of menopause compared to how much they were doing before menopause.[75] This drop in physical activity is a major, though not the only, contributor to the reduced metabolic rate that has been consistently reported in menopausal women. It also seems to be a major contributor to weight gain, because medical research shows that women who maintain or increase their level of physical activity during menopause tend to come out the other end without gaining weight, waist circumference or body fat.[76, 77] There is also some evidence that exercise helps to preserve a youthfully clinched-in waistline after menopause, with physical activity resulting in greater fat or centimetre losses from around the waist than from around the hips, particularly with more intense forms of physical activity such those that improve strength and cardiovascular fitness.[76, 78] This will be discussed in greater detail in Chapter 18. The bottom line is that if you keep eating and drinking the same amount after menopause as you did before, the menopause-induced reduction in metabolic rate means that you'll most likely gain weight, especially if you're not as active during the menopausal transition as before.

MENOPAUSE AND THE TSUNAMI OF SLEEPINESS

In talking with women about their experiences of menopause, many have described an insurmountable wall of fatigue that makes them feel tired just *thinking* about going for a walk or going to the gym. Given that reduced physical activity is emerging as an important contributor to weight gain in menopause, my research team and I are working to determine the reason for this tiredness. What we know is that the lack of oestrogen production by the ovaries leads to a temporary increase in the amount of a natural brain chemical called neuropeptide Y (NPY) in the hypothalamus,[38] the part of the brain that controls the Famine Reaction and the Fat Brake. This change may contribute to the tiredness of menopause, because we also know that an increase in the amount of NPY in the hypothalamus can induce a dramatic reduction in physical activity[1] similar to that observed in women going through menopause. By understanding more about the reasons for the sharp drop in physical activity and the fat gain that occur at the time when oestrogen is no longer produced by the ovaries, we may be able to develop new treatments to help women, particularly those at heightened risk of cardiovascular disease, get through the menopausal transition without gaining excess fat. It's important to note that we're still in the early stages of developing effective anti-obesity drugs; they are still years, if not decades, away. Additionally, weight loss drugs will never be effective unless they are combined with lifestyle changes that facilitate weight loss. That is, eating less and moving more.

Do you really need to eat as much as you think you need to eat?

While physical activity appears to reduce weight and waist gain in menopause, what if menopause makes you feel so tired that beefing up your activity levels is the last thing on your mind? That's where listening to your hunger signals and eating accordingly is *especially* important. Doing so will lead you to the perfect amount of food for you, an amount that will help you to reach and maintain your optimum biological weight, even though menopause is likely to reduce your metabolic rate. Let's take a look at this principle in action.

In the two years after her total hysterectomy (that is, removal of the ovaries as well as the uterus) at the age of 47, Bobbie gained 14.5 kilos. While she had been a willowy 60 kilos for her 1.75 metre frame for all of her adult life, Bobbie's weight peaked at 74.5 kilos and she found it impossible to get below 71.9 kilos despite eating healthy foods and exercising regularly. Bobbie's mystery was solved, however, when she started keeping a Success Diary. She realised that she just didn't need to eat as much as she thought she needed to eat. 'I am so surprised at the things I have found out about my body in just three days,' she told me in an email.

Being a schoolteacher I eat during recess at 11 o'clock and then I eat again during the lunch break at 1 o'clock. We have dinner at about 4.30 pm because that is when my husband returns from work. Then I go to the gym and when I return home I nibble and then nibble a little bit more. I have now realised that I eat because of habit and not because I am hungry. In the last three days (I am on school holidays) I have tried to listen to my body. I have breakfast, but I only eat lunch and dinner when I am hungry. My family still has dinner at 4.30 pm but I don't always join them at that time. I found that after a healthy satisfying breakfast I don't feel hungry until after 1 pm. I don't eat after the gym any more. I have always eaten healthily but I obviously never knew my body's needs. The first couple of days of using the diary I even found it difficult to identify whether I was feeling hungry or not because hunger was such a new experience!!! I find all of this amazing. I hope I am not boring you with the details but I am so excited, I feel I had to share it with someone who understands. THANK YOU.

Bobbie's exhilaration was warranted. Within four weeks of using a Success Diary she had lost 3 kilos, and within six months she had lost 4.9 kilos. The last time I communicated with Bobbie she had lost 7.4 kilos (in addition to the 2.6 kilos she had lost before starting her Success Diary) and had attained a lean, athletic weight of 64.5 kilos. Moreover, Bobbie had not regained weight since she started listening to her body over a year-and-a-half ago. This is what she wrote:

Dr Amanda, I am kicking some serious butt! And to think that before I met you I thought that I would never be able to lose this extra weight. It is amazing how many misconceptions exist out there. People would say that it is 'natural' to put on weight when you reach menopause and that you can never lose it. I actually started to believe it and I was becoming quite depressed. But then you happened and now I feel so much more in control and in tune with my body. Can I also add that my hot flushes are now rare? I don't think it is a coincidence. I no longer feel that the operation that I had robbed me of who I was.

ONE WAY TO DEAL WITH MENOPAUSAL HOT FLUSHES

Up to 75 per cent of menopausal women experience 'hot flushes', which many describe as beginning with a sensation of pressure in the head, like a headache, with the intensity increasing until a feeling of heat and burning comes over the face, neck and chest (flushing), followed by an outbreak of sweating, particularly on the head, neck, upper chest and back. Each hot flush lasts an average of four minutes, and they can occur as infrequently as once a week to as often as once or twice an hour in the most troublesome of cases. One of the most taxing things about hot flushes is that they not only make women feel hot and bothered, they can really interfere with a good night's sleep, thereby contributing to the feeling of tiredness that often occurs at menopause. Thankfully, hot flushes usually run their course within five years, and for the vast majority of women they're all over within 10 years.

Research suggests that hot flushes are caused when ovarian oestrogen production dwindles to rock bottom, leading to alterations in the sympathetic nervous system. The sympathetic nervous system is primarily responsible for the 'fight or flight' response you experience when you get a big fright. In menopause, the parts of the sympathetic nervous system that send nerve fibres to blood vessels and sweat glands in the face, neck and chest are overactive. On the one hand, this causes the blood vessels to dilate sporadically, thereby bringing more blood to the skin surface and resulting in flushing. Additionally, overactivity of these sympathetic nerves near sweat glands causes excessive perspiration.

One thing that may exacerbate menopausal hot flushes is weight gain and subsequent activation of the Fat Brake.

Indeed, one of the established remedies for hot flushes is to lose some excess weight. To understand why this may be so, remember that the Fat Brake fires up when you take in more kilojoules than you need to maintain your weight and/ or when you're carrying more weight than your Set Point, and that one of the effects of the Fat Brake is to rev up your metabolic rate,[6, 28, 32] thereby helping you to reverse your overindulgences. It does this by increasing the activity of thyroid hormones in your body, as well as by activating your sympathetic nervous system.[84] When your Fat Brake stimulates your metabolic rate, it actually increases your body temperature and can make you feel especially hot under the collar. Therefore, if you're experiencing menopausal hot flushes and you're also eating more than you need, resulting in your Fat Brake being activated, this can make them feel worse. In that case, using a Success Diary and eating only when you're hungry will not only help you to eat less and lose excess weight until you're no longer heavier than your current Set Point, thereby switching off your Fat Brake, it may also make your hot flushes noticeably less bothersome.

Finding the perfect balance between eating enough but not too much

While the reduction in metabolic rate that occurs with menopause means you'll probably need to eat less after the change in life than you did before, it's important not to eat too little. Over two years ago I received an email from a woman seeking my help to lose weight. 'PS,' she added, 'What do you think my chances are of losing this weight by October (five months away) in time for my son's wedding?' Before menopause, Maria had been a healthy 50 kilos for her petite 1.52 metre frame. She had never had to worry about her weight, even through three pregnancies. But with the onset of menopause at the age of 42, Maria gradually started to put on weight, and by the time she contacted me, at the age of 49, she had gained 5 kilos. In her attempts to lose weight over the years, Maria had got into all sorts of pickles over how much to eat. Most of her confusion came from trying to follow external recommendations about how much to eat. Can you recognise yourself in parts of Maria's story?

To tackle the creeping kilos, initially I just increased my exercise levels by going to the gym, and I also cut back on my kilojoule intake. I became more hungry and irritable – my weight dropped down a little but then I became very hungry and my hunger defeated me. I ended up eating like there was no tomorrow and I regained the kilos I lost plus a little more.

I went up a clothing size, so I increased the intensity of my gym workouts and tried a soup diet. I ate soup until I was dreaming soup and the weight just seemed to dissolve. I was thrilled until eventually the soup just didn't seem to satisfy my hunger. Again hunger won and I binged like crazy on lollies, cakes and white crusty bread. Yep, that dreaded yoyo cycle set in and my weight jumped beyond my previous high. The larger sized clothes that I'd bought were becoming somewhat snug.

I purchased a Slimming magazine from the supermarket that had a diet in it that was supposed to increase the metabolism of menopausal women. It stipulated that you must eat at least six times a day, and protein was to be included in as many of the meals as possible. I thought Great; this should keep my hunger under control. I found that in order to eat all of the allocated food as frequently as the diet stipulated, I was often eating even when I wasn't hungry, and I didn't even like much of the food I had to eat as I'm quite a fussy eater. I actually gained weight on that diet.

This pattern of yoyo dieting continued for the next few years. My middle son went away to live in Europe for two years and when he returned he gave me a massive warm hug. As he was hugging me he proceeded to tell me in a

joking way that I'd become much chunkier since he last
saw me. We laughed and joked about it, but deep down it
was truly getting to me. I felt increasingly frustrated by my
inability to lose the excess weight.

That was Maria 'before'. At times she was eating too little,
thereby activating her Famine Reaction and inadvertently
promoting bingeing and rebound weight gain. At other times
she was eating too much and subsequently gaining weight, even
when she was on the 'menopause diet'. Maria's confusion came
to an end when she started listening to what her body had to say
about eating instead of trying to follow external recommendations about what, when and how much to eat. Maria continues
her account:

A few months ago a health professional recommended
that I visit Dr Amanda's website. I was so absorbed by
the logical simplicity of losing weight by connecting with
your body as well as the scientific research behind it that I
emailed Dr Amanda to ask if it was possible for someone
like me – with just a few kilos in excess – to lose weight
on her program. Dr Amanda suggested I keep a Success
Diary for two weeks, rating both my hunger and satiety
before and after eating, measuring my waist and weighing
myself on day one then not again until the fourteenth day.
All she said was 'you'll see for yourself the results you can
achieve'.

During those two weeks, I paid extra attention to my
hunger levels before eating and to my satiety levels while I
was eating. I diligently wrote down everything I ate in my
diary as well as my hunger and satiety ratings. By the end
of the two weeks I was thrilled to have lost 0.6 kilos and
5 centimetres from my waist, all while eating what I felt
like when I felt like it and stopping when I felt elegantly
satisfied. I'm still jumping out of skin with the exciting
results.

Just 10 days after her son's wedding, Maria emailed me a photo of herself with her husband, two sons, daughter and daughter-in-law on the wedding day. I had to look closely to work out which woman was the mother of the groom. And what a vision she was! Dressed in an elegant taupe silk dress that fell just above her knee and was deeply clinched at the waist, Maria looked so young and fresh. Having lost 4 kilos in the five months since she first wrote to me, Maria was obviously extremely happy in her skin. Some weeks later I met Maria for a coffee, and she was a picture of radiance in a graceful fawn knit that accentuated her fabulous figure and wearing Murano glass jewellery, which highlighted the sparkle in her eyes and skin. Maria said that one of the benefits of being back at 51 kilos is that all of her old favourite clothes now fit her perfectly. But that's only part of it. 'I love the extra energy I seem to have since I stopped fighting against constant hunger. I feel empowered and liberated from guilt about eating,' she said. Maria has now maintained her optimum weight of 51 kilos for more than two years. She is so enraptured by the power and simplicity of losing weight and keeping it off in this way that now she works as a weight loss coach, helping others to do the same.

And what about Rowena, who gained four dress sizes in the aftermath of an earlier-than-expected menopause brought on by anti-oestrogen therapy for breast cancer? Rowena started using a Success Diary to connect with her body, and when I met her at a workshop I gave in Adelaide, she had dropped a dress size and was feeling positive about getting her body back. A year later she had dropped two dress sizes, with no sign of regaining weight. The women who have kindly agreed to share their experiences in this section of the book are proving that menopause needn't result in insurmountable weight gain. I'm personally relieved about that, because within the next decade I'll probably start feeling the change myself, and one of the worst things I can imagine happening is gaining excess weight. I'm not fazed by the idea of temporary tiredness or hot flushes or other menopausal symptoms, but I know that gaining weight would make me feel really cranky. You can bet your boots that when the first signs of menopause arrive, I'll arm myself with a fresh batch of Success Diaries so that I can learn how much I *really* need to eat as my hormones do their midlife thing.

So if you're cursing menopause, stop wasting your time. Take out your Success Diary and start attacking any −1s and 0s you catch in your Hunger column. Those −1s and 0s mean that you're eating when you're not yet comfortably and physically hungry, and they will thwart your weight loss efforts and contribute to menopausal weight gain quicker than you can say 'hot flush'. As your metabolic rate drops through the menopausal transition, you'll probably find that you just don't need to eat as much overall as you thought you did in order to keep hunger at bay. While eating less doesn't sound like much fun, the upside is that like Bobbie, Maria and Rowena, you may well be surprised to see that menopause doesn't have to result in intractable weight gain and that you *can* lose any excess weight effectively and sustainably.

Impaired thyroid function making you fat? Find another excuse

Another common contributor to weight gain is hypothyroidism (impaired thyroid function), which occurs when the thyroid gland fails to secrete sufficient thyroid hormones into the bloodstream. The thyroid gland is a butterfly-shaped gland located at the front of your throat, just under your larynx (the Adam's apple) and extending over either side of your windpipe. It produces the thyroid hormones T3 (otherwise known as triiodothyronine or 3,3',5-triiodothyronine) and the less active hormone from which it is derived, T4 (otherwise known as thyroxine or 3,5,3',5'-tetra-iodothyronine). Thyroid hormones act on almost every cell in the body to regulate several functions, notably the metabolic rate. In fact, if you didn't have any thyroid hormones in your system, your basal metabolic rate would drop by about 30 per cent.[79] In about 6 to 20 per cent of adults, particularly older women, the thyroid gland ceases to produce sufficient thyroid hormones and the result is hypothyroidism.[80] In developed countries, this is most commonly due to the autoimmune disease Hashimoto's Thyroiditis, where the body produces antibodies and white blood cells that attack and gradually destroy the thyroid gland. Other causes of hypothyroidism include iodine deficiency – now disturbingly common in Australia, the United States, Europe and other developed countries[81] – as well as dysfunction in parts of the pituitary gland or the hypothalamus which control the thyroid gland. Symptoms of hypothyroidism may include fatigue, depression, cold intolerance, hair loss, constipation, difficulties with concentration and unexplained weight gain. Thankfully, doctors can easily treat hypothyroidism with thyroxine tablets, which are a form of hormone replacement, or iodine supplementation, if the hypothyroidism is caused by iodine deficiency.

IODINE DEFICIENCY IN AUSTRALIA

In October 2009, Food Standards Australia/New Zealand introduced a new regulation requiring that any salt added to bread sold in Australia (whether produced locally or imported) be in the form of iodised salt as opposed to non-iodised salt. This public health initiative was introduced in response to research revealing that iodine deficiency had reached epidemic proportions among children in Australia.[82] This is particularly worrying given that iodine deficiency is known to be the commonest preventable form of intellectual impairment in the world. Bread – as opposed to iodised salt itself – was chosen as the most appropriate avenue for delivering sufficient iodine to people in Australia because excess salt intake is not good for health and because iodised salt can deliver risky levels of iodine to children. So, if you currently eat bread in Australia that lists salt among the ingredients, that salt will necessarily be iodised, and it's likely that you're getting sufficient iodine in your diet. If you have any concerns about your iodine intake, check with your health care practitioner as to how you can ensure you are getting adequate iodine intake from your diet.

Many people assume that the drop in metabolic rate that occurs with the onset of hypothyroidism – that is, before treatment has been initiated – will naturally result in a large weight gain. That is not so; not everyone who is newly diagnosed with hypothyroidism has gained a lot of weight. Part of the reason for this may be that while low thyroid function is known to cause a drop in metabolic rate, research suggests that it also causes a drop in appetite.[83] Could it be that the people who don't gain excess weight as their thyroid gland expires are those that are so in tune with their bodies that they actually eat less when their appetite decreases? More research is needed, but I'm inclined to believe that this may be the case. I've personally seen the effects, or lack thereof, of a deteriorating thyroid gland on body weight in people who have used a Success Diary and learned how to eat only when hungry. One such example is Raylene, 44, whom I introduced in Chapter 7 as the woman who lost all the weight she wanted to lose when she stopped eating six small meals or snacks per day, as the personal trainers at her local gym had suggested, and instead started eating according to what her body told her.

When I first met Raylene via email, she was so bright and bubbly. Every few weeks she would write and tell me about her weight loss adventure and how she was going in some other aspects of her life. She was working full-time as a receptionist in a busy medical practice while training to qualify as a health counsellor. But after several months, the tone of Raylene's emails began to change. Things at work seemed to bother her more than before, so much so that her frustration made its way into her normally chipper emails. Raylene counted down the days until her holiday in a Fijian resort with her husband, but when she got back from the long-awaited trip she seemed more worn down than ever. 'I am suffering badly from post holiday blues, I cannot get going at all, it is terrible!!!!!! I am sooooo glad I booked the rest of the week off as there is no way I would have done anything at all productive. We are already looking at where we can go next year, terrible, huh??? We have to have something to look forward to or we will go mad,' she wrote.

As it turns out, the cause of Raylene's fatigue and disgruntlement was hypothyroidism, which her doctor diagnosed with a blood test when she told him that she had been feeling unusually tired. Raylene's doctor told her that unexplained weight gain was another common symptom of hypothyroidism, but Raylene was unscathed by that one. Sure, during her holidays she had gained a kilo, but this was readily explained by 15 days of resort food. 'The food was just heaven, especially the breakfasts, so much fresh fruit and all sorts, and I ate heaps of lovely Indian food!!!' Moreover, within three weeks of returning from holidays, the extra kilo was gone. Of course, this didn't all just happen as if by magic. Raylene was scrupulous about making healthy food choices, about eating only when hungry, and about being active. This is what she wrote:

> I did eat a big breakfast every day at the resort, but then I rarely needed to eat anything until dinner time, so my intake was really not too bad overall, and we were active playing golf and walking all the time we were away. Now that we are back, my appetite is very low I must admit. I really don't feel like eating much, showing that my fat brake is working (it would have been working overtime on holiday!!). We have been eating a lot of salads since we have been back as that is what I have felt like eating.

So, if you're not feeling 100 per cent and you've got symptoms of hypothyroidism, as described above, you may like to ask your doctor to check your thyroid function. If you do happen to have hypothyroidism, keeping a Success Diary until you feel confident about eating only when hungry could mean the difference between being one of the people who gain 10 or more kilos when their thyroid gland gives up the ghost, and being one of the 'lucky' people like Raylene who successfully manage their weight. Additionally, the sooner your hypothyroidism is diagnosed and the sooner you start appropriate, medically supervised treatment, the less likely you are to gain disturbing amounts of weight. And once your condition is being treated, and you're being monitored regularly by your doctor, there's absolutely no reason why you can't manage your weight successfully. Many of my clients have told me that they gained excess weight around the time leading up to the diagnosis of hypothyroidism, but that hasn't stopped them from losing the surplus once they started using a Success Diary and eating according to their physical needs. One such example is 56-year-old Jocelyn, whom I introduced in Chapter 4 as the woman who shimmied easily into her new little black dress in size 12 after a few weeks of attentive exercise. Jocelyn lost 6 kilos, and 10 centimetres off her waist, to reach her ideal size 12 over the course of two-and-a-half years – including some ups and downs in the form of several overseas trips, some minor knee surgery and work stress – despite the fact that the Hashimoto's Thyroiditis (with which she was diagnosed six years ago) means that she'll need to take thyroxine tablets for the rest of her life. Here's what Jocelyn said about losing weight and keeping it off under these circumstances.

I have always struggled with my weight, but having hypothyroidism meant that I couldn't get any weight off no matter how hard I tried, and I gained about 15 kilos over a period of five years. I subsequently used a Success Diary for two years (not continuously, but on and off) and my weight loss was small but steady. In the second half of last year my doctor increased my dose of thyroxine, and since then I have lost weight quite easily. I need to do it all in order to lose weight – write down everything I eat in my Success Diary, use the hunger and satiety ratings, really try and listen to my physical needs, record my weight and measurements at regular intervals, walk at least an average of 10,000 steps daily (which means one or two half-hour walks a day and a lot of running around at work) and do some other exercise two or three times a week (swimming or weights or riding an exercise bike). If I don't consistently do all of those things, I seem to fall off the wagon completely. Maybe this is why, when other things in life intervene, I can't be so successful and my weight tends upwards again. I do, however, feel like it is within my power to control my weight, and the fact that I have Hashimoto's disease is not going to stop me. Also, even when my weight has fluctuated, the gains have not been as great as they were previously, and I have not had to crash diet in order to lose weight as I did in my youth. My doctor is very pleased with my progress – he weighs me once or twice a year and has noted the drop in my weight over the two-year period. I feel much healthier, I enjoy a wide variety of foods, and my friends tell me that I look great.

HOW YOUR BODY HELPS TAKE CARE OF YOUR WEIGHT EVEN IF YOU'RE TAKING THYROXINE

Because our bodies alter thyroid function in order to regulate metabolic rate and body weight despite wide fluctuations in daily food intake, people sometimes ask me how they can manage their weight if they're on a constant dose of thyroid hormone replacement therapy. For instance, when you eat more than you need, your Fat Brake reduces your appetite,[30] boosts your propensity to fidget or move about,[31] and increases your metabolic rate,[6, 28, 32] thereby helping you to burn off any excesses very efficiently. One of the means by which your Fat Brake boosts your metabolic rate is to increase the amount of thyroid hormones secreted by your thyroid gland.[84] This occurs because the part of your brain called the hypothalamus, which is the control tower of the Fat Brake and the Famine Reaction, produces and secretes increased amounts of a hormone called thyrotropin-releasing hormone (TRH). TRH then travels to your pituitary gland, which is located below your hypothalamus, at the base of your brain, and stimulates the synthesis and release into the circulation of another hormone, thyroid-stimulating hormone (TSH, also called thyrotropin). TSH travels through your bloodstream, and when it hits your thyroid gland it stimulates the production of thyroid hormones and their secretion into your circulation, in turn boosting your metabolic rate. The question then is: if your Fat Brake alters the secretion of thyroid hormones into your bloodstream to boost your metabolic rate, but you're taking a constant replacement dose of the thyroid hormone thyroxine, which means that your thyroxine levels don't change from one day to the next, how can your Fat Brake boost your metabolic rate and help prevent weight gain despite occasional overindulgences?

The answer is that your body has many ways of regulating the overall activity of thyroid hormones, one of which is to vary the amount of thyroid hormones produced by your thyroid gland and secreted into your bloodstream. To take another example, your body also regulates how much of the less active of the thyroid hormones, T4 or thyroxine, is converted to the more active thyroid hormone, T3. This activation step is mediated by a group of enzymes called deiodinases, which are found in your thyroid gland, your liver and your kidneys. So even if you're taking a constant dose of thyroxine, your body can regulate the amount of active T3 in your system by stimulating or inhibiting the activity of deiodinase enzymes as required. In addition, your body can regulate how effective thyroid hormones are when they reach your cells by adjusting the number of thyroid hormone receptors produced by your cells, and by increasing the ability of those receptors to interact with thyroid hormones. A hormone receptor is like a lock, and a hormone is like a key. Just as a key opens a door by interacting with a particular lock, hormones (such as thyroid hormones) have various effects on different cells when they interact with specific receptors (such as thyroid hormone receptors) on those cells. By means of these alterations in the activity of deiodinase enzymes, as well as the number and activity of thyroid hormone receptors, your body can tweak the effectiveness of thyroid hormones in your body even if the amount of thyroid hormone in your system doesn't change.

The result of this multilayered regulation of overall thyroid hormone action is that even if your thyroid gland no longer produces thyroid hormones and you're on a constant dose of thyroid hormone replacement medication, your body can still modulate your thyroid function and your body weight as needed. You've probably already noticed this yourself. When you eat a big, blow-out meal, do you feel any warmer than usual? That's your Fat Brake, revving up your metabolic rate to help you reverse your excesses, in part by increasing the overall activity of thyroid hormones in your body. When you decide to eat less and/or move more in order to lose weight, do you keep losing weight at the same rate for weeks on end, or does your weight loss sometimes slow down or stop altogether, even if you keep eating and exercising in the same way as when you started your regime? That's your Famine Reaction, reducing your metabolic rate to protect you from wasting away, in part by decreasing the overall activity of thyroid hormones in your body. With the ingenuity of your own body and a bit of help from modern medicine, there's no reason why hypothyroidism should interfere with your body's natural drive to attain and maintain an optimum healthy weight.

Over to you
Here's something you can do immediately to put the ideas in this chapter into action.

Stop making excuses about why you can't lose weight and start listening to what your body has to say. If you're carrying more weight than you need, it's likely that a voice of desperation has been quietly calling out to you for years, longing to be heard and telling you that you really don't need to eat so much. Once you start heeding your body signals instead of disowning them, you'll very likely feel better immediately and your weight will probably start going down.

Chapter 9

Step 1b. Another barrier to weight loss: eating until you feel oversatisfied

Never eat more than you can lift.
Miss Piggy, Muppet character from *The Muppet Show*

Eating when you're not hungry is the most common way to overeat, but another way to consume more kilojoules than you need is to regularly eat until you feel oversatisfied. Feeling oversatisfied can be as obvious as when you've eaten so much rich food that your stomach is stretched to capacity and you feel nauseous. This is how I felt the last time I indulged in an 'all you can eat' buffet. Like Miss Piggy, I couldn't resist helping myself to copious folds of soft-serve ice-cream with as many toppings as I fancied, despite having already eaten far too much! (It was such an unpleasant feeling that I now avoid such restaurants.) Feeling oversatisfied, however, is usually a much less extreme experience. You may have finished eating and still feel comfortable, but once you start doing other things you find that sensations in your gut keep intruding on your consciousness – not so much a feeling of tightness or discomfort, simply an awareness that there's food inside you. In your heart of hearts you know you've eaten more than you needed.

Everyone eats to the point of feeling oversatisfied sometimes. If you ask the most naturally lean person you know – the person who never diets and who never worries about their weight – if they ever keep eating after they feel satisfied, they'll probably say Yes and tell you about something they splurged on recently, maybe in a restaurant, at a party or the last time they went to the movies. Occasionally eating until you feel oversatisfied is not a problem. Remember, excess kilojoule intake activates your Fat Brake, which revs up your metabolic rate and cuts your appetite, especially your appetite for rich foods. This means that if you simply wait until you feel comfortably and physically hungry before eating again, you'll probably notice that occasional over-indulgences enable you to keep going without food for longer than usual, or enable you to keep going on lighter meals or snacks than you usually eat. Indeed, if you ask that naturally lean person you know what happens after they overeat, they will almost certainly say they instinctively eat less after their occasional overindulgences. Your Fat Brake is the reason why, despite oversatisfying yourself occasionally, your weight doesn't necessarily increase from one month to the next. If you eat to the point of feeling oversatisfied too often, however, this will put a spanner in the works of your weight loss adventure. It will stop you from losing weight and you may even start gaining weight.

Does this apply to you?

When it comes to your own weight loss adventure, could eating until you feel oversatisfied be your downfall? If you'd like to find out for sure, use my Diagnostic N°1b on the following page. If you discover that you're oversatisfying yourself too often, try to concentrate on changing this behaviour. And if you discover that you're *not* oversatisfying yourself too often, you'll know to focus your efforts on other forms of behaviour that may be preventing you from losing weight.

Dr Amanda's Diagnostic N°1b: Are you oversatisfying yourself too often?

To do this simple diagnostic test, use your Success Diary for 3 to 14 days as described in Chapter 5. For best results, aim to use your Success Diary for 14 days. That's because you may feel a bit uncertain in the first week as you experiment with reading your body signals and eating accordingly, but in the second week you'll feel more confident and your average result over both weeks will give you a good estimate of what you're currently capable of. You can use the same Success Diary that you used for any of the other Diagnostics in this book.

Once you've used your Success Diary for several days, your next step is to work out how many times per week you're eating until you feel oversatisfied. That is, how many times per week you're scoring a +4 in your Satiety column. If you've used your Success Diary for exactly 7 days, this is straightforward. You simply count how many +4s there are in the Satiety column of your Success Diary in that time. If you've kept your Success Diary for more or less than 7 days, here's how to calculate how many +4s you're scoring in a week on average, or how many +4s you'd be scoring in a complete week if you kept going at the same rate.

- Count the number of days you've used your Success Diary for the whole day.
- Count how many +4s you scored in the Satiety column of your Success Diary on those days.
- Divide the number of +4s you counted by the number of days on which you used your Success Diary for the whole day. This will give you the average number of +4s you're scoring per day.
- Multiply this number by 7 to get the number of +4s you score on average (or would score) per week.

For example, let's suppose that you've used your Success Diary for 14 days, but one day was a wipeout because, after writing down what you ate for breakfast and how you felt about it, you set off on a day trip and forgot to write anything else in your Success Diary. By the time you woke the next morning, having arrived home late the previous evening and crashed into bed, you'd forgotten how hungry or satisfied you felt before everything you'd eaten on your trip. So you've used your Success Diary for 13 full days. In those 13 days you count a total of four +4s in your Satiety column. So the number of times you're eating until you feel oversatisfied per week, on average, is:

4 times ÷ 13 days = 0.308 times per day
0.308 times per day × 7 days = 2.2 times per week

That is, you're scoring a +4 in your Success Diary approximately twice a week.

Interpreting your results

If you're eating to the point of feeling oversatisfied (that is, scoring a +4 in the Satiety column of your Success Diary) around twice a week or less, it's unlikely to be preventing you from losing weight effectively. If you're currently losing weight more slowly than you'd like, focusing on other aspects of your behaviour will probably bring you better results than attacking these lonesome +4s. You may like to skip straight to the next chapter.

If, on the other hand, you're oversatisfying yourself more than twice a week and you're not losing weight as fast as you'd like, reducing the number of +4s you score in your Success Diary to two or fewer times per week will help you get better results. Read on for ideas on how to conquer those +4s, taken from real life examples of others who've done it and who are now reaping the benefits.

Are you a prisoner of habit?

Sometimes eating too much is simply a habit, as was the case for 32-year-old personal trainer Samira.

I think eating more than I need is a habit, and old habits die hard. I grew up in a Lebanese family where it's customary to have lots of food choices at any one time, and my mother, who is a wonderful cook, would always be telling me that I should eat. So after moving out of home I adopted those habits – cooking large quantities, eating large quantities, and eating as a social thing.

When Samira began using a Success Diary, she noticed many +4s of oversatisfaction in her Satiety column; at least five a week. Noticing an unhelpful habit is easier than changing it, but Samira was determined. Feeling frumpy at 78 kilos for her 1.64 metre frame, Samira knew that she'd be much better able to motivate her clients to be fit and healthy if she herself felt lean and fit.

I am sick of food controlling me. I have decided that I should be the one in control of food. I don't ever want to feel that uncomfortable overfull feeling. It's not pleasant. It reminds me of how I used to eat, eating to excess, and I don't want to be like that or feel like that again. It reminds me of the OLD ME, and now I'm the NEW ME. Eating to excess is just eating to store fat, and I want to eat to be healthy and give my body the nutrients it needs. Also food is more enjoyable when you don't feel stuffed afterwards. I guess you have to control your greed, and really listen to your body. I used to eat from boredom and habit. Now when I'm home and bored I try to do something else with my time besides eat. I read, watch a movie, hang out with friends or exercise. Food is no longer something that I do to kill time.

Samira's body responded wonderfully to her commitment to challenging old habits. Four months after she started using a Success Diary and getting on top of the +4s, she'd lost 10 kilos and 14 centimetres off her waist and was able to shimmy into size 10 clothes. Now, more than 18 months later, they still fit.

Some habits die hard . . . so don't even try attacking them head-on

There are so many habits that can contribute to overeating and the feeling of oversatisfaction that comes with it. Some of these habits may be deeply ingrained, born of childhood conditioning, genetic programming or unmet emotional needs. These kinds of habits are almost impossible to break with the head-on approach. That's where the indirect approach works wonders.

Do you often feel oversatisfied because you're in the habit of cleaning your plate? This is a remarkably enduring habit that tends to stick with us throughout life. Shirley, 79, still automatically cleans her plate, often getting uncomfortably overfull in the process, because when she was young her mother used to tell her she should eat all her food and be grateful for it, because the starving children in China would give anything to have that food, and so it was wrong to let it go to waste. I can't remember my mother saying anything like that to me when I was young, but for some reason I do tend to eat whatever's on my plate. I don't even bother trying to change this habit; it's too hard. So instead I've made a habit of watching how much is put on my plate in the first place. When I'm at home and my husband serves me more food than I think I can comfortably eat, I put some back into the pot before sitting down to eat. I can always go back for seconds if I want, but it's not so easy to reverse the blah feeling that comes from eating more than I need. Nowadays my husband usually asks me to serve myself, because he knows how fussy I am about my portions. If I'm eating out, on the other hand, I often have to accept the plate of food I'm served. In this case, what works for me is to mentally draw a line through my food – or sometimes, if I can do so without making it obvious, I actually divide the food with my knife – estimating roughly how much it will take to make me satisfied. I find I get the same satisfaction from eating the amount I've allotted myself as I formerly would have got from cleaning my plate.

As I write this, I realise what a rigmarole I go through to control my portions. I might feel embarrassed about this if it weren't for the fact that it has been proved scientifically that portion sizes influence how much we eat. Research volunteers were invited to eat from a bowl of soup until they felt satisfied.[85] Unbeknown to any of the volunteers, some of them were eating soup from bowls that were slowly and imperceptibly refilling as their contents were consumed. Uncannily, these people ate a massive 73 *per cent more* than volunteers who'd eaten from normal soup bowls. What's even more fascinating is that the volunteers who'd eaten from the surreptitiously rigged bowls didn't feel any more satisfied or oversatisfied than those who'd eaten from normal bowls, demonstrating that we use visual as well as physical cues to determine when we've had enough to eat. All the more reason to control how much food is put on your plate before you sit down to eat.

Another habit that contributes to overeating and feeling over-satisfied is eating whenever there's food in front of you. A friend of mine, 65-year-old Elvin, has worked hard managing major corporations for the past 20 years, and now that he's retired he enjoys eating out in restaurants with his wife and their friends. He tells me his biggest problem is that for as long as they are seated at the table talking, he eats. He eats bread and butter before, during and after the meal, and then he nibbles on biscotti, chocolates or cheeses after dessert while they all sip their coffees and continue their conversation. Now this is a real monster of a habit to break, and I wouldn't even attempt to fight it head-on; it's extremely difficult to *not* eat delicious food when it's in front of us. However, there *is* a way to attack this habit from the side, and that's by keeping a safe distance between yourself and excess food. For instance, if the breadbasket or cheese board ends up right under your nose at the dinner table, you can always pass it to the other end of the table or ask someone to take it away, or only order as much bread or cheese as you feel you want to eat. As another example, once the meal is finished you could get up to do the dishes if you're at home, or clear the table to start a game of cards or something, or retire from the table to the sofa or another room . . . whatever it takes to get away from the temptation of a table full of delicious food and kilojoule-rich beverages when you're already satisfied. Another way to side-tackle the tendency to want to keep eating when there's food in front of you is simply to cut back on the number of times you say to friends, 'Let's meet up for a nice meal.' There are so many other things you can do socially that won't lead you down the path of overeating. There's golf; going to a beautiful beach or bushland area, or an interesting neighbourhood, and taking a walk; going to the movies; strolling around at a free community festival; or even training to jump out of a plane and parachute down to safety on your own – to give just a few examples. You can always go for coffee or a quick meal after the main event if you're hungry, but because the focus of the social gathering is something other than food, it's easier to stop eating once you've had enough.

Whatever strategies you use to avoid eating more than you need at meals, may your Success Diary be one of them. Elvin started using the notes program on his mobile phone to write a Success Diary, and every day for two weeks he sent me his daily diary entries via SMS. Within less than a week, the +4s that he was regularly recording after social meals when he started his Success Diary had dramatically decreased, and within two weeks he had lost a kilo.

Another habit that leads many people to eat until they feel oversatisfied is to snack after dinner in the evenings. This is another doozy of a habit to break, because snacking after dinner can be so incredibly pleasurable, and also because overeating is sometimes fuelled by pervasive emotions such as loneliness, anxiety or boredom. However, I've been surprised at the number of people who've told me that cleaning their teeth straight after dinner stops them from snacking. Presumably it works at least in part because many of us have been conditioned since childhood not to eat after cleaning our teeth at night, and this habit wins out over the habit of snacking after dinner. Also, cleaning your teeth replaces the taste of food with the fresh taste of toothpaste, and some find this is enough to distract them from thinking about food. Whatever the reason for this phenomenon, it's worth a shot to see if it works for you.

Do you stuff yourself as a reaction to dieting?

Sometimes overeating stems from trying to lose weight on a conventional diet. Conquering this kind of overeating is as simple as abandoning some of the techniques you learned in Diet Dungeon. When 24-year-old Helen started using a Success Diary, she noticed that she often kept eating until she felt over-satisfied. Sometimes this happened because she liked the taste of the food and she simply ate too much, but sometimes it would happen when she'd try to eat what she thought she *should* be eating when she was hungry, instead of what she wanted. 'Now, when I'm about to eat, I ask myself what I am really hungry for. If I want a toasted cheese sandwich, that's exactly what I have, because if I try to convince myself that I really only need some fruit and yogurt, I will eat the fruit and yogurt as well as the toasted cheese sandwich and end up feeling overfull.'

Helen lost 4 kilos in six months and reached 64 kilos, which is just right for her 1.67 metre frame. When you see or read about a lean young woman like Helen, it's tempting to think that weight management is easy for someone like her. But take a look at the email she sent me and you'll understand why I want you to know about her success. If Helen can do it, so can you.

From: Helen
Sent: Saturday 13th December 3:10 PM
To: Dr Amanda Sainsbury-Salis
Subject: Just a quick thank you

Dear Amanda,
  I just wanted to write you an email to thank you for changing my life in such an important way.
  I was an overweight child and obese as a young adult, consequently most of my life has been about battling with my weight.

After losing 20 kilos with a popular weight loss group when I was 19 I thought I had solved the problem but I was wrong. Post weight loss I could no longer lead a normal life if I wanted to stay thin.

I would breakdown in tears every time I had to go out for dinner because I knew it would result in more weight gain and I began to exercise obsessively and get furious if anything interfered with my gruelling regime.

This abnormal behaviour did not help my weight problem though and after a year of gradual gain I began cycles of starving myself, which would inevitably be followed by a binge. This went on for two years with me trying to hide my problem from people. Within 4 years I had gained 8 of the 20 kilos I had originally lost.

A year ago I read your book and at first I thought it must be too good to be true because the only way I had ever known weight loss to happen was through starvation and suffering. Six months later however I decided I had nothing to lose by giving it a go. The change has been gradual. Firstly I threw out my scales then I started drinking full cream milk (something I have longed to do since I was 12 years old when I was first forced to swap to skim milk because of my weight problem).

After this I worked on being able to gauge when I was full (I never had a problem gauging hunger). This took a long time because I was so used to eating carefully weighed portions.

In six short months, though, the bingeing has stopped, I no longer have a breakdown at the thought of going out to dinner and I have already lost 4 kilos.

So thank you Amanda, your wise words have given me the courage to change for good and now I know I will never have to be fat again.

Helen

True to her word, Helen has kept those 4 kilos – plus the 12 kilos she lost previously – off for more than a year. More importantly, Helen has made peace with her body.

> *After some experimentation I have realised that trying to get my weight below about 64 kilos makes me ravenously hungry which then leads to weight gain. I think for the first time ever I might have figured out the weight I am meant to be. I think if I really wanted to share something I've learnt through the many battles I've had with weight and body image it is this: don't think you have to look like a celebrity to be healthy and happy. When I aim to be too thin it is a constant battle, and one I can't win, but when I accept myself at a healthy weight the war ends and I realise I was fighting myself for no reason.*

The moral of the story is that when you feel hungry enough to eat, go for what you really feel like eating. To identify what you really feel like eating when you're hungry, the Three Yeses Test on page 117 can help. When, like Helen, you eat what you really feel like eating, you'll find it easier to feel satisfied without getting overfull, and this will help you to reach the weight you're meant to be.

You don't necessarily need to know why you overeat in order to stop doing it

Sometimes you may not know what drives you to eat until you feel oversatisfied. Fortunately, you don't need to understand why you're overindulging and clocking up too many +4s in your Success Diary in order to find a solution – but you do need to find the solution that works for you personally. Maree, 44, is a prime example of this.

Four years ago, Maree was felled by chronic fatigue syndrome. Although she continued to work throughout her illness so that she could pay her bills and maintain her position at work, sheer exhaustion meant that she had no energy left for anything else.

Exercise? Forget it. Shopping and chopping for dinner? You've got to be joking. Maree usually bought a takeaway as she dragged herself home from work and ate it before retiring for the night. She felt out of control about the way she ate and powerless to do anything about it. 'I think I might have starved to death in a previous life and the fear still remains with me,' she later said to me in an email. 'I'm not sure what word to use, I have a fear/phobia/paranoia about being hungry, so my normal way of eating is to eat more than I need and to eat the next meal before I'm actually hungry. The full feeling is emotionally comforting but physically uncomfortable, my body often says "no more", or "don't eat that because you will feel yucky afterwards", but my head or emotions take over and insist that I eat it.' The perils of her eating habits showed up when she could no longer fit into her size 12 clothes. Worst of all, Maree felt trapped in her illness: the more exhausted she was, the worse she ate; the worse she ate, the more weight she gained; and the more weight she gained and the worse she ate, the more exhausted she grew. On it went for months and then years. Maree grew out of her size 12s and then out of the new size 14 clothes she'd had to buy. When the sales were on, Maree went shopping with her 72-year-old mother. 'My Mum is a real clothes freak and she loves to shop. But when your Mum is smaller than you are and she can find more clothes that look good on her in the sales than you can, it's soul destroying,' she said. By springtime Maree had grown out of the size 16 clothes she'd found in the sales and it was time to go shopping again. This was her turning point. At 82.5 kilos for her 1.63 metre frame, she would either have to start shopping for clothes in the plus-size area of stores or lose weight. Shortly there-after, Maree registered for my advanced weight loss workshop on physical strategies for successful weight loss.

At the workshop I took Maree and the other participants through the simple diagnostic tests in this book, using the Success Diary that I'd requested they use for 3 to 14 days before the event. A week later, Maree emailed me about her experience of the workshop. 'I think the main thing I got out of the workshop was a firm grasp on what my biggest problem with weight is. I didn't identify with many of the issues that others brought up and this further highlights in my mind that my biggest problem is eating until I feel uncomfortable. Before the workshop I both knew and didn't know what a problem it was.' In her email Maree told me that although she was still getting used to reading her body signals, she had started losing weight and so she thought she must be on the right track. She finished her message with: 'It would be great to see some more information and strategies on how to pull back from eating too much – I think this is most people's biggest problem.'

Knowing that any strategies Maree found herself to help stop her from eating too much would be far more effective than anything I suggested to her, I put the question back on Maree. 'You have obviously had success in stopping from eating too much and to start losing weight already,' I emailed her. 'May I ask: what strategies did you use to come this far? I'd love to hear your views.' Over the coming months, Maree sent me several emails telling me about the strategies she was using to eat precisely as much as she needed, even through her gradual recovery from chronic fatigue syndrome, a couple of overseas trips involving a lot of socialising over food, and occasional lapses into incapacitating fatigue. Twelve months after the workshop, eating to the point of discomfort became the exception in Maree's life rather than the norm. 'I am really in tune with myself,' she wrote. 'In my day-to-day life I don't overeat and I have no problem stopping when I've had enough. In fact, I now hate that "being stuffed" feeling.'

Today, Maree is reaping the fruits of her efforts. She lost 12 kilos in as many months and has kept them off for eight months (and counting), and she is able to wear all her favourite size 12 clothes again. When she goes shopping with her mother, she can now find more clothes that look good on her than her mother can find for herself. One of Maree's latest finds is a long, black, sexy, clingy jersey-knit sheath dress with old-world peony roses on it. Recently she wore it to a family gathering and she knew she looked attractive. It was such a great feeling that she didn't even mind the blisters on her feet from her brand-new strappy, high-heeled sandals.

How did she do it, you ask?

I'm going to show you exactly how she did it, but only as food for thought, to inspire you to find your own strategies for dealing with any wayward +4s.

The first thing that Maree did to overcome overeating was to use a Success Diary. Although she had started recovering from chronic fatigue syndrome when she first decided to lose weight, her energy levels were still very low. In the past, Maree had lost weight by following a restrictive regime that necessitated preparing every meal at home and being very vigilant about what she ate. This approach was obviously not feasible in her current state of health, but using a Success Diary and focusing on how much she ate – without spending too much energy worrying about what she ate – felt do-able.

> *Your Success Diary has been of immense help. By writing down everything I eat and rating hunger and satiety I am seeing myself and my patterns more clearly. My diary still has the occasional 0 or –1 or +4, but I think I am getting better at controlling volume. I have decided to keep a diary until I reach my goal weight, no matter how long it takes, because I need to keep reminding myself that it's OK to get hungry and that overeating is not necessary – there is always more food if needed.*

As it turned out, Maree stopped using her Success Diary after three months, because by then she knew exactly when she needed to eat and exactly when she needed to stop.

The second thing that Maree did to overcome overeating was to control how much food was placed in front of her. This is what she said:

> *One of my guilty pleasures is the occasional chicken and wedges from the local chicken shop. They always give you*

way too many wedges. So now I ask them just to fill the bag halfway (I don't care about the charge). It's a bit of a challenge to get them to give me a smaller amount, but if I get a full bag I always start saying that I will only eat half, but most times I end up eating three-quarters of it or the entire bag. I actively try and get smaller quantities (just what I need to eat) of takeaway food, even if I am paying for more. Being excessively hungry when choosing what to eat is also a big danger for me, so I try to make sure I'm not starving when I go to a restaurant. I often order an entrée as a main meal, with the portion size of most restaurant entrées being a nice amount of food.

Maree knew that by far the best way to control the amount of food in front of her was to eat out less often, and early in her recovery she started cooking at home again. Even with home-cooked meals, however, she found she needed to come up with strategies to avoid overeating.

I am single so only have to prepare food for myself. I cook big batches of things and freeze them in individual meals for lunch at work or for dinner. My hunger varies quite a lot from day to day. In the past I would have prepared all of my meals in large sizes designed to satisfy me at my hungriest because I was worried about not being filled up – then eat all of it. I've now started preparing small meal sizes for my less hungry days, amounts that won't make me feel stuffed. I make sure there is always plenty of food to eat if I need it so my paranoia about being hungry isn't switched on, but I try to keep the options healthy.

Another strategy that Maree found helpful – one she implemented on the advice of a naturopath helping her with digestive problems – was to slow down and chew her food more thoroughly.

I was always a gobbler of food, always the first to finish. Eating slowing really helped me because I started to realise how unbroken-down the food I swallowed used to be and I now find the thought a bit disgusting. The slower, gentler delivery of food to my stomach felt so much nicer, my digestive troubles became less upsetting and it helped me to eat less. I found it very difficult to eat slowly and chew well if I had a fork full of food waiting to go in my mouth. So now I never fill my fork until I have totally finished my previous mouthful. For many years I've heard about the benefits of eating slowly and of chewing food well but had never really tried it before. It's amazing how much this small strategy has helped.

THE SCIENCE OF SLOWING DOWN

When you have a really good feed, the food acts in your gastrointestinal tract to trigger the release of 'satiety' or 'stop eating' hormones into your bloodstream. These gut-derived hormones – such as cholecystokinin (CCK), glucagon-like peptide-1 (GL-1), peptide YY (PYY) and pancreatic polypeptide (PP) – then act in your brain to switch off the signals that push you to eat, and this is what helps you to naturally end your meal. Intriguingly, new research shows that compared to wolfing down a meal in five minutes, eating the same meal over half an hour stimulates a significantly stronger increase in the circulating concentrations of the satiety hormones GLP-1 and PYY.[86] This difference persists for up to three-and-a-half hours after the meal and may contribute to a feeling of greater satisfaction from the same number of kilojoules, and – if you're listening to your body and only eating as much as you need to feel satisfied – it may contribute to greater weight loss.

Reading about Maree's weight loss adventure, you may think that it was all pretty straightforward, but that is almost never the case. One example of the challenges Maree faced during her journey to a healthy weight occurred while she was on holidays for a couple of weeks after Christmas. 'I wasn't feeling very well and was very tired – I have identified that feeling serious or prolonged tiredness is one of my biggest risk times. I ate out or had takeaway food for two weeks, almost never cooking. I overate and reached a level of +4 often.' It's how Maree responded to her holiday splurge that made all the difference to her success. Instead of succumbing to all or nothing thinking and negative self-talk, she continued to do as much as she could and reminded herself of the things that she was doing well. 'I did keep exercising, though. Walking a lot and swimming at the beach. The interesting thing is: what I now consider "overeating" used to be the way I ate every day. Overeating in the old days meant a lot more food. So while I was eating more than I needed and not eating very good things, I still had your principles in the back of my mind and was exercising so the net effect is that my weight stayed the same.' Since then Maree has had several lapses into fatigue, but she's developed an excellent coping strategy. 'If I get very tired I can now recognise it, and I let myself go for a few days because I understand what is going on, and it actually works better to let myself go, emotionally I feel comforted, and then pretty soon I start feeling yucky from eating wrongly and my urges naturally correct themselves.'

While in some months Maree lost 4 kilos, in other months she didn't lose any weight at all. Losing weight in bursts is a strategy you'll read about in Chapter 19, because deliberately taking a break from losing weight can mean the difference between reaching your healthy weight and giving up and putting it all back on again. Another thing you may have noticed in Maree's success story is that exercise was part of her plan. In Chapter 18 you'll read about being active enough to lose weight even though you may be feeling dead-tired. 'The big thing that I have come to realise is that weight loss and regaining your vitality is a process,' Maree said. 'You start as a beginner doing easy things, then gain confidence to try a little more and so on. I think I am at the advanced stage now, I really have my diet in hand, my health is improving well and my physical fitness is great.'

Over to you

Here's something you can do immediately to put the ideas in this chapter into action.

The beauty of listening to your body in order to lose weight is that you already have all the answers inside you, neatly packaged inside your genes. If you just give it the chance to do so, your body will tell you what you need to do in order to be your optimum healthy weight.

If Diagnostic N°1b revealed a few too many +4s in your Success Diary and you're not losing weight as quickly as you'd like, then bringing those +4s into line will help you to lose weight more effectively. So my question to you is this: What are the things you can do to make it happen?

Chapter 10

Are you eating too little to lose weight and keep it off? Peta's story

The second day of a diet is always easier than the first.
By the second day you're off it.
  Jackie Gleason, American comedian, actor and musician,
                                                    1916–1987

If you're heavier than your optimum biological weight, it's because at some stage in your life you ate more than your body needed. The solution, therefore, is to create a kilojoule deficit by either cutting back how much you eat or beefing up how much activity you do, or both.

The best way to create a kilojoule deficit is to eat enough to satisfy your physical needs, no more and no less; to choose mostly nutritious foods; and to do some form of physical activity. In their pursuit of weight loss, however, many people eat so little that they end up feeling physically hungry. Maybe this has happened to you? You may have felt so distractingly hungry between those carefully counted diet meals and snacks that you ended up watching the clock until your next scheduled diet ration. Or you may have woken up to a raging hunger in the middle of the night and found it difficult to get back to sleep as you tossed and turned and fantasised about what you'd allow yourself to eat at breakfast. Or maybe you didn't notice feeling particularly hungry; it's just that when you finished eating your meals you still felt mildly irritable, longing for something else to fill the gap – preferably something substantial such as bread with butter and cheese, or chocolate. It's like: I've had my diet, now I'll have my lunch. When you repeatedly feel hungry or dissatisfied while you're trying to lose weight, it's a sign that your Famine Reaction has been activated. Remember, the Famine Reaction not only makes you feel hungrier and makes you crave substantial foods,[1-3] it can also make you feel lethargic[1, 4] as well as slowing your metabolic rate [1, 4-7] and messing around with your hormones so that you tend to store fat and lose muscle and bone.[2, 8, 38, 41-49] With your Famine Reaction raging inside you, it's almost impossible to continue losing weight or to keep it off.

Every yoyo dieter has experienced their Famine Reaction, even if they don't know it by that name, but they make the mistake of thinking that if they just try hard enough they'll be able to overcome it. Time and again they fall off the wagon, only to pig out and gain weight. Peta, 43, knows this scenario all too well, having spent much of her life binge eating and thinking that she would forever be addicted to food. It was only once she realised that she needed to eat *more* when she felt physically hungry that she was finally able to get out of Diet Dungeon and walk to her freedom.

Having lost a total of 47 kilos through various means, Peta recently featured in a magazine article about weight loss, complete with before and after photos. When she was visiting Sydney recently, Peta and I met for coffee. The magazine had just hit the newsagent shelves and Peta brought a copy with her to show me. As we sipped our coffee at a corner table and looked at Peta's glossy 'after' photos, we agreed that women seeing them would probably find it hard to believe that she had ever had a problem with food or her weight. At 63 kilos and 1.65 metres tall, she looked amazing in a tiny, silver, spaghetti-strap top and figure-hugging gym pants. Peta told me how reluctant she had been to appear in that magazine, let alone write her story for my book, because doing so had stirred up a lot of painful memories that are still almost too tender to touch. However, I'm glad she did decide to share her experiences. If you're making the mistake of eating too little to lose weight, Peta's story may give you the inspiration you need to break that habit, as she did.

I was troubled by eating and weight issues from an early age. I was a 'chubby' 9-year-old when my preoccupation with dieting and weight loss began. I did the Scarsdale diet and the grapefruit diet to recall a couple. I was in a diet club by the age of 14, where I learned that I could binge for the first half of the week and diet for the last half, and step on the scales at the meeting and be clapped for weight loss. For most of my teenage years I fluctuated between 60 and 70 kilos in typical yoyo fashion.

I still recall the first time I binged at 14 years of age and the guilty pleasure I felt. The inevitable weight gain ensued and my response was stricter dieting. I participated in the 40-hour famine and learned how to fast. Bingeing became a regular feature of my life for the next 7 years, and once I left home I would fast for up to 5 days to control my weight after a binge.

The physiological and emotional toll this created became evident and I would spend entire weekends in bed. I either starved myself drinking nothing but coffee, or I slept and ate. My dream to travel through Europe was similarly dogged by this problem as I binged in European style – gelati in Rome, pastries in Paris and bratwurst in Munich! The contrast between my friends and me was stark. They were absorbed by our travelling adventures, whilst I was obsessed with my size and fighting the impulse to binge on most days. I was shocked to realise that for the past 7 years I had not eaten normally – I was either in diet mode or in binge/overeat mode. I NEVER sat at a table and just had dinner like others; I was ALWAYS on the way up or down.

I eventually consulted a therapist for my disordered eating and was introduced to the 12-step addiction model for food and weight problems. This initially worked well for me – I ate well, lost weight slowly and had emotional support. Therapy taught me about patterns and dynamics and I enjoyed the journey of self-understanding. However, despite my success with this path I still knew that I was not truly free. Within the addiction model the power of the substance remains intact no matter how long one is free. Thus an alcoholic may have been sober for 20 years yet still believe they are only one drink away from being a 'drunk'. Similarly with food, a 'relapse' can be devastating and thus it was for me. After many years of weight stability I relapsed into bingeing and for the first time ever my weight ballooned to 110 kilos.

These were the most difficult and depressed years of my life, yet at the same time they launched my personal quest to understand more and to comprehend what had gone wrong. Through cognitive behavioural therapy I learned to pick myself up and dust myself off and get on with life more readily after each binge. My bingeing became less frequent at times, and over a number of years I gradually dropped from 110 kilos to 69 kilos. But I wanted to lose a little more weight. And most disturbingly, my bingeing persisted. I longed for total freedom.

It was at this time that I attended one of Dr Amanda's workshops, but only because there was a PhD after her name! I would never have bought a book with the word 'diet' in the title. I was stunned to learn about the Famine Reaction and the Fat Brake. Sure enough, when I examined my recent past and looked at my overall history, my patterns did indeed fit this new knowledge. If I looked at recent infrequent binge patterns, they usually occurred when I had dropped a kilo or so, and as I approached my normal weight range every kilo I lost would trigger a Famine Reaction and a binge! This stunned me – I was still thinking 'once an addict always an addict', which is a 12-step mantra. Instead of seeing myself as personally or emotionally flawed in some way, this new knowledge showed me that I wasn't. Knowledge of the Fat Brake helped me to understand why I had been through periods of weight stability without rigid control over what I ate, as well as how a healthy person naturally regulates their weight without external controls. I took away with me an understanding of the perfection of this apparatus that is the body.

Over the following months I experimented with the new ideas I had learned from Amanda. The next time a 'binge urge' overwhelmed me I made my first attempt to eat my way out of it. I was quite afraid, sure that I was kidding myself, sure that this was a binge by any other name, because one day I seemed to do nothing but eat every hour or two all afternoon and all evening, even after eating a proper lunch and dinner. I ate chocolate sultanas from a bag I kept dipping into, I ate crumpets with butter and honey, and I ate a big banana as well as a lot of pistachio nuts. My eyes said, 'STOP, you've eaten way too much,' but my stomach said, 'Yum, that's good, we feel good.' And then . . . as urgently as the desire to eat had come on, it stopped. The growling hunger, the nagging persistent drive for more – they just stopped, like someone had turned the switch off. Over the next few days I ate somewhat more than usual (although not as much as that first day), and when I weighed myself the next week I had not gained any weight at all. I was weight stable and had eaten like a horse or so it seemed. Eating my way out of a binge had worked! This was a real breakthrough for me personally and eventually led to my absolute and total freedom.

It has now been five years since I did Dr Amanda's workshop and I am so in tune with my body that it is difficult for me to even remember the past and the way I used to think. In fact, it has not been easy for me to write this and to revisit those many years of suffering where I just did not understand the trap I was in. Today I am a wonderful weight (I've gone from 69 to 63 kilos since the workshop), I look as if I never had a weight or an eating problem in my entire life, I make no menu plans nor use any external controls over what or how much I eat, and I don't drink diet drinks or skim milk any more. I have no scales and I have total food freedom. I have the freedom I always sought and a body that wakes up each morning full of life and flexibility and energy. I don't plan to exercise, I just do. When I have not been very physical for a while this drive to move takes over and I move for fun and strength, not for weight loss!!!!! Most of all, the greatest gift is my total lack of fear. I NEVER worry about how to maintain my weight, nor do I worry about so-called relapses. The 12-step approach suggested I could never be normal around food, that I was somehow 'allergic' to sugar or other favourite binge substances. Amanda's work showed me that there was in fact very little wrong with me and that I could have my life back again.

Through Amanda's work, the last piece of knowledge that I needed to be completely well became available to me. Instead of worrying about what I should or should not eat, what I weigh or what meeting or group I should attend 'to make sure I'm OK', my life evolves with a better class of issues that can really make a positive difference to my life and the lives of people around me.

Over to you

Here's something you can do immediately to put the ideas in this chapter into action.

Do you recognise yourself in any of Peta's story? If you've ever felt driven to eat foods you normally try to avoid or to eat food in larger quantities than you usually allow yourself, it's quite likely that inadequate food intake at certain times may be the culprit. If so, making sure you are eating enough overall will help you to break this vicious cycle and reach your own equilibrium, just as Peta has done so successfully.

While the recommendation to eat according to your hunger and true cravings rather than denying them has impeccable scientific credentials and is used in clinical practice to break the cycle of overeating or binge eating, many people worry that doing so will stop them from losing weight and may even cause them to gain weight. In the next two chapters I'm going to walk you through the logistics of eating enough to have a healthy relationship with food while also enabling your body to peacefully and efficiently assume the weight and size it's biologically meant to be.

Chapter 11

Step 1c. One way to eat too little for weight loss: waiting until you feel ravenous before eating

Try not to get too hungry. Hunger signals are a bit like our bladder signals. If we wait too long to respond, we're more likely to have an accident!

Dr Rick Kausman, Australian pioneer of the non-dieting approach to healthy weight management

If you've ever followed a diet on which you wound up feeling ravenously hungry between meals, you may believe that in order to lose weight you actually *need* to get ravenously hungry. This is not so. In fact, medical research proves that the less you eat in order to lose weight, the stronger your Famine Reaction becomes, the hungrier you get and – wait for it – *the less efficiently you lose weight.*[21] Part of the reason for this is that the less you eat, the greater the degree to which your Famine Reaction slows your metabolic rate, and the more you then need to restrict what you eat in order to lose weight. Additionally, when you get ravenously hungry before eating, you're more likely to break out and overeat. If you've ever stood in front of the fridge inhaling copious quantities of whatever rich foods you could get your hands on after a hard day's dieting, you know exactly what I mean.

Does this apply to you?

Everyone sometimes gets caught unawares and ends up ravenously hungry before eating. For instance, maybe you do something a bit more energetic than usual – checking out the January sales or snorkelling over a reef – and by the time you get around to eating you're shaking like a leaf. Getting ravenously hungry on the odd occasion is not a problem; our bodies are designed to cope with that. But if you're trying to lose weight or keep it off, then getting ravenously hungry too often will sabotage your progress. If you've been struggling with your weight for a long time, getting too hungry before eating can become such a way of life that you don't even realise you're doing it. Take my diagnostic test to find out if you're letting yourself get too ravenous for your own good.

Dr Amanda's Diagnostic N°1c: Are you letting yourself get ravenously hungry?

To do this simple diagnostic test, use your Success Diary for 3 to 14 days as described in Chapter 5. Remember, it takes only about three minutes a day to use a Success Diary, and you can use the same pages from your Success Diary for all the diagnostic tests in this book. For best results, aim to use your Success Diary for 14 days so that you get an accurate estimate of what your current eating patterns are.

Once you've used your Success Diary for several days, your next step is to work out how many times per week you're letting yourself get ravenously hungry before eating. In other words, how many times per week are you scoring a –4 in your Hunger column. If you've used your Success Diary for exactly 7 days, you simply count how many –4s you scored in the Hunger column in that time. If you've kept your Success Diary for more or less than 7 days, here's how to calculate how many –4s you're scoring in a week on average, or how many –4s you'd be scoring in a complete week if you kept going at the same rate.

- Count the number of days you've used your Success Diary for the whole day.
- Count how many –4s you scored in the Hunger column of your Success Diary on those days.
- Divide the total number of –4s you counted by the number of days on which you used your Success Diary for the whole day. This will give you the average number of –4s you're scoring per day.
- Multiply this number by 7 to get the number of –4s you score on average (or would score) per week.

For example, let's suppose that in the past seven days you've used your Success Diary for only four days, because your routine was disrupted over the long weekend. In those four days you count a total of one –4 in your Hunger column. So the number of times you're getting ravenously hungry before eating per week, on average, is:

1 time ÷ 4 days = 0.25 times per day
0.25 times per day × 7 days = 1.75 times per week

That is, you're scoring a –4 in your Success Diary less than twice a week.

Interpreting your results
If you're getting ravenously hungry (that is, scoring a –4 in the Hunger column of your Success Diary) around twice a week or less, you're on the right track for permanent weight loss. Avoiding ravenous hunger will help you keep your Famine Reaction under control as you lose weight, thereby helping you to lose excess weight as efficiently as your body is able to do so. If you feel confident about avoiding too many –4s as well as avoiding the temptation of going on a diet that leaves you feeling ravenously hungry between meals or snacks, you may like to skip straight to the next chapter.

If, on the other hand, you're getting ravenously hungry more than twice a week, then reducing the number of –4s you score in your Success Diary to two or fewer times per week will reduce your risk of a Famine Reaction and of breaking out and bingeing, thereby helping you to lose weight in a way that is sustainable in the long term. Read on for examples of how avoiding too many −4s has helped others to lose weight more effectively.

Feeding your hunger rather than denying it will bring instant benefits

If you make a conscious decision to steer clear of too many −4s in your Success Diary, you'll obviously enjoy the instant benefit of freedom from ravenous hunger. But what you may be surprised to realise is that by making the decision to stamp out ravenous hunger, you're likely to lose weight. A great example of this is 41-year-old Leonora.

From: Leonora
Sent: Saturday 17ᵗʰ May 8:56 PM
To: Dr Amanda Sainsbury-Salis
Subject: Finally relief from the famine reaction!!

Hi Amanda,

I was in your workshop in Melbourne last Saturday and although I had sort of started following your principles before the workshop, once I started entering details into the diary a remarkable thing happened. For the first time in many years I stopped being constantly hungry! I have spent years either completely denying my hunger or being in a state of constant extreme hunger and it has finally stopped. In only a week! I hope I stay this way. I am certainly going to continue using the diary for a while to make sure everything is working. I am eating less and feeling completely satisfied. So I'm looking forward to finally shedding these kilos!

Thank you,
Leonora

When I replied, I asked Leonora to keep me posted on her progress.

> *From: Dr Amanda Sainsbury-Salis*
> *Sent: Monday 19th May 8:51 PM*
> *To: Leonora*
> *Subject: Re: Finally relief from the famine reaction!!*
>
> *Dear Leonora,*
> *It is marvellous to hear of your great experiences in just one week, and I encourage you to keep eating enough to satisfy your hunger. What is also great to see is that when you started allowing yourself to eat enough to keep your hunger at bay, you started eating less while feeling completely satisfied. What a power it is to feed your body's needs rather than deny them. You are now working with your marvellous body instead of against it.*
> *When you look in the Hunger column in your Success Diary, do you see all −2s and −3s? I encourage you to strive for that, so that when you weigh in again after your first two weeks of using your Success Diary you will see good results.*
> *Will you let me know how you get on at your next weigh-in? I'd love to hear your news.*
> *Sincerely,*
> *Amanda*

Thirteen days after she came to my workshop and started using a Success Diary, Leonora wrote to tell me that she had lost 1.5 kilos. Leonora's experience is a great example of the fact that rather than leading to weight gain, as you might think it would, eating when you feel physically hungry – as opposed to letting yourself get ravenously hungry – helps weight loss along by decreasing your interest in food and preventing the drop in metabolic rate that the Famine Reaction induces.

Feeding rather than denying hunger brings emotional as well as physical relief

My friend Holly has lost 13 kilos since she came to one of my workshops two-and-a-half years ago and started eating according to her body signals. Before that time, Holly had spent over 25 years trying to lose weight. Currently weighing 101 kilos for her 1.69 metre frame, Holly still wants to lose some more weight, but the weight she has already lost seems to be gone for good. 'I feel as though I want to make things happen faster but I'm happy that I've not put back on what I've lost,' she said. Holly recently told me of the significant effect that listening to her body has had on her emotional stability.

The concept of eating when I'm hungry has by far been the most valuable and most foreign strategy I've ever implemented in all my years of losing and gaining weight. All those dieting classes I've attended over the years have wired my brain into thinking that hunger is a natural part of losing weight, and that ignoring it and becoming emotionally strong about those physical feelings is just something you have to do if you want to lose weight. And then of course, when you are unable to do it any more for reasons I now understand as the Famine Reaction, all those emotions around feeling strong and successful come crashing down and turn to feelings of being weak and out of control. So by implementing the strategy of eating when I'm hungry, I just don't have to deal with the ups and downs of dieting. This, to me, has been the most helpful thing that I have learned from you, and the 13 kilos that I have lost over the past two-and-a-half years are also of course a big bonus.

Feeding your hunger rather than denying it can help you to lose more

Not allowing yourself to get ravenously hungry – that is, avoiding –4s in your Success Diary – will bring you greater physical and emotional contentment and help you to lose weight, but it does more than this. It can also help you to lose *more* weight and keep it off for *longer* than if you try to lose weight by denial.

For most of her adult life, 50-year-old Astrid has been fit and muscular, consistently weighing in at around 58 kilos. It wasn't until she had a baby at the age of 40 that she put on any excess weight.

> When I got to 67 kilos I panicked and joined a diet club. I lost 8 kilos in as many weeks and promptly put it all back on again plus more. After that I tried another organisation that provided low-kilojoule meals. I lost 3 kilos in three weeks and abandoned it as I felt dreadful eating so much processed food. Once again I put on the fat I had lost plus more. Then I tried the weight loss program offered by my personal trainer. I lost 4 kilos in as many weeks and then put this back on and more. On each of the occasions that I abandoned my diet it was because I got so hungry that I overate, felt that I had failed and then gave up. When I reached 72 kilos I was so desperate that I entered an Ironman race consisting of a 4 kilometre swim, a 180 kilometre bike ride and a 40 kilometre run. I trained for about 15 hours per week and got down to 68 kilos even though I was eating like a horse. After the race I couldn't train due to injuries and I ate my way through a very worrying time with my son and ended up at a massive 83.7 kilos, significantly more than I weighed full-term just before giving birth.

In almost a decade of dieting, the maximum weight that Astrid had been able to lose was 8 kilos, and each time the kilos came back, plus more. However, after reading my book *The Don't Go Hungry Diet*, Astrid lost 20 kilos in 10 months and has kept all but 3 of them off for over 9 months, which included a one-month holiday where she ate exactly what she wanted to eat, as well as a broken knee, an encounter with swine flu and a chest infection. Exercise is an important aspect of Astrid's success, but she attributes her success mainly to feeding rather than denying her hunger.

> *The REALLY important thing I learned from your book is to eat when you are hungry, but make sure it is nutritious. That seems to be the key to losing weight for me. In the past I used to think that to lose weight I had to feel hungry a lot of the time, but in actual fact if I get too hungry it is a disaster waiting to happen. So now I eat when I am hungry and I ignore any other prescriptions I hear about how much and what to eat and when. Last year I wore size 16s, and now I am a size 8 or 10. It has been great to have to completely change and downsize my wardrobe twice! I genuinely feel as if I have given myself an extra 15 years of life. I feel, and other people say I look, closer to 38 years old rather than 50! I treasure the lesson your book taught me.*

Over to you
Here's something you can do immediately to put the ideas in this chapter into action.

If you're in the habit of letting yourself get too hungry too often, do what Leonora, Holly and Astrid did and use your Success Diary until you become expert at losing weight by avoiding ravenous hunger and eating enough. Try it for yourself and see how much easier losing weight and keeping it off can be.

Chapter 12

Step 1d. The most common way to eat too little for weight loss: failure to 'go all the way'

Please, sir, I want some more.

From *Oliver Twist*, by Charles Dickens

Eating when you are physically hungry is such an instinctive response that once people notice too many −4s of ravenous hunger in their Success Diary, they are usually able to eradicate them swiftly and pretty well for good. A far more common way to eat too little for weight loss, however, and a mistake that people find it trickier to avoid, is habitually finishing meals or snacks before feeling genuinely satisfied. I call this a failure to 'go all the way'. If you've ever finished eating a carefully kilojoule-counted diet meal and felt that you could easily eat the same again, you know how unsettling it is not to eat enough. What most people don't realise is that repeatedly failing to go all the way not only feels awful but can also interfere with your ability to lose weight. In Chapters 8 and 9 I wrote about 'satiety' or 'stop eating' hormones, which are released from your gastrointestinal tract into your bloodstream after you eat. These hormones then act on your brain to reduce your appetite. If you don't eat enough, however, you don't get a strong enough rise in blood levels of satiety hormones and you never fully extinguish your desire to eat. You may find yourself thinking excessively about food and dreaming about all the things you'd like to eat. You may feel on edge and irritable, because one of your body's most basic needs has been left unmet. You may find it difficult to resist snacks, especially energy-dense treats such as Florentine slice or nougat. If you *repeatedly* stop eating before you feel properly satisfied, this can trigger a Famine Reaction that will set you up for a binge and prime your body to shunt the food you eat towards fat. On the other hand, when you allow yourself to continue your meals and snacks until you feel genuinely satisfied, you're better able to relax and get on with your life without constantly thinking about food. You're much less inclined to reach for snacks when you don't feel hungry. You'll find that overindulging in excessive quantities of foods that make you feel bad about yourself is something you can put behind you. The overall result is that you can lose weight more effectively. So let's find out if failing to 'go all the way' is hindering *your* weight loss progress.

Does this apply to you?

When people embark on the journey of losing weight by connecting with their body, they are often reluctant to eat to the point of genuine satiety for fear of putting on weight. Most people don't realise how detrimental this can be to their weight loss progress, and they don't realise when they're doing it, either . . . until they see it in black and white in the following diagnostic.

Dr Amanda's Diagnostic Nº1d: Are you failing to 'go all the way'?

To do this simple diagnostic test, use your Success Diary for 3 to 14 days as described in Chapter 5. For best results, aim to use your Success Diary for 14 days.

Bonus offer

If you've come this far without trying any of these diagnostic tests, I'd like to give you a special incentive for doing this one. If you use your Success Diary for a minimum

---

of three days and then do this Diagnostic N°1d, you may well discover that you can actually eat *more* at each meal or snack than you thought you could, all the while losing weight more effectively to boot. Not eating enough at a meal or snack is a mistake that so many people trying to lose weight make that I'd hazard a guess that you make it, too. And remember, once you've used your Success Diary for three or more days, you can use the same Success Diary for all 10 diagnostic tests in this book – that's '10 for the price of one'.

How to do it
Once you've used your Success Diary for several days (and good on you for taking up the challenge), your next step is to work out how many times per week you're failing to go all the way when you eat. That is, how many times per week are you scoring a +1 in your Satiety column? If you've used your Success Diary for exactly seven days, you simply count how many +1s there are in the Satiety column of your Success Diary in that time. If you've kept your Success Diary for more or less than seven days, here's how to calculate how many +1s you're scoring in a week on average, or how many +1s you'd be scoring in a complete week if you kept going at the same rate.

- Count the number of days you've used your Success Diary for the whole day.
- Count how many +1s you scored in the Satiety column of your Success Diary on those days.
- Divide the total number of +1s you counted by the number of days on which you used your Success Diary for the whole day. This will give you the average number of +1s you're scoring per day.
- Multiply this number by 7 to get the number of +1s you score on average (or would score) per week.

For example, suppose that you've used your Success Diary for 16 consecutive days. In those 16 days you count a total of 11 +1s in your Satiety column. So the number of times per week you're failing to go all the way when you eat, on average, is:

11 times ÷ 16 days = 0.69 times per day
0.69 times per day × 7 days = 4.83 times per week

That is, you're scoring a +1 in your Success Diary approximately five times a week.

Interpreting your results

If you're finishing meals or snacks when you're not quite satisfied (that is, scoring a +1 in the Satiety column of your Success Diary) around twice a week or less, you're going great guns. Keep doing what you're doing, because it will help you keep your Famine Reaction at bay so you can lose weight as effectively as your body is able to. If you feel you've got this skill honed, you may like to skip straight to the next chapter.

If, on the other hand, you're failing to go all the way more than twice a week, reducing the number of +1s you score in your Success Diary to two or fewer times per week will not only help you to feel more physically content, it will also help you to manage your weight more effectively in the long term. Read on for examples of the benefits of going all the way.

Brooke broke her diet, went all the way and never looked back

At 51 years of age, Brooke had been a member of her local diet club for 10 years. With her healthy eating habits and lithe figure (around 77 kilos and 1.78 metres tall), Brooke was the envy of all her friends. Some would say she's 'lucky', but Brooke knew otherwise. For the past decade she'd kilojoule-counted every single thing she had eaten, endeavouring to remain within her diet's allowance. Yet, despite her constant counting, Brooke's weight constantly oscillated.

'Whenever my weight crept up a few kilos to where I wasn't comfortable, I would "go on a diet" to lose it again,' she wrote to me in an email. Brooke's diet consisted of reducing her daily food intake from maintenance levels to weight loss levels, the latter being determined by her diet club. The trouble was, although her diet club's diet was sensible and nutritionally balanced, sometimes Brooke just needed to eat more. 'I have sometimes gone to bed absolutely starving because I have tried to stick with my diet and "do the right thing",' she wrote. 'Then I end up not sleeping well due to my nagging hunger.' Indeed, if you've lost weight and your Famine Reaction has been activated, even the most sensible of diets can leave you feeling famished. When she couldn't 'white-knuckle it' any longer, Brooke would give in to her hunger. 'I might have an extra slice of toast with peanut butter at breakfast and an extra yogurt at afternoon tea as I usually come home from work at 5.30 pm feeling very hungry. Then I might have an extra piece of fruit at suppertime.' Hardly excessive eating, as you can see, but certainly more than her weight loss rations would allow. If Brooke had three days within a week where she exceeded her diet's allowance, she felt as though she had failed miserably. 'On "hungry days" I thought there was something wrong with my ability to diet and regarded myself as hopeless at dieting and hopeless at using willpower. Then I would think, "There's no point to this as I can't do it how it's supposed to be done" and then I would proceed to eat anything and everything I had denied myself.'

At other times, Brooke would manage to resist her hunger and force her weight down to where she wanted it, but then she would struggle with the maintenance phase of her diet. 'It was hard to gradually increase my food intake so as not to put on weight,' she wrote. 'Thus, it would only take a few months before the extra food would be converted to fat and additional weight.' This is a typical sign of the Famine Reaction at work. When you push against it by sticking to your diet's allowance no matter how hungry or unsatisfied you feel, your Famine Reaction 'pays you back' by slowing your metabolic rate so that you pack on the weight again with impressive efficiency.

Having battled against extra kilos and her Famine Reaction for many years, Brooke gave up. 'I am now frightened to go on any sort of diet again (I could do with losing 3 kilos) as I am afraid of putting my body into that slow metabolism mode again and having to re-train my body after the diet.'

Brooke didn't need to give up her desire to shed those extra kilos. In fact, all she needed was to learn how to go all the way. However, although Brooke understood intellectually that eating more in hungry times might be the answer to her predicament, she was apprehensive about abandoning the kilojoule counting that now came so easily to her. After all, counting kilojoules for a decade had at least helped prevent her weight from escalating to an unhealthy level, and she was worried about what might happen if she let go of this habit.

After discussing her dilemma with me via email and over the phone, Brooke decided to continue counting kilojoules as she had done for years. But instead of forcing her body to comply with her diet's rigid allowance, she would allow her body to tell her what, when and how much to eat . . . and then simply watch how much food she tallied up each day. Being a person who thrives on structure and guidelines, Brooke felt comfortable with this approach. Four weeks after letting her body help her count her kilojoules, Brooke emailed me to let me know how she was getting on.

From: Brooke
Sent: Saturday 26ᵗʰ January 7:43 PM
To: Dr Amanda Sainsbury-Salis
Subject: Still discovering amazing things!

Dear Amanda,

Thank you for your last email. You gave me some things to think about. I am astonished that, at 51 years of age and spending 30 years watching my health, following various diets and thinking I knew a reasonable amount about it all, I am learning SO MUCH from you.

Thanks to you, I now give myself permission to be hungry and eat 'guilt free'. Here is an example from the last week. On Tuesday, I woke up starving. I took the dog for a 40-minute morning walk and felt quite listless. I ate a 'larger-than-usual' breakfast (a good-sized serving of porridge, milk, 2 pieces of toast and peanut butter and 2 cups of coffee). Normally this would cause me to think that I'd blown my diet and then I would eat 'whatever' for the rest of the day. But on Tuesday I allowed myself to be hungry and to eat. By 11.15 am I was hungry again and had a small tin of baked beans and a yogurt. At 1 pm I was hungry again and had a sandwich, a salad and a breakfast bar. At 4.30 pm I ate three small hot cross buns and an apple and at 7 pm I ate chicken and veggies for tea. I felt nicely full, but not upset with myself. I didn't binge eat, I didn't blow it, I simply ate because I was hungry. I knew when to stop eating AND I didn't fret about having a so-called 'bad' day. In the past, this would be the start of a number of days of 'bad eating' as I would be completely convinced that I was hopeless.

However, on Wednesday, I didn't feel hungry and easily ate much less. Today also, I have eaten very little simply because I haven't been at all hungry. This has taken no willpower at all and in fact I don't even feel like eating anything much at all.

I am just amazed at how your approach and its impact on my psychology make all the difference to the way I think about what I am doing. I have finally realised that I do have some hungry days and some not-so-hungry days and it doesn't mean that I am in any way a failure. In fact, eating more on some days and less on others makes me feel like I am succeeding beautifully.

Brooke was certainly succeeding in her weight loss adventure. Four weeks after deciding to eat however much she needed in order to feel satisfied, she had lost 1.2 kilos and 2 centimetres from her waist. 'I can't wait to continue the journey,' she said. Almost a year-and-a-half later, I had the pleasure of hearing the outcome of Brooke's journey.

> *From: Brooke*
> *Sent: Monday 4th May 2:38 PM*
> *To: Dr Amanda Sainsbury-Salis*
> *Subject: Birthdays and looking good*
>
> *Hi Amanda – you may remember me – Brooke – I wrote to you on a number of occasions last year as I tried to put the ideas in your book into practice, whilst still following the diet program that I have followed for years.*
>
> *Well here we are, maybe 12 months since I last emailed you. I turned 53 just two days ago and I feel great!!!! In the last 17 months, since reading your book, I have lost 7 kilos and kept it off!!! When I first contacted you, my set point was 76.6 kilos. Through following your ideas, loosely sticking to my diet program (not counting too strictly) and leading two health challenges with colleagues, I gradually lost 7 kilos. My weight is now very firmly settled at around 69.5 kilos, which is where I have been for five months now and with very little effort. I am not dieting, just monitoring my hunger and of course, eating healthy foods and exercising. Your research and ideas have really helped me change the way I think about my body and how it works.*
>
> *Thanks for your monthly newsletter and happy birthday to you, too!*
> *Kind regards,*
> *Brooke*

It's now been more than 18 months since that email from Brooke, and she's still maintaining her weight within a range of 67.5 to 69.5 kilos. By satisfying her hunger and going all the way rather than denying her physical needs, she has finally licked her internal struggle with excess weight.

Going all the way makes it easier to resist eating when you're not actually hungry

One thing I've noticed among people who frequently stop eating before feeling genuinely satisfied is that they often also eat when they are not yet physically hungry. Whenever I see a Success Diary with a lot of +1s in the Satiety column, there's almost always a lot of −1s in the Hunger column as well. If you scrimp on your portion sizes because you're trying to lose weight – to the point that you often feel unsatisfied when you finish eating – you may knock the edge off your hunger, but you don't actually stop it dead in its tracks so that you can get on with your life and forget about eating for a while. The result is that you may feel compelled to eat tasty little titbits even when you aren't actually hungry. This is an insidious habit that can keep you stuck in Diet Dungeon interminably. If you simply ate slightly larger meals or snacks, large enough to make you feel genuinely satisfied, you would fully extinguish your desire to eat and be able to go for much longer before getting the urge to poke around the kitchen looking for something to eat. By then you'd probably also be hungry enough for another decent-sized meal or snack. Indeed, when I suggest to clients who struggle with excessive +1s that they focus on eating until they feel genuinely satisfied at a level of +2 to +3, any non-hungry snacking often magically disappears. If you're clocking up too many +1s in your Satiety column and you're also scoring a few too many −1s or 0s in your Hunger column, going all the way will probably help you to consume fewer kilojoules overall by minimising non-hungry eating, and this will help you to lose weight more effectively.

Let me take you somewhere safe

If feeling unsatisfied is such a way of life for you that you often find yourself feeling edgy and irritable because you haven't eaten enough, you probably have a lot of fear about eating until you feel genuinely satisfied: fear that you may gain weight, fear that you won't be able to stop yourself eating if you cut yourself some slack, or fear of feeling out of control as you venture into unfamiliar territory. If so, take my hand and I'll walk you through it. Once you've visited True Satiety After Every Meal or Snack and you've seen the effects on your weight, you'll realise that it's actually the safest place to go with your appetite, and you'll soon feel 100 per cent confident about going there on your own.

The first thing you need to do as we set out on this voyage to True Satiety After Every Meal or Snack is to arm yourself with a Success Diary. Remember, you won't need to use your Success Diary forever; it's only for a few weeks or months until you feel confident about losing weight by connecting with your body.

Now that you've got your Success Diary in tow, the next time you eat a meal or snack, take note of how satisfied you feel when you think it's time to finish eating. If you had to write down a number to match your level of satisfaction at that point, what number would it be? If you're still feeling a bit edgy or you're already thinking about what you'd like to eat at your next meal or snack, you most probably haven't eaten enough; you're probably experiencing a +1. In the beginning you may not recognise +1s when they occur, but you'll get better at it. And when you do spot a +1 when you're thinking about finishing your meal our snack, all you need to do is look around and find something that will extinguish your desire to eat. This is where the Three Yeses Test on page 117 will help; it will lead you to exactly the food or foods you need to eat in order to feel pleasantly satisfied at that moment. Maybe what you really need to eat is more of what you just had? Or maybe what you need is some cheese and crackers? The French custom of eating cheeses after dinner was obviously invented by people who weren't quite satisfied after their meals. Or would a slice of toast do it for you? Or perhaps what you're looking for to fill the gap is a mouthful of something fatty and sweet, such as a couple of fresh dates with a dob of peanut butter or tahini?

Whatever it is that will fill the gap and make you feel really good, go for it!

So how do you feel now? Are you feeling comfortable and relaxed? Not oversatisfied, but content and ready to face whatever's next in your day? This is a +2 or a +3, and you'll get better at recognising what it feels like to you. If you keep aiming for this feeling every time you eat, you'll be astounded at the difference it will make to your ability to manage your weight.

If you want to lose weight faster, don't try to fix your satiety scores if they're not broken

Mindy, 42, has lost almost 6 kilos in the three months since she started using a Success Diary. In the beginning she was eating more than she needed at least once a day (by eating when she wasn't hungry or eating until she felt oversatisfied), but within three weeks she had got used to listening to her body and was scoring all 2s and 3s. This, in addition to making sure she ate sufficient fruit and vegetables and maintaining her active lifestyle, contributed to her gratifying results. Recently, however, a few −1s and 0s of non-hungry eating have crept back into Mindy's Hunger column, and although she's still scoring all +2s and +3s in her Satiety column (she has really mastered the art of stopping before she has eaten too much), her weight loss has stalled. Keen to get her weight moving steadily downwards again, Mindy emailed me to ask whether, in addition to reining in her non-hungry eating, she should also try to end her meals and snacks when she feels just satisfied (a +2 on the satiety scale) as opposed to elegantly satisfied (+3). Many people who wish to speed up their weight loss have asked me the same question, the idea being that finishing a meal or a snack on the lighter side of satisfied would reduce their overall food intake and therefore accelerate weight loss. This, however, is not a tactic I would recommend, as you'll read in my response to Mindy's question below.

From: Dr Amanda Sainsbury-Salis
Sent: Thursday 27th May 10:25 PM
To: Mindy
Subject: Re: I've stopped losing weight

Dear Mindy,

With regards to aiming for all +2s instead of a mixture of +2s and +3s in your Satiety column, I don't recommend that as a weight loss strategy. The reason for this is that doing so can lead you to eat just that little bit less than you really need, even though you may still rate your level of satiety as a +2 rather than a +1. If you regularly feel even just slightly unsatisfied after eating, it can make it really hard to eat only when hungry (and therefore lose weight), because you can feel driven to eat even though you're not actually hungry. So I would keep going for the mixture of +2s and +3s that you are so successfully achieving now. From your Success Diary I can see that you have really mastered the art of knowing when to stop eating, so there's no need to 'fix' that because you're already doing brilliantly.

On the other hand, your plan to stamp out those -1s and 0s in your Hunger column by focusing on eating only when hungry sounds excellent; that will undoubtedly help you to get your weight moving in the direction you want. Go for it! I look forward to hearing how you get on.
Sincerely,
Amanda

So, if you're comfortably scoring either all +3s in the Satiety column of your Success Diary, or a mixture of +2s and +3s, let it be.

Needs and pleasure go together

When I lived in Switzerland, I once heard the expression *Les plaisirs d'homme sont les besoins d'homme*, meaning that the things we get pleasure from are the things that meet our needs. If you're stuck in Diet Dungeon, you may think that eating enough to feel pleasantly satisfied would lead to weight gain, but in fact the opposite is true. The reason why eating until you feel truly satisfied is so pleasurable is that it helps your body to do what it's biologically programmed to do, and that includes being an optimum healthy weight for life.

Over to you

Here's something you can do immediately to put the ideas in this chapter into action.

If Diagnostic N°1d revealed a few too many +1s in your Success Diary, it's time to start yielding to the pitiful voice inside saying 'Please, sir, I want some more'.

Give that little voice what it's begging for, and you'll be amazed at how much more human you'll feel. You'll probably also be astounded at how much easier it will be to keep going until you reach the weight you're meant to be.

Chapter 13

Which key strategies will ensure *you* stay out of Diet Dungeon?

Education is learning what you didn't even know you didn't know.

Daniel J. Boorstin, American historian, professor, attorney and writer, 1914–2004

In concluding this Step 1 of mastering the art of eating according to your physical needs, I'd like to ask you two questions.

How long have you been struggling with your weight?

What has that struggle cost you in terms of your health, your happiness and your relationships?

If you're tired of starting a brand-new Diet To End All Diets on the first day of every week, month or year, only to crash and burn shortly thereafter, with your dream in tatters, how would you like to leave all that behind you?

As you've seen from the case studies in this section of the book, one thing that's helped many others to escape from Diet Dungeon and break the endless cycle of dieting is to use a Success Diary and learn the *real* reason why they can't lose weight effectively or sustainably.

So what's the real reason why *you* can't lose weight or keep it off?

You may assume it's because you're eating too much, so you therefore try to fix it by eating less and less with every new weight loss attempt. But what if eating too much when you're trying to shed fat is *not* the problem, and the real reason you can't reach a healthy steady weight is that you're not actually eating enough at certain times, either waiting until you're ravenous before eating or not going all the way when you do, or both. If this applies to you, then – like Peta, Leonora, Holly, Astrid and Brooke, who stepped free of decades of dieting by eating more at certain times, not less – wouldn't you rather know about it now, so that you could spare yourself another 10 or more years of struggle?

Or you may assume that the reason you can't escape from Diet Dungeon to reach your ideal weight or stay there is that you don't exercise enough, so you therefore try to fix it by increasing the frequency, duration and intensity of your exercise, to the point that you no longer have time for your normal social life, and so relationships will just have to wait until after you reach your goal. But what if your inability to slim down for good had nothing whatsoever to do with exercise, and the real reason was that you were quietly sabotaging your efforts with all those healthy meals and snacks that you eat when you're not hungry? Wouldn't you rather know about it now, so that you could fix the problem at its source, rather than struggling on with gruellingly unsustainable exercise routines and missing out on other important aspects of life?

Or you may assume that the reason you have so much trouble losing weight is that you're no good at resisting all the 'foods to avoid' you've seen listed in the various diets you've followed over the years, and so you try to fix this by cutting out entire food groups to the point that you can no longer eat a meal outside the home without going on a guilt trip. But what if your lack of weight loss was not because you sometimes 'slipped' and had mashed potato and peas with your dinner, but because you usually eat until your stomach feels ever so slightly uncomfortable because you rarely eat exactly what you feel like eating? Wouldn't you rather know about it now, so that you could save your energy for the important things in life, rather than constantly dreaming about all of your favourite foods and how to avoid them?

Whatever your weight loss challenges, your Success Diary and the Diagnostics in this section will enable you to identify exactly which of my 10 key strategies you need to focus on to lose weight and keep it off once and for all, without the endless restrictions you knew in Diet Dungeon. Many Professional Dieters think they already know how much they need to eat in order to lose weight or keep it off and that a Success Diary is only for novices. But as we've seen in this section, the amount you need to eat in order to reach your optimum biological weight is a tricky target to hit, because it changes all the time depending on what your Famine Reaction and your Fat Brake are up to, how active you are, and what your hormones are doing. On the other hand, if you listen to your body and eat accordingly – keeping a Success Diary and using Diagnostics Nᵒs 1a, 1b, 1c and 1d until you know how to do this – your body will direct you to exactly the amount of food you need to eat in order to attain and maintain your ideal healthy weight, now and through almost anything that life will throw your way.

Eating according to your physical needs is the first and most important step you can take towards escaping Diet Dungeon and reaching your ideal biological weight for life, but it only works when you eat the right foods. Let's move now to Step 2 and take a look at the types of foods you need to eat in order to lose weight by connecting with your body. While it does take a degree of focus and organisation to eat in this way, it's a lot more liberating than you may expect.

Step 2: The power and simplicity of nutrition for weight management

In order to lose weight, the number of kilojoules you ingest must be smaller than the number of kilojoules you burn off. The greater the shortfall, the faster you lose weight. Therefore, if you're losing weight by listening to your body, it's vital to choose foods that make you feel satisfied and that keep your hunger at bay on the minimum number of kilojoules. Many people assume that this means eating only non-starchy vegetables and lean sources of protein with very few carbohydrates and little added fat. But if you've ever tried to eat in that way, you've probably noticed that while it fills your belly and contains fewer kilojoules than a home-cooked roast dinner with all the trimmings, it doesn't truly satisfy you, because it often leaves you with a lingering desire for a packet of salt and vinegar chips or churros with chocolate sauce. So what *are* the foods that help you to feel *genuinely* satisfied on the minimum number of kilojoules? There is a lot of debate about, and ongoing research into, the satiating power of different ratios of various macronutrients, but most nutrition experts agree on a few general principles that apply universally. These are summarised overleaf.

THE THREE NUTRITIONAL GUIDELINES FOR PERMANENT WEIGHT LOSS
To lose weight and keep it off, most nutrition experts agree that you need to eat:

1. A large variety
2. of mainly whole foods
3. with plenty of vegetables and fruit.

In *The Don't Go Hungry Diet*, I covered the science underpinning these three simple nutritional guidelines for permanent weight loss. The main aim of the present book is to show you how to apply these principles in your day-to-day life. In the following chapters I'm going to give you practical tips and inspiration to help you put these guidelines into practice, drawing on recent scientific studies and real-life success stories. You'll meet people who have discovered various ways to adjust their diet in line with these principles and who have therefore lost weight efficiently *and* sustainably. It's not necessarily easy, but I'm going to show you some very simple, practical ways to do it. And the good news is that you *can* eat fun foods from time to time or enjoy an occasional alcoholic drink and still lose weight and keep it off. But before then, let's quickly recap the 'why' behind these three nutritional guidelines for permanent weight loss.

What is the science underpinning these three nutritional guidelines?

If you're not eating a wide enough variety of foods (for example, if you cut out most foods high in fat or carbohydrate), or if you're eating a lot of variety but your food choices are highly processed, it's practically guaranteed that your diet will be deficient in some essential nutrient or other. In fact, over 50 per cent of adults in developed countries are deficient in one or more essential nutrients.[87, 88] This is not only a risk factor for the development of diseases such as osteoporosis and cancers; it also spells bad news for your weight. Even when you're eating more kilojoules than you need, studies have shown that if your diet is deficient in just one nutrient, your body can go into a kind of Famine Reaction that pushes you to eat until you meet your needs for that one nutrient.[22-27] This will make it harder for you to reach the weight you're biologically meant to be, and even harder to maintain it once you get there. As you lose weight and approach your optimum biological weight, you'll undoubtedly come up against your Famine Reaction at least once. The last thing you want is to go into avoidable battles with your Famine Reaction because your diet is lacking in essential nutrients. By eating a wide variety of minimally processed foods, as outlined in the following chapters, you will help ensure you're getting the nutrients you need[89, 90] and thereby help keep your Famine Reaction in check as you progress towards your ideal weight.

Another reason why it's important to avoid too many processed foods if you want to lose weight and keep it off comes from studies on the effects of excessive saturated or processed fats on the brain. If you're eating heavily processed foods such as deep-fried takeaways or commercial cakes and biscuits every day, your diet will be high in both saturated fats and processed fats such as cheap vegetable oils. While eating processed fatty foods from time to time is not a problem, research shows that *continuously* high intakes of the kinds of fats they contain actually changes the balance of natural chemicals (neurotransmitters and hormones) in your brain such that the Fat Brake no longer works as effectively. This is particularly so if you have a genetic propensity to gain weight. For instance, long-term overconsumption of a diet rich in saturated fats or vegetable oils decreases the ability of leptin (a hormone that helps to activate the Fat Brake by telling the brain when the amount of body fat has increased) to act on its receptor in the brain.[91-94] (A hormone such as leptin exerts effects on cells by interacting with a receptor on those cells, similar to the way in which a key opens a door by interacting with a lock on the door.) And once leptin can no longer switch on the Fat Brake when needed, the body can come to accept a higher weight as its new Set Point. This is part of the reason why you can weigh 93 kilos or more, like I used to weigh, and still have a Famine Reaction after losing just a few kilos, even though it's glaringly obvious that you're in no danger of wasting away. The good news is that switching to a healthier diet can reverse this effect and restore leptin's ability to function as it should.[94] In the following chapters I'm going to show you simple ways to reduce the amount of heavily processed foods in your diet without feeling deprived, thereby enabling your body to shed excess weight and adopt progressively lower Set Points.

As well as eating a wide variety of mainly whole foods and cutting back on processed foods, it's vitally important to eat plenty of vegetables and fruit. In fact, the importance of eating vegetables and fruit for permanent weight loss can scarcely be overemphasised. As you'll see in the next chapter, vegetables and fruit are your 'short cut' to eating in a way that enables you to lose weight and keep it off by simply listening to your body.

Chapter 14

Steps 2a and 2b. Fruit and vegetables – the easiest way to eat well

Some things you have to do every day. Eating seven apples on Saturday night instead of one a day just isn't going to get the job done.

Jim Rohn, American entrepreneur, author and motivational speaker, 1930–2009

If you want to lose weight and you're watching how much you eat, the single thing that's most likely to determine whether or not you lose weight is whether or not you're eating enough vegetables and fruit every day. Whenever someone asks me to help them to lose weight, the only rigid prescription I give is 'use your Success Diary every day and aim for *all* 2s and 3s, and try to eat at least two serves of fruit and at least five serves of vegetables every day'. You'll notice that these are the first two steps outlined in my kick-start weight loss guide in Chapter 5. Many people start losing weight within two weeks of following this simple prescription, particularly if they're physically active as well as watching how much and what they eat. On the other hand, whenever I read the Success Diary of someone who has eaten according to their physical needs but has eaten scarcely any vegetables or fruit, they usually haven't lost any weight, even if they've done loads of exercise. In short, your intake of vegetables and fruit can make or break your weight loss success.

Eating more fruit and vegetables doesn't mean eating *only* fruit and vegetables

Before you start thinking, 'Oh great, how am I ever going to feel satisfied eating an apple at afternoon tea time' or, 'I loathe eating salad, it never fills me up', remember that this is the Don't Go Hungry Diet, not a conventional diet. Although you'll most likely need to increase your fruit and vegetable intake to get your two or more serves of fruit and five or more serves of vegetables every day, you still need to keep hunger at bay in order to lose weight efficiently and sustainably. So if you've eaten a fruit- or veggie-rich meal or snack and you're not quite satisfied, you simply need to keep eating the types and amounts of mostly nutritious foods that make you feel genuinely satisfied.

Vegetables and fruit are the heavyweight champions

Why are vegetables and fruit so critically important for weight loss? One reason is that they tend to be less energy-dense than other foods, meaning that for a given weight they contain fewer kilojoules. For example, whereas a 100 gram packet of fat-free rice crackers contains 1730 kilojoules (410 calories), the same weight of Greek salad with oily dressing contains just over a quarter the amount of energy (470 kilojoules or 110 calories). As another example, whereas a low-fat orange and poppy seed muffin weighing 120 grams contains 1260 kilojoules (300 calories), an equivalent weight (half a cup) of tinned black cherries in syrup contains only one-third as much energy (390 kilojoules or 95 calories). These differences in energy density are important for weight management because the *weight* of the food you eat – not just its kilojoule or nutrient content – seems to contribute to how satisfied you feel after eating it.[95, 96] In a crossover study designed to test the effect of energy density on appetite, research volunteers ate in a laboratory for two days in each of two separate test sessions. During each of the two-day sessions, the foods they ate differed in energy density. In the first session, for example, the volunteers were given a pasta salad for lunch and a chicken casserole for dinner, and in the second session the same volunteers were similarly given a pasta salad for lunch and a chicken casserole for dinner but with one important difference: the vegetable content of the two dishes was higher (and the pasta content lower), which reduced their energy density by about 25 per cent. This difference went unnoticed by the volunteers, who didn't know that the study was about energy density and who perceived the meals in both sessions to have the same kilojoule content and rated them as being equal in taste and pleasantness. The volunteers were requested to eat as much as they wanted at each meal, and the researchers then recorded how much they ate over each of the two-day sessions. Interestingly, the volunteers ate the same *weight* of food in both sessions, demonstrating that the weight of food eaten is an important factor determining when we stop eating. However, because the foods in the second session were about 25 per cent less energy-dense, the volunteers consumed about 25 per cent fewer kilojoules per day in the second session. Their average daily energy intake for the second session was 5700 kilojoules (1400 calories), as against 7500 kilojoules (1800 calories) for the two days they ate the energy-dense versions of the same dishes. Intriguingly, despite the significant decrease in kilojoule intake in the second session, the volunteers didn't report feeling any hungrier or any less satisfied than in the first. The conclusion drawn from this study is that vegetables can help you to feel satisfied on fewer kilojoules – and therefore help you to lose weight more effectively and keep it off – because they are relatively heavy for the number of kilojoules they deliver.

Fibre power

Another reason why vegetables and fruit are so important for weight loss is that they provide high amounts of dietary fibre, which bulks out your gut contents and slows down the absorption of nutrients from your digestive tract, thus helping you to feel fuller on a smaller number of kilojoules. In part, this is because dietary fibre stimulates the release of hormones that make you stop eating ('satiety' or 'stop eating' hormones). For instance, when the food you eat reaches your intestines, it triggers the release of satiety hormones, such as cholecystokinin (CCK) and peptide YY (PYY), from cells that line the inner walls of your intestines. CCK and PYY travel through your bloodstream and exert effects on your brain that induce a feeling of satisfaction, thereby helping you to stop eating. Interestingly, meals that are rich in dietary fibre lead to greater or more prolonged rises in the concentrations of CCK, and possibly also PYY, in the bloodstream than meals with the same kilojoule content but a low fibre content.[97] The bottom line is that if you're eating a diet rich in vegetables and fruit and the dietary fibres they contain, you're likely to keep hunger at bay and feel satisfied on a smaller number of kilojoules.

How many serves of vegetables and fruit do you need to eat for health and weight management?

In order to substantially reduce your risk of such serious health problems as cardiovascular disease, stroke, hypertension, certain cancers, excess weight, type 2 diabetes mellitus, cataracts and macular degeneration of the eye, it's recommended that you eat at least two serves of fruit and at least five serves of vegetables every day, choosing from a wide variety of types and colours, raw or cooked. This is the conclusion that the National Health and Medical Research Council of Australia came to after an extensive review of the scientific literature on fruit and vegetable intake and health.[89] Note that the recommendation is to eat *at least* two and *at least* five serves of fruit and vegetables respectively, meaning that you don't need to be stingy with your portion sizes. To lose weight by connecting with your body there is absolutely no need to weigh or measure any of your portions, because your body will show you exactly how much you need to eat. However, to be certain that you are eating at least two serves of fruit and at least five serves of vegetables every day, you do need to know what constitutes a serve.

HOW MUCH IS TWO SERVES OF FRUIT AND FIVE SERVES OF VEGETABLES?

One serve of fruit is 150 grams of fresh fruit or:

- One medium-sized piece of fruit, such as an apple
- Two smaller-sized pieces of fruit, such as two apricots, two plums or four dried apricot halves
- One cup of canned or chopped fruit, such as fruit salad
- One-and-a-half tablespoons of dried fruit, such as sultanas or raisins
- Half a cup (125 millilitres) of 100 per cent fruit juice

(If you're watching your weight, it's best to limit dried fruit and fruit juices to occasional treats, because they are significantly less satisfying than other forms of fruit. I'll talk more about the dangers of liquid kilojoules in Chapter 15.)

One serve of vegetables is 75 grams or:

- Half a cup of cooked vegetables, such as steamed peas, beans or broccoli
- Half a cup of cooked legumes, such as dried beans, peas or lentils
- One cup of salad vegetables
- One medium-sized potato

I've met a surprising number of people who think that eating two serves of fruit and five serves of vegetables means having a few sultanas in their fruit scone at morning tea and a few strawberries on their custard tart after lunch, plus five different *types* of vegetables on their plate at dinnertime, even if the quantities are small (a tablespoon of peas, a tablespoon of steamed carrots, five string beans, a few streaks of caramelised onions with their steak, and a potato). Not so. Getting the recommended intakes of fruit and vegetables means bulking out your diet with decent weights of plant matter.

One example of how to get your daily dose of health-giving fruit and vegetables would be to snack on a couple of pieces of fruit, such as a bunch of grapes (one serve of fruit) and a couple of kiwifruit (one more serve of fruit), throughout the day, have at least two cups of salad at lunch (two serves of vegetables), then have a stir-fry at dinner including at least one-and-a-half cups of chopped cooked veggies such as onions, carrots, capsicum, beans and bamboo shoots (three more serves of vegetables).

Or it may work better for you to incorporate them into your meals. During the day I don't particularly enjoy eating fruit and vegetables; my preferred lunch is a toasted sandwich or a wrap and a caffé latte from one of my favourite cafés, and my preferred daytime snacks are energy-dense foods such as wholemeal crackers with nut paste or cheese, a bowl of muesli, or a small tin of tuna and a chunk of bread. However, at breakfast and dinner I go to town on fruit and veggies. Every day begins with a large fruit salad made of whatever seasonal fruit we have at home, or tinned fruit and a banana if I want an occasional break from all that chopping (two serves of fruit). This means that even if my family or I don't touch a single piece of fruit for the rest of the day, at least we're protected by the invisible force field of our morning minimum. In the evenings I work five serves of vegetables into my dinner alongside whatever main course I may be eating. For example, if I'm having grilled lamb chops, I might enjoy them with one-and-a-half cups of steamed broccoli, cauliflower and zucchini (three serves of vegetables), half a cup of caramelised onions sautéed in tinned tomatoes (one more serve of vegetables), and an ear of corn on the cob (another serve of vegetables). By the time I eat those five serves of veggies, I usually don't have much room for more energy-dense foods such as rice, pasta or desserts.

It doesn't matter when you eat your fruit and veggies, just as long as you eat them at some stage during the day. As you can see, it takes a bit of forethought to get your daily fix of both, but you'll find lots of practical tips and recipes at: www.gofor2and5.com.au

Increase your fruit intake and reap the rewards

If you're currently eating fewer than two serves of fruit per day and you're struggling with your weight, increasing your intake to two or more serves per day will help you to lose weight more effectively. If you've lived through a generation of outdated diets that either limit fruit intake or relegate certain types of fruit to the list of 'bad' foods to avoid, you may find it difficult to believe that eating more fruit could help you to lose weight. However, new research indicates that fruit – not just vegetables – is important for successful weight management.[98, 99] For instance, when volunteers participating in clinical weight loss trials are encouraged by researchers to increase their fruit intake, they usually lose more weight than volunteers who aren't encouraged to eat more fruit. Additionally, the majority of studies show that people who eat fruit regularly are more likely to weigh less, and are less likely to gain excess weight, than people who eat less fruit. These scientific insights into fruit and weight management match what you see in real life.

When 47-year-old Andy started her Don't Go Hungry Weight Loss Adventure, she found it relatively straightforward to increase her vegetable intake to the recommended five or more serves per day. However, she wasn't so keen on fruit. She'd usually only eat about one serve of fruit every other day, such as the occasional sprinkling of berries or the odd prune or sliced banana on her breakfast cereal. Andy is not alone; adults in Australia eat an average of only one to two serves of fruit per day.[89] Having noted this in her Success Diary, and having heard me talk about the importance of fruit and vegetables for weight management at my advanced weight loss workshop, Andy developed a bag of tricks that helped her to eat more fruit. She tried different ways of eating them at breakfast or at morning tea, such as blending soft fruit like strawberries, bananas, mangoes and frozen berries into smoothies with milk and a touch of sugar; she started eating fruit that she liked, such as pears and peaches, as snacks for morning and afternoon tea; she made deals with herself whereby she wouldn't allow herself to eat any little treats, such as chocolate or a dessert, unless she'd already eaten two or more serves of fruit that day; and she put asterisks in her Success Diary to highlight how many serves of fruit she had eaten, aiming for two or more asterisks every day. Within a few weeks Andy was eating at least two serves of fruit a day. This change alone had important effects on her diet. By the time she had satisfied her between-meal hunger with a morning or afternoon snack of something like chopped fresh mango with yogurt, she usually had no appetite remaining for the couple of buttered scones or the handful of biscuits she might otherwise have eaten. As a result of this change, the energy density of Andy's diet decreased and its nutritional value increased. This, combined with eliminating the −1s and 0s of non-hungry eating that she'd noted in her Success Diary, as well as using a pedometer to boost her step count to 8000 or more steps per day, helped Andy to lose 4.6 kilos in eight weeks.

Eating more vegetables can transform your diet

Similarly, if you're currently eating less than five serves of vegetables per day, increasing your vegetable intake will help you lose weight. When 48-year-old Thea started her Don't Go Hungry Adventure she wasn't doing too badly with her regular fruit intake but her vegetable intake was modest. A typical day from her Success Diary at that time reads as follows. Breakfast was a couple of slices of wholemeal toast with butter and jam and a cup of tea, followed by a mid-morning snack of an apple. Lunch was a couple of small multigrain bread rolls filled with chicken and salad and followed by a muesli bar. For dinner she had beef curry with rice followed by fresh strawberries and a scoop of ice-cream, and supper a couple of hours later consisted of another slice of wholemeal toast with butter and jam. As you can see, Thea was eating a pretty nutritious diet, but she was only eating about two serves of vegetables per day on average. This is typical of adults in Australia, who eat an average of two to three serves of vegetables per day, half the number of serves that are recommended for good health.[89] I could also see that Thea was eating once or twice a day when she wasn't hungry (that is, she was scoring one or two –1s or 0s in the Hunger column of her Success Diary every day). In the letter that she sent me with her Success Diary, Thea remarked that after 19 days of using her diary she was still the same 76 kilos she had been when she started. After discussion with me via email, Thea decided to tweak two things about how much and what she ate. The first thing was to eat only when she felt hungry, and the second was to increase her vegetable intake. These two simple dietary changes had a marked effect on Thea's kilojoule intake. By the time she had eaten something like hummus with vegetable chunks or minestrone soup with borlotti beans for her lunch, and larger salads or serves of steamed or stir-fried veggies with her dinner, and because she was now only eating when she was hungry, she no longer had enough appetite to eat as much of the more energy-dense foods she used to eat, such as toast with butter and jam, bread rolls, muesli bars, homemade muffins, crispbread, gingernut biscuits, or beef curry and rice. She still ate these types of nutritious and nurturing foods every day, but in smaller quantities, and that's what helped her to create enough of a kilojoule deficit to start losing weight. Within six months of making these changes, as well as joining a gym and working out on a regular basis, Thea had lost 6 kilos and had to wear a belt to stop her jeans from falling down.

Scope out regular sources of vegetables and fruit

Whenever I go away for a holiday or a conference, one of the first things I do is scope out possible sources of vegetables and fruit at my destination. I learned the importance of this through hard-won personal experience. When I was eight months pregnant with our first child, my husband and I booked ourselves in for a long weekend away in a secluded bed and breakfast in Sydney's Blue Mountains. It was wintertime, and freezing cold outside, but the house was charmingly cosy with its log fire and spa bath. Alas, when I awoke on our first morning away from the hustle and bustle of the city, I was dismayed to realise that there was no fruit on the breakfast menu! There was a choice of fruit juices and small amounts of fruit coulis drizzled over porridge and swirled through yogurt, but no fresh fruit to speak of, just loads of energy-dense foods such as bread, butter, jam, honey, eggs, cereals, yogurt and pastries. Without any fruit to dilute my morning kilojoules, I ate much heavier breakfasts during our mountain retreat than I usually do. The same was true of my lunches and dinners at the romantic little mountain restaurants we chose; it was invariably tricky to get vegetables in sufficient quantities, and so I ended up filling up on more energy-dense foods such as salmon with baby chat potatoes in butter and sometimes dessert. By the time we got back to Sydney some three nights and four days later, I was all swollen from the fluid retention that comes from eating more than you need. That was a learning experience. Why would I want to spend all that money to go on a trip if it meant coming back feeling like Ten Tonne Tessie? Nowadays, any trip away from home starts with a visit to a local supermarket or store to stock the fridge with fruit, and I make sure I'm not too hungry before setting out for a meal so that I have sufficient time to look around and find an eatery that serves plenty of vegetables.

Does this apply to you?

If you're concerned about your weight, you probably already eat fruit and vegetables regularly. But are you eating them every day and in large enough quantities in order to lose weight and keep it off? If you're not eating enough – and you'll find out for sure with the simple diagnostic tests on the following page – the good news is that increasing your fruit and vegetable intake will transform your diet so that you can start losing weight by listening to your body.

Dr Amanda's Diagnostics N°s 2a and 2b: Are you eating enough fruit and veg to lose weight and keep it off?

To do this acid test for adequate fruit and vegetable intake, use your Success Diary for 3 to 14 days as described in Chapter 5 and then select three days at random. Avoid the temptation of saying 'that day doesn't count because I was on call' or 'having a binge'; if you've filled in a page of your Success Diary, it's as good a day to pick as any other. (When I do this diagnostic test at my workshops, I invite participants to ask their neighbour to pick three days from their Success Diary for them, because this helps to ensure a random selection of days.) Now go through your entries and count up how many serves of fruit and how many serves of vegetables you ate in total in those three days, then divide your results by three to get the average number of serves of fruit and vegetables you ate per day.

Interpreting your results

If you're eating an average of two or more serves of fruit and five or more serves of vegetables per day, well done and keep it up! By eating this way you're not only helping to reduce your risk of chronic diseases, such as cancers and type 2 diabetes, you're also making it easier to attain and maintain your optimum biological weight without having to count kilojoules or feel hungry or deprived.

If, on the other hand, you're eating less than two serves of fruit and five serves of vegetables per day on average, then increasing your intake will help you to eat fewer kilojoules without feeling hungry or unsatisfied. If you're eating according to your hunger signals as described in Step 1, then this single dietary change will most likely get the ball rolling on your weight loss, particularly if you're also doing some form of physical activity. Read on for easy ways to incorporate more fruit and vegetables into your life.

The taste and convenience factors

Many people simply don't enjoy preparing and eating vegetables and fruit as much as they enjoy eating more energy-dense foods such as pizza, pasta or something fast on toast. But once you get used to eating them in adequate quantities, and once you've seen the effects of this on your appetite and your weight, you won't want to do without your daily dose of vegetables and fruit. It needn't take a lot of time, either. Here are my favourite short cuts for making sure I eat vegetables and fruit every single day, no matter how tired or busy I may be.

Super-easy vegetable ideas

- I always keep a packet of frozen peas in the freezer. Whenever I have one of those nights when cooking is the last thing I want to do, I just pour some into a glass bowl, cover it loosely, whack it in the microwave for a minute or two, season with a little butter and salt, and dig in for a delicious two or more serves of vegetables. Add some scrambled eggs and toast and you have a satisfying meal. Frozen vegetables have almost as many nutrients as farm-fresh vegetables, so any variety you enjoy eating is good.

- I like to keep ring-pull tins of green beans in the cupboard for midnight snacks. If I'm a bit hungry and anxious at night and I just can't get back to sleep, I can drain one of those tins and eat it without fear of waking anyone with the noise of the microwave or the stove. Tinned green beans are soft enough to feel (almost) like comfort food, to me at least, and they soothe dead-of-night hunger and anxiety without spoiling my appetite for breakfast. While farm-fresh or snap-frozen produce is superior to tinned produce in terms of nutritional value, eating tinned vegetables is still better for your health and your waistline than not eating enough vegetables.

- Another instant and comforting source of vegetables is ready-to-eat vegetable soups in ring-pull tins or tetra packs. My favourite is a spicy lentil and bean soup; I always keep a few tins of it in my kitchen drawer full of 'war supplies'. When

I've got a big afternoon ahead, a tin of that soup takes less than three minutes to heat on the stove yet gives me at least four serves of vegetables and enough energy to keep going like a Duracell bunny. I'm always on the lookout for tasty tinned vegetable soups that contain real foods and no bizarre-sounding additives.

- Baked beans are another handy stand-by that I keep in my stocks of 'war supplies'. I've heard a lot of bad-mouthing of baked beans on account of their high salt content or the numbered additives or mysterious 'natural flavours' they sometimes contain. (Many people don't realise that natural flavours may contain naturally derived monosodium gluta-mate, or MSG, in quite a high concentration.) However, a number of common brands of baked beans contain no numbered additives. Moreover, if you're in need of quick comfort and it's a choice between dial-a-pizza or baked beans on toast, the latter will leave you satisfied on fewer kilojoules and give you at least one serve of vegetables into the bargain.

- Dried wasabi peas are a handy snack to keep in the pantry. Often when I'm feeling edgy and peckish I'll pour some into a bowl and start crunching my way through them. There's something about the burning taste of wasabi that helps take my mind off niggling worries, while also adding a serve or two of veggies to my day. Look for varieties of wasabi peas that don't contain numbered additives.

- Roasted chickpeas provide another clean and convenient means to snack on vegetables. Crispy and substantial, you can buy them from stores that stock Mediterranean snack foods.

Moderately easy vegetable ideas

- Take a Lebanese cucumber, wash it, peel it, slice it and voila! In 40 seconds flat you've got over a serve of vegetables. For even faster preparation and more nutrients, don't peel it. This is one of those vegetables that I never have to sweet-talk myself or my kids into eating.

- Keep some fresh asparagus in your fridge, and when you need veggies in a hurry, rinse a bunch under the tap, pop it in the microwave (loosely covered), zap for a minute or two (or steam it over a small amount of water in a saucepan until tender if you prefer not to use a microwave), sprinkle with black pepper and eat. Delicious! I learned this one from my clever mum.

- Invest in a large salad spinner, then wash and spin a mixture of loosely broken lettuce leaves, rocket and herbs such as fresh basil, coriander and mint; then drain off the water and store it in your fridge for several days. You can also throw in some whole washed cherry tomatoes. Whenever you need salad, just reach into your salad spinner and grab a handful or three.

- Keep a bottle of to-die-for salad dressing in your fridge door. I like to make up a bottle of my own with equal parts olive oil and white balsamic vinegar, flavoured with lemon juice, crushed or roasted garlic, French mustard, honey and salt; sometimes I buy a bottle of tasty natural salad dressing from a gourmet shop as a treat. When the dressing tickles your taste buds, eating salad is a pleasure rather than something you 'have to do'.

Advanced vegetable options

- I regularly make a big batch of hummus and keep it frozen in small glass bowls about the size of one cup. If I grab a bowl of it from the freezer as I run out the door after breakfast, by lunchtime it's thawed and I can enjoy it as a quick and easy meal or snack with a handful of wholegrain crackers or some mountain bread. It contains at least one serve of vegetables and it doesn't even feel like I'm eating vegetables.

- Whenever I make a freezable veggie-based dish, such as borlotti beans in a tomato-based sauce with carrots and potato, or red lentil soup, I always make a large quantity and store a few meal-sized portions in the freezer. That way, my husband and I always have a veggie-rich meal on hand that can be quickly thawed and reheated in the microwave, even if we come home late with our children and we're all tired and hungry.

- When I make a Bolognese sauce for pasta, I push as much veg into it as I can without completely de-masculinising it. For every half-kilo of ground beef I use about two medium-sized brown onions, two large cloves of garlic, four sticks of finely sliced celery, four medium-sized grated carrots, two large grated zucchinis, four 400 gram cans of crushed tomatoes, and two handfuls each of red and green lentils. I cook it up in my giant pot, and then freeze it in meal-size serves. On days when I just can't face all that chopping, I use onions, garlic, tinned tomatoes and about three handfuls each of red and green lentils.

- We prefer to eat dinner at home as much as we can. Compared to eating out, it's a cheaper way to get plenty of vegetables.

Eating vegetables when eating out

- I often order a substantial salad, such as a chicken Caesar salad or an Asian-inspired salad with prawns, as a main course. Add some bread or rice to fill the gaps, and I find this a delicious and satisfying way to eat three or more serves of vegetables in a single meal.

- If I feel like a main course such as veal piccata or chicken in some kind of sauce, I always order an additional salad or serve of steamed vegetables, sometimes both. While most meat- or fish-based restaurant mains include vegetables, the quantities are often less than a serve. And if someone suggests that we share the salad or vegetables, I usually refuse! Instead, I suggest that we order two salads (preferably different varieties), or a salad and a side of steamed vegetables, to share between two.

- I eat my vegetables first, and then fill the gaps with more energy-dense foods such as meat, polenta or dessert. This often means leaving some of my main course unfinished.

Super-easy fruit ideas

- Don't leave home without a banana or an apple. If you get hungry while you're out and about, they make a super-convenient snack and are often filling enough to stop you from eating something you may later regret.
- Keep a packet of frozen berries in the freezer. Whenever you feel like a fruity treat, thaw some in the microwave or in a saucepan on the stove for a few minutes and serve with plain yogurt or on their own. Sheer decadence!
- I always keep a few tins of fruit in the drawer of 'war supplies' in my kitchen, or in the fridge, for occasions when I run out of fresh fruit – or steam! My personal favourites are tinned black cherries, fruit salad, and apricots or peaches.

FRUIT AND VEGETABLE JUICES: FRIEND OR FOE?

If you're concerned about your weight, juices are *not* a short cut to adequate fruit and vegetable intake; they are a short cut to even more frustration about your weight. While a 375 millilitre serve of 100 per cent fruit juice is recognised as three serves of fruit and will certainly give you a lot of vitamins, minerals and antioxidants (especially if it's freshly squeezed), it doesn't give you the same benefits for weight management as eating three pieces of whole fruit. This is partly because most of the fibre is removed, and so juices just don't have the same satiety value as solid fruit. In Chapter 15 I'll talk more about the effects of liquid kilojoules on weight management.

Moderately easy fruit ideas

- Buy the best-looking and tastiest fruit of the season and arrange it on a platter on your kitchen bench or dining table. If it looks attractive, you'll soon start eating them. I learned this trick from a stylish friend. One summer's day when my family and I went to lunch at her house, I spotted a dish of delicious-looking peaches on her kitchen bench. They looked so inviting that I wanted to pick one up and start eating it, even though I've never been a fan of fuzzy peach skin. Inspired, I went out and bought some myself, washed them and arranged them on an attractive platter on the kitchen bench. To my great surprise, our seven-year-old son – who is rather pernick-ety about his fruit choices – grabbed one and happily started eating it! My family and I now regularly enjoy peaches in the all-too-short summer fruit season.

- Start the day by making fresh fruit or fruit salad a part of your breakfast; that way it's 'over and done with' and you're protected for the rest of the day, no matter where you go or how hard it may be to find or eat fruit there.
- Stew up a batch of apples or rhubarb or poach some pears and keep a supply in the fridge. They'll keep for a couple of days, and whenever you feel like something cold and sweet with a meal or snack, dive in. There's nothing wrong with adding a bit of sugar to your stewed fruit if it makes you more inclined to eat it.

Over to you

Here's something you can do immediately to put the ideas in this chapter into action.

Cast aside the restrictions you learned in Diet Dungeon – the forbidden fruit, the low-fat dressings, the 'free list' vegetables and the limitations on serving sizes – and rediscover the pleasures of vegetables and fruit.

What vegetables and fruit did you love eating when you were younger, before being indoctrinated with the restrictive 'shoulds' and 'shouldn'ts' of conventional diets?

What vegetable-rich or fruit-rich recipes have you seen on television, in magazines or in books and thought, 'Hmm, that looks nice'?

Can you find or create a to-die-for salad dressing?

You may find, as many people have, that increasing your fruit and vegetable intake and eating according to your physical needs is all it takes for you to start shedding excess weight. However, there's a common mistake that many people make that could prevent you from losing weight in this way, and that's the subject of the next chapter.

Chapter 15

Step 2c. When it's time to tame the parties in your mouth

'Tis not the eating, nor 'tis not the drinking that is to be blamed, but the excess.
John Selden, English jurist and scholar, 1584–1654

If you focus on eating at least two serves of fruit and at least five serves of vegetables every day, this is often enough to bring your whole diet sufficiently into line that you can start losing weight, as long as you're listening to your hunger signals and eating accordingly. But what if you make this change and you're not losing weight? The most common reason for this is excessive intake of foods or beverages that deliver a lot of kilojoules relative to their degree of satiating power or the number of nutrients they contain. By far the most destructive diet-wrecking substance I see is alcohol, which affects the parts of the brain that control appetite and thus contributes to excessive kilojoule intake unless you watch your intake extremely closely. When someone asks me why they haven't lost any weight despite diligently eating only when hungry and stopping before feeling overfull, as well as eating adequate amounts of fruit and vegetables, the culprit is usually found to be excessive alcohol intake. In some cases, however, excessive intake of desserts, sweets, chocolates and fried takeaway-style foods may also be contributing to the lack of weight loss. It's extremely important to have some fun in your diet as you're losing weight; if you don't, you're going to give up long before you reach the weight you're meant to be. We'll look at that in more detail in Chapter 17. But in the meantime, let's take a look at whether too many highly processed foods or liquid kilojoules such as alcohol are stopping you from losing weight, and if so, at how to tame those parties in your mouth gently so that you can lose weight at a motivating pace and without feeling deprived.

Effects of alcohol on health and weight management

Many weight loss regimes stipulate that if you want to lose weight, complete abstinence from alcohol is the way to go. If you're not particularly fond of alcohol and you can happily take it or leave it, becoming a teetotaller is a great idea. Alcohol not only comes with significant health risks, as outlined in the box below, it also puts a spanner in the works of appetite regulation and can thwart your progress faster than you can say, 'That's enough for me, thank you'.

REVISED AUSTRALIAN GUIDELINES TO REDUCE THE HEALTH RISKS FROM DRINKING ALCOHOL

I often hear people espouse the health benefits of regular consumption of alcohol, particularly red wine. Recent scientific evidence, however, suggests that the health benefits of alcohol have probably been overestimated and that the benefits only occur with low levels of intake (approximately half a standard drink per day).[100] On the other hand, there is strong scientific evidence linking alcohol consumption to life-threatening diseases, injury and accidents.[100] For instance, regular alcohol intake significantly increases your risk of long-term cognitive impairment and depression while heightening your chances of developing dementia. Additionally, alcohol is a well-recognised carcinogen (cancer-causing substance) and has been linked to the development of cancers of the mouth, liver and breast, for example. Regular alcohol intake is also associated with the development of nutritional deficiencies, diabetes, cirrhosis of the liver, haemorrhagic stroke and some types of cardiac failure. The more you drink, the greater your risk.

While there's no level of alcohol consumption that's completely 'safe' or 'risk-free', the National Health and Medical Research Council of Australia recently released new guidelines that will enable healthy people to *minimise* their risk of alcohol-related death from diseases, injury or accidents.[100]

Guideline 1: For healthy men and women, drinking no more than two standard drinks on any day reduces the lifetime risk of harm from alcohol-related disease or injury.

Guideline 2: For healthy men and women, drinking no more than four standard drinks on a single occasion reduces the risk of alcohol-related injury arising from that occasion.

Guideline 3: For children and young people under 18 years of age, not drinking alcohol is the safest option.

Guideline 4: For women who are pregnant, planning a pregnancy or breastfeeding, not drinking alcohol is the safest option.

What is a standard drink of alcohol?
A standard drink contains 10 grams of alcohol. Here is a list of some some common drinks and how they stack up.

- A can or stubbie of low-strength beer = 0.8 standard drinks
- A can or stubbie of mid-strength beer = 1 standard drink
- A can or stubbie of full-strength beer = 1.4 standard drinks
- A small glass (100 millilitres) of wine (with 13.5% alcohol) = 1 standard drink

- A 30 millilitre nip of spirits = 1 standard drink
- A can of spirits (approximately 5% alcohol) = 1.2 to 1.7 standard drinks
- A can of spirits (approximately 7% alcohol) = 1.6 to 2.4 standard drinks

Alcohol and other liquid kilojoules are not as satisfying as kilojoules in solid form

The main reason why alcohol makes it harder to lose weight is that it's a kilojoule-containing *liquid*, and kilojoules in liquid form just don't give the same degree of satisfaction as kilojoules in solid form. When research volunteers were given a bowl of fresh watermelon chunks to eat and were then invited to eat a lunch of chicken sandwiches until they felt comfortably satisfied, they ate significantly fewer sandwiches than when they hadn't eaten any watermelon before lunch but had drank an equivalent volume of water instead.[101] This is not surprising when you see the amount of watermelon they were given to eat – around four cups, containing approximately 740 kilojoules (175 calories). Indeed, you've no doubt noticed yourself that if you eat something such as a salad as an entrée, this reduces how much of your main course you can eat without getting uncomfortably full. However, when the volunteers *drank* the same number of kilojoules in the form of watermelon juice instead of eating them as watermelon flesh (that's about 500 millilitres of watermelon juice, equivalent to a regular takeaway-sized juice), they ate almost as many chicken sandwiches as when they had consumed only water before their meal. In other words, the watermelon juice didn't have anywhere near as much power to satisfy their drive to eat as the watermelon flesh. In fact, on the day that the volunteers drank the watermelon juice with their lunch, they consumed a total of 12 per cent more kilojoules over the course of the day than when they ate the watermelon flesh. Similar effects were shown with solid versus liquid forms of other foods, with a chunk of cheese or pieces of coconut meat being appreciably more satisfying and resulting in daily kilojoule intakes up to 19 per cent lower than when an equivalent number of kilojoules were drunk as milk or coconut milk, respectively.[101] The take-home message is that if you're watching your weight, it's prudent to *eat rather than drink your kilojoules wherever possible.*

TRY THIS EXPERIMENT

While the biological basis for the ability of liquid kilojoules to increase the overall daily kilojoule intake is not clear, it's easy to see this phenomenon in action in your own life. If you regularly drink a glass of fruit juice with your breakfast, for example, try replacing it with an equivalent amount of fresh fruit. Half a cup (125 millilitres) of 100 per cent fruit juice is equivalent to one serve of fruit, so if you usually drink a small glass (250 millilitres) of juice at breakfast, replace it with two serves of solid fruit such as an orange and a small mango. Then sit back and watch out for some interesting effects on your appetite.

How long does it take you to get hungry for your morning snack or lunch compared to the time at which you usually get hungry enough to eat? And when you tuck in at your next snack or meal, how much do you need to eat in order to feel satisfied compared to how much you usually need to eat? Once you notice the effects of whole fruit versus fruit juices on your appetite and your weight, you won't want to drink juices unless they're particularly dear to you. It's for this reason that I almost never drink fruit or vegetable juices myself. If I'm going to come to grief over my weight, I'd much rather it happens because of Easter eggs or Swiss chocolate truffles!

Alcohol and the aperitif effect

Like other liquid kilojoules, alcohol leads to passive overconsumption because you consume the kilojoules from what you drink on top of all the kilojoules you would normally eat in order to feel satisfied.[102] In addition, research shows that drinking alcohol within an hour of a meal can lead to active overconsumption, pushing you to eat more than you would if you didn't drink.[102, 103] This aperitif effect may be due to the acute effect of alcohol on the parts of your brain that control perceptions of pleasure, such that foods you'd otherwise find relatively easy to refuse suddenly appear irresistible.[102] (The same could be said for the effect of alcohol on the perceived desirability of the person sitting opposite you at dinner.) Additionally, alcohol may affect the parts of your brain that control how satisfied you feel, so that it takes more food for you to feel satisfied after a shot of alcohol than it would without alcohol. In light of these effects, if you enjoy a tipple of something alcoholic on a regular basis and you're eating according to your physical needs as described in this book, you'll end up consuming more kilojoules than you would if you weren't drinking alcohol. Since the aim of the weight loss game is to create a kilojoule deficit by consuming fewer kilojoules than you burn, this can make or break your success.

Alcohol interferes with weight loss

Many people find it difficult to believe that alcohol could interfere significantly with weight loss, but it does. When 50-year-old Carmen attended one of my introductory workshops and took on the two-week challenge of losing weight by connecting with her body, she did almost everything 'by the book'. She used her Success Diary every day and scored literally *all* 2s and 3s. 'I didn't score a single −1, 0 or +4 in my diary in the past two weeks, honestly!' she told me in an email two weeks after the workshop. She ate fruit and vegetables every day. 'I eat bananas, apples and pears etc, but in the first week I also ate more exotic fruit and berries. As for veggies – I make a lot of stir-fries with onions, red and green peppers and leeks, and I also regularly eat steamed vegetables such as potatoes, sweet potatoes and broccoli. I probably eat around five serves of veggies and two serves of fruit on average per day,' she reported. Additionally, Carmen prepares most of her food at home, as she's not keen on heavily processed foods, and she's a devoted fan of regular exercise. 'I do something active nearly every day – walk, play golf, cycle, swim etc,' she told me. With such a wholesome lifestyle, and being so closely attuned to her body signals, why is it that Carmen didn't lose a single gram in her first two weeks of using a Success Diary? This is the question that Carmen put to me in her email. She was still the same 80 kilos at the end of her two-week challenge as she was when she'd started – about 8 kilos more than she needed on her 1.7 metre frame. Where could the problem lie?

The problem turned out to be alcohol. 'I had between six and eight glasses of wine per week in the past two weeks,' Carmen told me in a subsequent email. 'That is the hard bit – I like a glass of wine with my meal,' she wrote. While Carmen's alcohol intake was well within the limits for reducing the risk of long-term alcohol-induced diseases as discussed above, it was too much to allow her to lose weight. Indeed, when Carmen pruned her alcohol intake back to two to four glasses of wine per week instead of six to eight, she lost a kilo in two weeks.

HOW MUCH ALCOHOL WILL STOP YOU FROM LOSING WEIGHT?
Alcohol gives you kilojoules without satiety and can make you eat more than you would if you didn't drink (the aperitif effect). Because alcohol alters what your body tells you about how much to eat, if you want to lose weight by listening to your body it's important to limit alcohol intake to approximately **4 standard alcoholic drinks or fewer per week**. For many people, the amount of alcohol that obstructs weight loss will be less than this: up to two standard drinks per week. If you like a regular drink, it's important to try different levels of intake until you find your critical alcohol limit, the level of consumption below which you need to stay in order to lose weight or keep it off. You'll undoubtedly discover that in order to lose weight you'll need to keep your alcohol intake lower than you do while you're maintaining your weight. For example, while Carmen maintained her weight on an

alcohol intake of six to eight glasses of wine per week, she needed to cut this back to two to four glasses per week in order to lose weight. If this sounds onerous to you, you might prefer to lose weight in short bursts, interspersed with regular weight loss holidays where you can drink a bit more while maintaining your weight. Stay tuned and I'll tell you all about this tactic in Chapter 19.

When you've had one too many cupcakes

Excessive alcohol intake is the most common reason why people don't lose weight despite eating well. Sometimes, however, eating too many highly processed foods can also stop you from losing weight. In addition to a wide variety of nutritious foods, 53-year-old Olivia normally eats some kind of sweet food, such as a slice of cake, a Danish pastry, a few chocolates or a dessert such as rocky road, every day, sometimes twice a day. She doesn't like deferring gratification and has never been in the habit of doing so. While there's absolutely nothing wrong with having a bit of your must-have fun foods on a regular basis while you're losing weight (doing so will actually make your weight loss more sustainable in the long term), the amounts that Olivia was eating were preventing her from losing any weight at all. Although she was eating precisely according to her hunger signals (every single entry in her Success Diary was a 2 or a 3), and although she was eating almost two serves of fruit and almost five serves of vegetables every day, her weight stayed the same. Losing weight would require cutting back on sweets and desserts, because compared to the number of kilojoules they bring, they don't bring as much physical satisfaction as more nutritious foods such as wholemeal bread, porridge, fruit and lamb. Cutting back on the treats would therefore help Olivia to reduce her kilojoule intake sufficiently to lose weight.

The question is: how can you cut back on nutrient-poor, kilojoule-rich foods when you've got a strong drive to eat them? That's a tough one. Apart from environmental and psychological factors that can drive us towards rich, processed foods, new research shows that genetic differences give some of us a stronger drive to eat than others. People born with mutations that block the function of certain genes (such as the gene for leptin) have an extremely strong desire to eat, and this results in massive obesity, which becomes clearly apparent in childhood. While this form of inherited obesity is relatively rare, it's now known that many people have slight variations of the same genes, and this results in those genes having a somewhat impaired function, probably contributing to an increased drive to eat and an increased propensity to gain excess weight. Indeed, the greater the number of these variant genes you have, the more you eat and the more you weigh.[104, 105] (I must have one or two of those bodgie genes myself. Whenever we have ice-cream at home and I do the dishing up, my husband is always amazed at what I consider to be satisfying-sized servings, and when he does the dishing up his servings seem unsatisfyingly small to me. This is precisely why I rarely keep ice-cream in our apartment, or any other fun foods that I know I can't be trusted with.)

Olivia experimented with different strategies for cutting back her intake of desserts. What didn't work was trying to cut them out altogether. 'Yesterday I told myself that I'd eaten too much the day before, so today I would eat plainly. I immediately went out and ate two packets of chips, which I don't even like very much!' What did work for Olivia was eating bigger, more nutritious breakfasts (such as fruit salad with Greek yogurt, two pieces of ciabatta bread with ham and Brie, and two coffees, rather than a less leisurely breakfast of cereal with fruit and yogurt), as well as shopping for and preparing nourishing snacks to eat when she was hungry, such as hummus with wholemeal bread or crackers, fruit, or homemade wholemeal muffins with nuts. Within two weeks of making this change, Olivia noticed some shifts. Besides losing half a kilo, she no longer felt compelled to finish fun foods that happened to be in front of her. In a meeting she attended during those two weeks, Olivia noticed that there was one lonesome biscuit left on a plate . . . and she felt quite OK about leaving it there.

Does this apply to you?

Are too many kilojoule-rich, nutrient-poor processed foods, or liquid kilojoules such as alcohol, stopping you from losing weight at a satisfying pace? Use this simple diagnostic test to find out.

Dr Amanda's Diagnostic N°2c: Could reducing your intake of fun foods or liquid kilojoules help you to lose weight more efficiently?

To do this diagnostic test, use your Success Diary for 14 days as described in Chapter 5. If you lose weight and/or centimetres at a satisfying pace in those two weeks, you're on the right track and there's no need to rein in your intake of fun foods or liquid kilojoules, at least not in terms of your weight. (For your health, it's a good idea to check that you are also eating a wide variety of nutritious foods, including at least five serves daily of vegetables and at least two serves of fruit, and that you are not exceeding the level of alcohol intake recommended for reducing your risk of disease and accidents.)

If, on the other hand, you don't lose weight and/or centimetres in those two weeks despite scoring practically all 2s and 3s in your Success Diary and eating at least two serves of fruit and at least five serves of vegetables every day, it's time to examine how many treats you're having. Take a close look at the food and beverage choices in your Success Diary. You'll probably spot some fun foods or liquid kilojoules that are extremely dear to you, the ones that you'd go out to hunt for if they weren't in your home, office or car, or otherwise within easy reach. These are the occasional pleasures that you need to keep in your diet, because eliminating them will make your diet unsustainable. But you'll probably also spot some fun foods or liquid kilojoules that have simply scored a free ride into your Success Diary. These are the treats that have weaselled their way into your diet without a personal invitation from you, and without bringing much nutritional or hunger-busting value with them. That piece of caramel slice you didn't really want or enjoy, but ate simply because a colleague made a batch and was offering it around at morning tea time. That glass of wine with your lunch that you didn't particularly appreciate, but drank just because your companion poured it for you and it was there. Those chocolates you ate after dinner, not because you had a particular craving for chocolate at the time, but because they'd been left in your home after the season's festivities and you were procrastinating about doing something else. That juice you drank every day at breakfast, not because you love it to bits and would feel deprived if you drank water or ate fresh fruit instead, but because it's a habit. Those wedges with sour cream and sweet chilli sauce that you ate at the pub before going home to dinner, not because you had a particular craving for wedges with sour cream and sweet chilli sauce at that time, but just because you were ravenously hungry and hadn't given yourself enough time to prepare healthy snacks to sustain you until dinnertime. That iced coffee you drank with your treasured bi-weekly scone from the café across the road, not because you particularly love iced coffee, but simply because you were thirsty – even though you would just as happily have drunk a pot of tea with a splash of milk. You get the message. Now have a look for all the freeloading kilojoule-rich, nutrient-poor foods or beverages in your life that you could just as happily do without if they weren't right in front of you. Do whatever it takes to evict these freeloading kilojoules from your life in the next two weeks – remove temptation from your home and all the places you frequent, change your hobbies, change the route you travel to work – and you'll undoubtedly notice a much better outcome for your weight and/or waist. Read on for ways to cut back on freeloading kilojoules without feeling deprived.

Crowd them out gently

When it comes to cutting back on freeloading kilojoules, it's better to crowd them out of your life gently by replacing them with other foods or habits than to try to eliminate them directly.

The reason for this is that whatever you focus on tends to dominate your thoughts. If I ask you right now to *not* think about a purple elephant with pink spots, what is it that you see in your mind's eye right now? See what I mean? The same is true of fun foods or alcohol. If you've got a two-cupcake-a-day habit, for instance, and you feel it's stopping you from losing weight, then focusing your attention directly on cutting back on the cupcakes will only serve to make you obsessed with cupcakes, until you finally crack and end up eating more than you ever wanted to eat before.

When I was a PhD student in Geneva, sudden severe pains in my abdomen and lower back led me to visit the doctor, where I learned that I had gallstones. (Yes, all those years of bad eating and gaining and losing weight, plus a family history of gallstones, caught up with me.) I was put on a waiting list to have my gallbladder and gallstones removed, probably in a few months' time. The doctor gave me stern instructions to eat as little fat as possible while I was waiting for my chole-cystectomy, and to especially avoid concentrated sources of fat such as butter and *gâteau au chocolat*. The reason for this was that dietary fat is known to make the gallbladder contract, and with my gallbladder so laden with chalky, fatty stones, any movement could dislodge a tiny piece and lead to painful, dangerous blockages. With that, I became obsessed with fat. I scoured the supermarket shelves for foods with a low fat content (which is when I discovered that lollies such as jelly babies contain zero fat). My misery at not being able to eat fat grew and grew, as did my temptation. Finally I cracked and I had a big slice of *gâteau au chocolat* at a party, even though I've never actually liked chocolate cake that much. Just as my doctor had warned, a piece of gallstone must have dislodged itself and blocked my common bile duct, because I went bright yellow, like one of those naughty children in *Charlie and the Chocolate Factory*, as a result of bile salts and waste products from my liver spilling into my bloodstream. The doctor took one look at my jaundiced skin and eyes, said, 'What did you eat?' (how did he know?), and told me to go immediately to the emergency department of the hospital, where he teed up an emergency cholecystectomy.

The moral of the story is that whenever you try to lessen a particular behaviour by focusing your attention directly on that behaviour, this almost always backfires. The behaviour you're trying to avoid transfixes you and comes to dominate your consciousness, and as you try to chase it out it usually ends up trampling you, much as an elephant (of any colour) might do if you tried to shoo it aggressively from the room. On the other hand, if you focus on introducing new behaviours to replace the ones that are no longer helping you, the elephant will gradually feel uncomfortably crowded and will probably shuffle out of its own accord, with significantly less likelihood of trampling you in the process. This is perhaps part of the reason why telling people to increase their vegetable and fruit intake has been scientifically demonstrated to result in more weight loss than telling people to decrease their fat intake.[95] So if too many fun foods or liquid kilojoules such as alcohol are hampering your efforts, it's best to crowd them out of your life gently by replacing the behaviours you don't want with behaviours that will give you a better result. In the table on the following page you will find some examples of how you might do this, taken from my own experiences and the experiences of people I've helped.

Getting over the addiction: the less highly processed foods you eat, the less you want to eat them

Did you ever feel that you were addicted to quick-fix foods, just as a drug addict may feel addicted to drugs? I've certainly felt that way myself. Some years ago I was sitting in a restaurant with a group of friends. I was very hungry, but we'd ordered our meals and dinner was on its way. Even though I knew I'd be eating a proper meal in 10 minutes or so, I felt compelled to excuse myself 'to go to the ladies' room' and then duck out to the nearest convenience store and buy myself a chocolate bar, which

Instead of telling yourself . . .	Try saying . . .
I'll only have two standard alcoholic drinks this week.	This week I'm going to treat myself to two glasses of wine with my dinner on Friday night, and every other night I'll enjoy a tall glass of sparkling mineral water with lemon and the feeling of being in control of my weight.
I'm not going to drink at the function tonight.	Tonight I'll stick to a diet soft drink or two and then drive everyone home.
I'm going to stop drinking juice with my breakfast.	I'm going to enjoy some delicious whole fruit with my breakfast every day.
I'm going to stop eating a bar of chocolate every day.	Every day I will go to the shop if I feel like it and buy myself an individual 25 gram serve of whatever chocolate I fancy.
I'm not going to eat so many desserts this week.	This week I'm going to treat myself to a slice of cassata ice-cream cake at my favourite restaurant on Saturday night.
I'm going to stop eating so many fatty takeaway foods at lunch.	I'm going to eat at least two serves of fruit and at least five serves of vegetables every day.
I'm not going to eat so many Danish pastries and things like that at morning or afternoon tea.	I'm going to eat enough wholesome foods at breakfast to power me through until lunch, and I'm going to keep nutritious snacks such as hard-boiled eggs and mountain bread on hand in case I get hungry.
I'm going to stop eating so much rubbish.	I'm going to consciously choose tasty foods that are as close as possible to their natural state and that provide my body with valuable nutrients.
I'm going to stop eating as a way of rewarding myself for completing onerous tasks.	I'm going to reward myself for completing challenging tasks by sitting down to read the newspaper with a coffee with a dash of milk or a cup of tea.

I then scoffed in secret before rejoining my dinner companions and eating my meal. I felt embarrassed about my behaviour, but new research provides possible explanations for it.

Constant exposure to and overconsumption of highly processed fatty, sugary foods trigger similar changes in the brain to those seen in drug addiction, and these changes drive the development of compulsive overeating and excessive weight gain.[70] In a telling experiment, adult laboratory rats were given unlimited access to bacon, sausages, cheesecake, pound cake, frosting and chocolate, as well as their normal healthy diet, for about 20 hours a day for 40 days. Much as you may have noticed in situations where fun foods are freely available to you, the rats quickly came to prefer the more processed foods. (This is all the more reason to sanitise your home, car, office and any other place you frequent of all secret stashes of foods such as cake with frosting!) Not only did the rats prefer the fun stuff, they also started eating it compulsively, as demonstrated by the fact that they kept eating it even in adverse conditions that normally put rats off their food. Needless to say, the animals gained significant amounts of excess weight within the 40-day period. This drive to eat compulsively was probably due to a decrease in the amount of dopamine D2 receptors in a part of the brain involved in the development of addictive behaviours – a change that is also seen in the brains of people who are addicted to drugs, as well as in people who have a body mass index in the obese range. This finding helps to explain the addictive quality of fun foods, whereby the more processed foods you eat, the more you may feel you need a regular fix of them just to feel normal.

The good news, however, is that this addiction-like brain change seems to be reversible. When drug addicts abstain from the drug to which they are addicted, the levels of the dopamine D2 receptor in their brain increase towards normal. A similar increase has been reported in people who have lost excess weight.[70] In fact, many people who have changed their diet and lost weight end up actually disliking many of the more processed foods they used to eat compulsively. For instance, while I still love a bit of chocolate from time to time, I don't eat chocolate compulsively any more, like I used to, nor do I eat it in ample quantities just before dinner. Moreover, many of the foods I used to binge on – takeaway pizza, hot chips, takeaway ice-cream sundaes and lollies from convenience stores – no longer hold much appeal for me at all. As another example, when 31-year-old Nellie decided to lose weight by listening to her body, she weighed over 130 kilos and felt driven to eat energy-dense foods containing a lot of sugar or fat relative to the amount of nutrients they provide. Some of her regular favourites were fried chicken and chips, chocolate-covered ice-creams and store-bought muffins. When she started eating more nutritious foods, however, Nellie's cravings for fun foods rapidly diminished and the weight started falling off.

From: Nellie
Sent: Thursday 20ᵗʰ November 3:44 PM
To: Dr Amanda Sainsbury-Salis
Subject: Progress report

Dear Amanda,
*   It has been 9 weeks since I began my new way of life, and after stepping on the scales this morning, I was quite excited and wanted to tell you that I've now lost 11 kilos. Although I have been going to the gym 3–5 times a week for strength training and cardio, it feels like my weight is coming down effortlessly. I know that sounds ridiculous in light of my going to the gym so regularly, but based on my previous attempts to lose weight with just as much exercise, this is easy. Another thing I've noticed after being on this diet for over two months is how rotten I feel whenever I eat anything sweet and stodgy. It gives me similar symptoms to a hangover! NO THANK YOU VERY MUCH! Previously I've never been able to stick to any diet for long enough to realise what a negative effect those bad foods have on my body after not eating them for so long and then going back to them. I now get queasy just at the thought of eating junk. I still love my chocolate but I can't eat as much of it as I did before without feeling yuck, so like you I only eat the best I can afford. Now that I've begun to eat mostly 'real' foods and have cut most of the crap from my diet, I also find that my body does not require such large portions so often (because it is not starving due to malnutrition!). I've gotten to the point where I no longer have to pay such close attention to my levels of hunger or satiety, my body self-regulates and I eat accordingly. I always used to watch 'skinny' people and wonder how they could eat so little and be full. I now find that I'm doing the same. I'm not skinny yet but my body has learnt to appreciate 'real' wholesome food. Thank you for opening my eyes.*
*   God bless you,*
*   Nellie*

If the prospect of cutting back on the amount of fun foods you're eating feels like an insurmountable feat, keep in mind that the more you persist at cutting back gently by replacing them with more nutritious options, the easier it's likely to become.

Choose your favourites and savour them to the full

As you go through the process of gently crowding out free-loading kilojoules from energy-dense, nutrient-poor foods or liquid kilojoules, you'll undoubtedly become aware of certain treats that are very dear to you. These are the treats that simply cannot be crowded out of your life, the ones whose absence makes the heart grow fonder, the ones for which you'd don your hunting gear and go out on a search mission if you didn't have any on hand. Once you've identified these treasured treats, it's important to include them in your diet in a way that gives you maximum pleasure and therefore makes your diet sustainable in the long run, but that doesn't stop you from losing weight or keeping it off.

As an example, there are a lot of freeloading kilojoules that I'm quite happy to keep out of easy reach and do without, and that's why I never or rarely consume them. These include kilojoules from alcohol, fruit and vegetable juices, most cakes (including *gâteau au chocolat*), biscuits, potato chips and lollies. However, there are some liquid kilojoules and treats that I simply cannot do without, notably caffé lattes and chocolate. One of my current favourite forms of chocolate – besides Swiss chocolate truffles and Easter eggs – is a chocolate lick: a little pot of molten chocolate from my favourite chocolate café. I know that if I don't have some of my favourite treats regularly I'll cave in under the pressure and end up eating too much of something else I don't enjoy nearly as much. But I also know that if I have my favourite treats too often, my clothes will start getting tight on me. So I've reached a happy equilibrium by allowing myself a caffé latte every day if I feel like it (and if I'm a bit peckish), as well as a treat such as a chocolate lick or a couple of Swiss chocolate truffles two or three times a week if I've got an appetite for it. I've learned through trial and error that this is enough to satisfy my cravings, but not enough to send my weight back up to the 93 kilos I used to be. Because I can't be trusted with treasured treats at home, I make a point of going out to buy them in individual servings when the urge takes me.

Staying safe with treasured treats

When you're on a date with your treasured treat, remember to stay safe. If one of your true loves is cheesecake, but every time you have it you can't stop eating until you've demolished several sizeable slabs, the best option is to buy it in a restaurant or a café as a single sit-down serving rather than as a whole cake 'for visitors'. Given the addictive-like quality of fun foods for many people, please don't try to perform superhuman feats like buying a whole bottle of your favourite wine or a whole packet of your most prized chocolates and then endeavouring to have 'just one glass' or 'just one or two when I really feel like it' if you know it will hard for you to stop drinking or eating that particular thing. It's far better to go out and buy an individual serving only when you really feel like it. It's much more expensive to do that, and that's a good thing, because the added expense is another barrier to get through. You have to *really* want the prize; otherwise, it's just another source of freeloading kilojoules.

Finding your own critical limit

There is no set level of fun food consumption below which you're guaranteed to lose weight and above which you're guaranteed not to lose weight. That's because the amount of fun food you can eat while still keeping your weight on target depends on many factors, such as what your favourite treats are, what else you usually eat and drink, your activity levels, any health conditions you have and any medications you are taking, your age, your sex and your genetics. I've known women in their early twenties who can eat fried foods such as wedges with sour cream or doughnuts five days a week while still losing weight by listening to their bodies, and women in their fifties or sixties who can't eat more than a few spoonfuls of dessert once a week without stalling in their weight loss efforts. The thing is to experiment with different levels of fun – starting perhaps with one or two treats a week – and see how you go. If you're losing weight and/ or centimetres at a satisfying rate, there's no need to rein yourself in, at least as far as weight loss goes.

Fun foods and hunger

When you enjoy fun foods or beverages, it's *especially* important to ensure that you're not consuming more than your physical hunger signals decree. Remember, any kilojoules consumed when you're not yet comfortably and physically hungry, or which take you to the point of feeling oversatisfied, are in excess of your physical needs and will be stored as extra bulk on your body. If you're tucking into a chocolate lick and a caffé latte an hour after lunch and you're not in the slightest bit hungry at that time, or if you weren't quite satisfied after lunch but the chocolate lick and latte bring you to the point of feeling oversatisfied, the damage will be greater than if you'd eaten something like an apple. So, whenever you consume anything containing kilojoules – *especially* kilojoule-rich fun foods, such as a slice of your favourite cake – be sure that you're either physically hungry at a level of –2 or –3 when you start eating, or if you're eating it as the continuation of a larger meal or snack, be sure that you've got enough of an appetite to eat it without ending up feeling oversatisfied.

Over to you
Here's something you can do immediately to put the ideas in this chapter into action.

If your weight or your waistline is doing what you want it to do, there is no reason to change what you eat and drink, at least in terms of managing your weight. But if you're using your Success Diary every day and scoring practically all 2s and 3s, and eating at least two serves of fruit and at least five serves of vegetables every day, and you're not losing weight or centimetres, it's time to examine your intake of fun foods and liquid kilojoules – especially alcohol.

Are there any treats that are getting a free ride into your life, without a personal invitation from you? The ones you're eating or drinking not because you particularly love them, but just because they're there? If you simply change your environment so that you're not so exposed to these freeloading kilojoules, you'll consume significantly less of them and you'll probably lose weight more effectively. What's more, you won't even miss them, because you weren't actively seeking them in the first place.

As you eliminate freeloading kilojoules from your life, you'll undoubtedly discover which treats you absolutely adore, the ones you can't do without, the ones you actively seek out even if they're out of easy reach. Make a date to enjoy some of these treasured treats *safely* and on a regular basis – often enough to keep the lid on your cravings, yet not so often that they stall your progress. You might like to try enjoying some once or twice a week as a starting point and see how you go at your next weigh and measure. If you're losing weight and/or centimetres at a satisfying pace, there's no reason to prune back.

If you are to lose weight and keep it off, your body needs nutrients without excess kilojoules. The simplest way to get maximum nutrients into your diet without excess kilojoules is to gently crowd out all but your most beloved of treats with a bounty of fruit and vegetables, nutrient-rich foods and activities that make you feel good about yourself. Sometimes, however, that's not enough. Sometimes you need something more, and that's the subject of my next chapter.

Chapter 16

Step 2d. The importance of eating a wide variety of foods

The most delightful pleasures cloy without variety.
Publilius Syrus, Roman author, 1st century BC

As I outlined at the start of Step 2 on nutrition for weight loss, if you're not getting enough goodness into your diet, your body will go into a type of Famine Reaction that will push you to eat until it gets its fill of vital nutrients.[22-27] So, getting as many nutrients into your diet as you can will help you to keep your Famine Reaction under control and allow you to lose weight and keep it off without feeling like you're fighting a constant war against yourself. Focusing on eating fruit and vegetables and fewer processed foods will help, but sometimes you also need to take stock of how much *variety* you're getting in your diet. I've met a lot of people – women in particular – who have got into the habit of eating only a limited range of wholesome foods for fear of gaining weight and are therefore slowly starving their bodies of vital nutrients. This strategy usually backfires, because it almost always induces nutritional deficiencies that can make it extremely difficult to lose weight and keep it off. Not only that, nutritional deficiencies and the Famine Reaction they fuel can prevent you from fulfilling your biological potential. Let's take a look at a real-life example of this principle in action.

Food for fertility

Having lost 25 kilos and kept it off for more than two years, 41-year-old Michelle, a music teacher, decided to apply her teaching skills to helping others to achieve their optimum weight. That's when I met her, in a course for weight loss consultants that I was lecturing in. During a break between lectures, I had an opportunity to talk with Michelle. Although she was now a petite and slender 55 kilos for her 1.52 metre frame, she had to exert a lot of effort to stay that way ('white-knuckling it', as I call it). 'When I feel hungry, I eat the bare minimum of the least fattening foods to try and last until the next meal or snack. I often go to bed a bit hungry and think it's a good thing because that way I'll burn up more fat,' she told me. In addition to restricting how much she ate, Michelle restricted the *types* of foods she ate. She had banished almost all high-fat foods from her life, including many wholesome and nutritious foods such as tahini and peanut butter. Now that she knew about the Famine Reaction and its wily ways, however, Michelle realised that a prolonged Famine Reaction could well be the reason why it was so difficult for her to maintain her weight. As the students cleared the lecture theatre for lunch, Michelle stayed back to ask my opinion about something that had been troubling her. 'My husband and I have been trying to conceive for over a year. My doctor tells me that gaining a few kilos would probably help me to get pregnant. Having learned about the effects of the Famine Reaction on sex hormones in your lecture, I was just wondering what you thought of that idea.'

I could understand how hard it would be for Michelle to accept the idea of gaining weight after all the effort she had put into getting it off in the first place. I also knew the clear-cut effects of the Famine Reaction on fertility. As we stood there, my mind travelled back to the time my colleagues and I made one of our most startling discoveries. We were working with a strain of mouse called the *ob/ob* mouse, which has a naturally occuring mutation in the gene for leptin. Leptin is produced predominantly by body fat (white adipose tissue), and one of its functions is to tell your hypothalamus that you're well fed, thereby helping to keep the Famine Reaction quiet. When you lose weight, the amount of leptin in your bloodstream decreases dramatically, and this is one of the triggers that activate the Famine Reaction.[14, 106] Thus, *ob/ob* mice and people who don't produce any leptin endure a chronic Famine Reaction and its effects: a voracious appetite, lethargy, a reduced metabolic rate, and hormonal changes that favour the accumulation of body fat while simultaneously weakening lean body tissues such as muscle.[107] In addition, people or mice with insufficient leptin have impaired fertility. In our mission to find new ways to alleviate the Famine Reaction so that more people can attain and maintain a healthy weight, my colleagues and I were testing the effects of blocking the Y4 receptor, which is found in the brain and which we thought might mediate some of the effects of the Famine Reaction. However, our obese mice didn't lose any weight or fat in response to our experimental treatment. I remember feeling quite dejected about this at the time; all that work for no outcome. With a sigh, I resolved to go back to the drawing board and devise another way to block the Famine Reaction. It was at this point that I noticed something very odd. A female *ob/ob* mouse to which more than six months earlier we'd given the experimental treatment and which we had then paired with a male mouse was now nursing a litter of tiny pups! This was totally unexpected. None of the female *ob/ob* mice that hadn't received the treatment became pregnant; they were totally infertile. It was the most dramatic and clear-cut experiment I'd ever taken part in, even though it produced a result I wasn't looking for. It demonstrated that the infertility of these chronically 'famished' mice was due to the action of the Y4 receptor, and that blocking Y4 had the effect of switching off that part of the Famine Reaction that represses fertility.[108] For many years it had been known that situations that activate the Famine Reaction, such as heavy exercise or poor nutrition, reduce sex hormone concentrations and significantly depress ovulation and fecundity.[41] With our team's new discovery, now we knew why. I then fully understood the importance of switching off the Famine

Reaction if you're trying to conceive. With this in mind, I gave Michelle the following advice. 'If my fertility were on the line, I'd do everything in my power to wash any trace of the Famine Reaction out of my system. I'd make sure I always ate enough, and I'd eat a wide variety of wholesome foods, including the "fattening" ones you don't currently let yourself eat. Gaining a few kilos may also help.'

That evening, Michelle went to a pizzeria with her husband and had salad and a *pizza quattro formaggi* (four-cheese pizza), something she hadn't eaten in more than nine months. In the ensuing weeks Michelle reintroduced many other wholesome foods into her diet. 'Yes, I started eating things I was avoiding because of their high calorie count, such as full-fat marinated feta cheese, avocado, tahini, peanut butter and butter,' she told me in an email two months after the course. 'For the first few weeks after the course I was craving these foods. Now I feel like them less often but will definitely eat them if I feel like it. Not only that, I also enjoy them *senza* guilt! A wonderful change, thanks to you. In retrospect, I think my body was deprived of good fats and oils and needed to stock up.' As well as eating a wider variety of wholesome foods, Michelle now ate enough to satisfy her physical hunger.

> *If I need a snack I might have a piece of toast with peanut butter or raisin toast with twice as much butter as the tiny scrape I used to have before, or a few wholemeal crackers with feta cheese instead of six token nuts like I used to eat. Before, I would have had the nuts to try and tide me over until dinnertime but I would not have felt satisfied. Now I eat a snack until I feel more satisfied and I probably eat less at dinner than before. So the total number of calories I'm eating is probably similar to what I was eating before, I'm just arranging them differently. Or, I might be eating more. It's hard to tell because I have finally stopped counting them. Another great change.*

You may expect that eating in this more liberal way would have seen Michelle heading straight back towards the 80 kilos she used to be. It didn't, because Michelle used a Success Diary for a couple of weeks to be certain she was reading her body signals correctly, she remained vigilant about eating mostly nutritious foods, and she kept exercising almost every day. In fact, after eight weeks of this she actually lost a kilo. 'I was 53.9 kilos when I weighed myself yesterday morning!!' she told me in her email. 'A weight I don't remember being since I was a teenager. As you know I was mainly aiming to maintain my weight, but since following my body's lead I have lost more without much effort.' Indeed, maintaining her weight became a lot easier for Michelle.

I am less grumpy than I used to be. Last year when I was trying to get my weight back down to 55 kilos I felt like a grumpy old menopausal bitch! I actually thought I was going through perimenopause. After learning about the Famine Reaction and its effects on hormones I know that it was probably just a result of depriving myself. So I am much happier now. I have also noticed that I don't get dizzy as much in yoga classes when I stand up. I used to get very light-headed, probably because my metabolism was slower. Now I have more energy, and I even started jogging again yesterday. I now know why it was so hard to lose weight and keep it off. I was just working against myself and inducing a pretty constant long-term famine reaction. Now I eat when I am hungry, whatever time it may be. I make choices in terms of nutrition rather than calories. I eat a lot more fruit because it is full of good things, rather than thinking it has more calories than a carrot stick. I put butter on steamed veggies to make them taste better and because I now know it helps with the absorption of nutrients.

As you can see from Michelle's story, eating a wider variety of foods, in the quantities she needed, made it noticeably easier for her to keep off the 25 kilos she had lost.

As I started writing this story, I emailed Michelle to ask how she had been doing with her weight management adventure over the past year. I had secretly wondered whether eating more liberally might have released the stranglehold the Famine Reaction may have had on her fertility. It made my day to receive the following reply from Michelle.

From: Michelle
Sent: Friday 5th March 2:28 PM
To: Dr Amanda Sainsbury-Salis
Subject: Re: Michelle's Success Story

Hi Amanda,
Funny you should email last Sunday. At 1:17 pm on that day I lost 4 kilos in a matter of hours, giving birth to our beautiful, healthy baby daughter!! Can fill you in more soon. I think the change in diet helped my body to get pregnant due to not being in a Famine Reaction.
Michelle

While it's impossible to know if Michelle's successful pregnancy was directly due to the change in her diet, one thing's for certain: if you're struggling with your weight and slowly starving yourself of nutrients by not eating a full range of wholesome foods, then eating a more varied diet could not only help to switch off any Famine Reaction that may be persuading your body to hold onto fat, it will also help your body to function as it's biologically programmed to do. More and more research now links nutritional deficiencies with heightened incidences of diseases such as spina bifida, thyroid dysfunction, diabetes and osteoporosis. By eating a wide range of nutritious foods, you'll help ensure that your body gets the nutrients it needs,[89, 90] and everything about you – from your immune system to your thought processes – will work so much better.

Does this apply to you?

To get an indication of whether your diet is nutritionally adequate, use the following two-minute diagnostic, which was developed by eminent international nutritionist Professor Mark Wahlqvist together with Dr Gayle Savige and Dr Bridget Hsu-Hage of Monash University in Melbourne.[90] Their research shows that eating 30 or more different foods every week will optimise your chances of getting all the nutrients you need in adequate doses. It worries me deeply that whenever I invite participants at my workshops and seminars to try this diagnostic, only 10 to 15 per cent are getting adequate variety in their diet. So how does your diet stack up? Try this simple Diagnostic and find out.

Diagnostic N°2d: Are you getting enough variety in your diet?

To do this diagnostic, go through the foods in the following list and think about whether you've eaten any of them in the past seven days. Disregard whether you ate the listed foods some time last month, or whether you're going to eat some of them tonight – just think about whether you've actually eaten any of them in the past week.

If you've eaten a reasonable amount of a listed food in the past week, put a tick in the box next to it. Commonsense will tell you what's a reasonable amount. For example, if the only time you ate kiwifruit in the past week was when you ate two slices of it as a garnish on your pavlova, it doesn't count.

When you get to the end of the list, count up how many boxes you ticked.

Grains and cereals
- ❐ Barley
- ❐ Corn (e.g. corn on the cob, creamed corn, popcorn)
- ❐ Oats (e.g. porridge, muesli)
- ❐ Rice (e.g. brown rice, white rice, rice crackers)
- ❐ Rye (e.g. rye flakes, rye bread)
- ❐ Wheat (e.g. wholegrain or white bread, foods made with wheat flour, Weet-Bix)

❐ All other grains and cereals (e.g. buckwheat, millet, quinoa, sago, semolina, tapioca, triticale)

Fruit
❐ Apples
❐ Bananas
❐ Berries (e.g. raspberries, strawberries)
❐ Citrus (e.g. oranges, lemons)
❐ Dates, kiwifruit, passionfruit
❐ Grapes (including raisins, sultanas)
❐ Melons (e.g. honeydew, rockmelon/cantaloupe, water-melon)
❐ Pears, nashi
❐ Stone fruit (e.g. apricots, avocados, cherries, nectarines, olives, peaches, plums, prunes)
❐ Tropical fruit (e.g. guavas, jackfruit, lychees, mangos, papaya, pineapple, star fruit)

Vegetables
❐ Flowers (e.g. broccoli, cauliflower, endive, chicory, lettuce)
❐ Leafy greens (e.g. spinach, cabbage, brussels sprouts, silverbeet)
❐ Marrow-like (e.g. cucumber, eggplant, marrow, pumpkin, squash, swede, turnip, zucchini)
❐ Onion (e.g. spring onions/shallots, garlic, leeks)
❐ Peppers (e.g. capsicums)
❐ Roots (e.g. carrots, sweet potatoes, potatoes, bamboo shoots, beetroot, ginger, parsnips, radishes, water chestnuts)
❐ Stalks (e.g. celery)
❐ Tomatoes, okra

Legumes/pulses
❐ Beans (e.g. green beans, fresh peas, including snow and sugar-snap peas, dried peas)

❐ Adzuki, baked beans, haricot, black beans, black-eye beans, borlotti beans, cannellini beans, chickpeas, kidney beans, lentils, lima beans, lupins, mung beans and sprouts, pinto beans, soya beans and sprouts, soya milk, bean curd

Nuts and seeds
❐ Almonds, brazil nuts, cashew nuts, chestnuts, coconut, hazelnuts, peanuts, peanut butter, pecan nuts, pine nuts, pistachio nuts, pumpkin seeds, sesame seeds, tahini, hummus, sunflower seeds, walnuts

Meat
❐ Game animals (e.g. kangaroo, rabbit)
❐ Game birds (e.g. quail, wild duck, pigeon)
❐ Lamb, beef, veal
❐ Organ meats (e.g. liver, brain)
❐ Pork (including ham and bacon)
❐ Poultry (e.g. chicken, turkey, duck)

Seafood
❐ Crustaceans (e.g. prawns, lobster, crab, shrimps)
❐ Freshwater fish
❐ Oily fish (e.g. anchovies, tuna, salmon, sardines, herring, mackerel, kipper, pilchards)
❐ Roe (caviar)
❐ Saltwater fish
❐ Shellfish and molluscs (e.g. mussels, squid, oysters, scallops)

Dairy
❐ Milk, yogurt (without live culture), ice-cream, cheese
❐ Live cultures (yogurt with live culture, e.g. acidophilus, bifidobacteria)

Eggs
❐ All varieties

Fats and oils
❐ Oils
❐ Hard/soft spreads

Fermented foods
❐ Miso, tempeh, soya sauce
❐ Sauerkraut
❐ All other varieties

Beverages
❐ Non-alcoholic (e.g. tea, coffee, cocoa)
❐ Alcoholic (use in moderation, if at all)

Herbs and spices
❐ Use regularly

Yeast
❐ For example: Vegemite, Marmite, brewer's yeast

Fungi (mushrooms)
❐ All varieties

Sugar/confectionery
❐ Jam, honey, syrups, sugars, soft drinks, all other varieties (use sparingly)

Water
❐ Including mineral water

Today's date   ....
Your score   ....

Next week's date ....
Your score   ....

Interpreting your results
If you scored 30 or more, well done and keep it up! Try not to exclude whole food types (such as grains and cereals or wholesome higher fat foods). This will help ensure that you get an optimum mix of nutrients into your body.

If you scored less than 30, it's likely that you're getting less than your fair share of the nutrients you need. This can make losing weight and keeping it off unnecessarily difficult, because it can trigger a kind of a Famine Reaction that pushes you to eat more in an attempt to meet your nutritional needs, not to mention weakening many of your vital functions. If you're eating fewer than 30 foods per week, a highly effective way to increase your score is to simply make a date with yourself to do this diagnostic again in one week's time. I guarantee that you'll be amazed at what you can achieve, both in terms of increasing the variety in your diet and how you feel.

Variety kills cravings

A key benefit of increasing the nutritional value of your diet by choosing a wide variety of wholesome foods is that it will seriously cut cravings for energy-dense, nutrient-poor foods. Many people who are concerned about their weight make the fatal mistake of cutting out whole food groups. Michelle's weight management tactic of severely restricting wholesome fat-rich foods is extremely common, as is the practice of cutting out most grains and cereals (except in the case of a binge, when it's often kilojoule-rich, nutrient-poor varieties such as croissants or biscuits that make a comeback). Research shows, however, that as soon as you put restrictions on certain foods, your cravings for those foods escalate.[109] Part of the explanation for this phenomenon is psychological (we want what we can't have), and part is physical. For instance, grains and cereals are a major source of B vitamins, and if you try to cut them out of your diet, then B vitamin deficiencies can send you on the prowl for a fix. The trouble is, when it's a choice between being deficient in particular nutrients and having enough to function properly, your body doesn't care in the short term where those nutrients come from, just so long as it gets them. Moreover, the quickest source usually wins. If you get them from a serve of nutrient-rich quinoa that you've cooked into a delicious meal for your dinner, that's great. If you get them from a large slab of carrot cake at your colleague's birthday celebration (as well as two additional slabs that you ferreted out of the fridge after your colleagues had left for the evening, as I've known myself to do in the past), that's fine for your body in the short term, too. Indeed, while the white flour in the carrot cake is much lower in B vitamins than quinoa or other less processed grains, it still contains some goodness, so if you eat enough of it you'll get the B vitamins you need. On the other hand, if you make a habit of eating a wide range of wholesome, nutrient-rich foods, you're less likely to have nutritional deficiencies, and splurges, pig-outs, mini-binges and full-blown binges will trouble you less and less.

As a case in point, I'd like to introduce you to one of my friends from high school days, Chris. I'd always appreciated Chris as a teenager, and he was one of the people I looked forward to catching up with at our 20-year high school reunion. Unfortunately, neither of us could make it to the event. However, several months later Chris ordered three copies of my book *The Don't Go Hungry Diet* from my website. I sent him his parcel, and we chatted over a couple of emails. A year later Chris ordered seven more copies of my book. I think he must have liked it! I didn't have much time to wonder what on earth he was doing with all those books, because shortly after I received the following email.

From: Chris
Sent: Thursday 27th August 1:01 PM
To: Dr Amanda Sainsbury-Salis
Subject: Re: Your Receipt #10898427

Hi Amanda,
    Hope that all is well. As you will see, I've placed an order for some of your books to give to my family and friends. I am living in Asia but will be in Sydney from the 12th to the 15th of September, and then I travel to Port Macquarie for National Youth Champs for touch football.

Obviously I have been training hard so the exercise has to take some credit but I have been using the general principles you espouse, not least eating a wide variety of whole foods. So, I'm now down around 68 kilos, which is not bad for 1.69 metres. I was 88 kilos five years ago and had lost a bit of weight before I read your book last year, but I'd say that I've moved from 80 kilos to 68 kilos in the 18 months since then. Hope that all is well and regards,
  Chris

I was curious to learn why Chris felt that eating a variety of whole foods had helped him to lose weight, so I arranged a time to talk with him over the phone. (I just love food; it's the best social glue in the world. We hadn't spoken in over 20 years and our first conversation was about food!) Chris told me that before he read my book he was eating healthy foods but hadn't considered how limited a range it was. For instance, he realised that he was missing out on variety by eating the same breakfast cereal every day. Chris had also tried a meal replacement formula derived predominantly from milk. He had started drinking this in place of regular food in order to lose weight five years ago, after a visit to his doctor revealed that the back pain he had assumed was muscular in origin was actually reflux (a condition that is significantly more prevalent among people carrying excess weight and that often disappears after weight loss) and that he was 20 kilos above his estimated ideal body weight. On top of this, his blood cholesterol levels weren't great, either. Chris started out taking the meal replacement formula three times a day, then progressively reduced it to twice a day, then once a day and then stopped taking it, adding back in a normal meal each time. His meals were nutritious, based on non-starchy vegetables and lean meats, but again they were limited in variety. While this strategy had certainly helped Chris to lose 16 kilos in four months, improve his cholesterol levels and get fast relief from reflux, slowly but surely the weight crept back. He had increased the amount of physical activity he was doing compared to how much he was doing before he started losing weight, and therefore he thought logically that the weight should have stayed off. Without his realising it, though, the lack of variety in his diet was working against him. From time to time, Chris got the urge to eat biscuits, chocolates or sweets and didn't feel satisfied when he did so. So within a year he had regained 8 of the 16 kilos he lost on the meal replacement program.

Chris said that since reading my book *The Don't Go Hungry Diet* and introducing a wide range of whole foods into his diet, taking care to choose minimally processed foods and to eat food that was as close as possible to its original condition, the weight came off steadily He made the comment that one of the reasons for his previous poor cholesterol levels was the amount of highly processed food he ate while living and working in Asia. He noted that the biggest selling brand of instant noodles in the country had some 25 different ingredients listed, many of which were numbers. When he compared this with the list of ingredients for the closest competitor, which he said didn't even come close in terms of taste or market share, the ingredient list was less than half as long. So he went back to all the good advice his mother used to give him and concentrated on eating simple foods. 'That's why I love eating foods like mountain bread, because when you look at the ingredients list all it says is "flour, water",' he said.

Chris's dietary changes had a big impact on both his weight and his cravings. 'Now I can quite happily have one or two biscuits or sweets or an ice-cream, walk away and not feel like eating it again for another month,' he told me over the phone. This, combined with his decision to find time to exercise by coaching and refereeing touch football, despite his six-days-a-week career as an engineer, means that Chris has kept those 20 kilos off for more than a year.

If you're currently eating the same old foods day in, day out, then increasing the variety of wholesome foods in your life could help you to cut cravings and lose weight for life – just as it did for Chris. Then when *your* next high school reunion rolls around, you can rock up feeling your physical best and swan around flirting with all the people you used to have a crush on.

Food variety and special diets

If there are certain foods you can't eat owing to allergies, intolerances or personal preference, increasing the variety in your diet may sound like an impossible feat. For example, if you follow a vegan diet, there will be lots of boxes in Diagnostic N°2d that you didn't tick this week and that you wouldn't tick next week, either. Fortunately, there are so many different foods available in this country that even if you can't eat certain foods there are always plenty of other foods from which to get your nutrients – as long as you keep your eyes open for different types of wholesome morsels.

Throughout her life, 64-year-old Cheryl had suffered from food allergies. As a child she frequently had an upset stomach and skin rashes that itched abominably, and as she progressed into adulthood the stomach upsets and skin irritations came with her. Cheryl's body was reacting to harmless substances in the foods she ate as though they were disease-causing pathogens, triggering the immune cells in the walls of her intestines to produce immunoglobulin E antibodies in an attempt to neutralise the offending substances. Cheryl was seriously allergic; these substances were able to enter her circulation, from where they triggered dreadful allergic reactions in her skin. But Cheryl didn't realise this at the time. It was only after decades of periodic suffering that, at the age of 52, she became conscious of the fact that every time she ate anything containing beef, lamb or pork, she'd get stomach cramps, diarrhoea and the most awful itching imaginable. Eliminating these three foods from her diet reduced Cheryl's allergic reactions, but still they persisted. Four years later, Cheryl's body was ready to be heard once and for all. She came down with debilitating stomach cramps and circular weals of swollen, reddened, itchy skin on her torso, arms, hands and upper thighs. A visit to her doctor revealed extremely high circulating levels of immunoglobulin E. 'You have some allergies to sort out,' he concluded.

With guidance from a naturopath, Cheryl tried eliminating not only red meat but also dairy products, wheat (gluten), shellfish, some tropical fruit, the cabbage family, and nightshade plants such as potato, tomato, eggplant and capsicum from her diet. 'Low and behold, all the allergic reactions abated,' she told me in an email. 'My naturopath and GP suggested I try proving the strength of my new diet by challenging myself with foods I now had to avoid. Results were always a return of the allergic reaction, which included debilitating gastric and skin responses.' Cheryl found it easy to follow this new way of eating, because avoiding the incapacitating symptoms she had put up with for so many years was extremely motivating.

Having sorted out what not to eat in order to feel good, Cheryl turned her attention to her next challenge, her weight. When she retired from full-time work two years ago, she weighed 91 kilos and was 'sick and tired of feeling tired and sick'. At 1.64 metres tall and with a family history of diabetes and heart disease, Cheryl knew she needed to lose some weight. But would the restricted range of foods she was able to eat hinder her ability to lose weight by listening to her body? Knowing the importance of dietary variety for health and weight management, Cheryl examined the foods she *could* eat and tried to eat as many different types as possible in each group. Although she doesn't eat red meat, Cheryl conscientiously eats a variety of protein-rich plant foods. 'I use nuts, seeds and legumes because these are good sources of protein for me. I also conscientiously multiply food types within groups. For example, I use a lot more types of vegetables than the food variety quiz gives me opportunity to score. My husband and I grow most of our own food and we try to eat as many types of plant foods as possible,' she told me. As for grains and cereals, Cheryl knew that many of the commercial gluten-free products available were too highly processed to allow her to lose weight if she ate them too often, so she opted instead for minimally processed gluten-free grains and seeds such as amaranth, quinoa, buckwheat, soy, flaxseed, and sunflower and pumpkin seeds. 'While I've developed a great many recipes that use these ingredients to replace bread-like products, on occasion I can and do use gluten-free commercial products if I feel I want to. Not daily, but when I feel like it,' she said. Cheryl scored 24 in the food variety quiz in Diagnostic Nº2d, a fantastic score given that there are many common foods she can't eat. And it was enough dietary variety for her to lose weight. She had already been keeping a food diary to help sort out her allergies, and when she added a couple of extra columns in which to record her hunger and satiety levels and aimed for all 2s and 3s, she lost 17 kilos in 6 months.

Two years later, Cheryl has kept 12 of those kilos off and is a steady 80 kilos. She still wants to lose another 5 kilos or so, but she's not in a rush. 'I am very confident about losing more – and not impatient. I know I have the tools to help me and I have no pressure to win road races!' While Cheryl says that learning to recognise and follow her body's signals about how much to eat is one of the key things that helped her to shed all this excess weight and keep it off for so long, she knows that if she hadn't first identified and avoided the foods that made her feel awful, she wouldn't have been able to do it. When she felt miserable, itchy and insanely irritable, going out for a walk or spending a couple of hours in her garden, for example, were the last things she felt like doing. Once she no longer had to worry about debili-tating allergic symptoms, Cheryl found it much more do-able to introduce an appropriate exercise routine. And that, she says, is the other key to her success.

If there are foods you can't or don't eat, this doesn't have to be a problem for your weight, because there are always plenty of other wholesome and nutritious foods that you can eat instead. Just go for maximum variety among the foods you *can* eat. When you eat the foods that feel good to your body (and avoid the ones that make you feel bad), it's so much easier to reach the weight you're meant to be, because you'll have so much more energy to do the things you need to do to get there. And let's face it, losing weight and keeping it off takes focus and attention. You need to keep your environment free of the kryptonite foods and bever-ages that make you go weak; you need to plan a little in advance so that you can get fruit, vegetables and nutritious foods into your body when you're hungry; you need to be conscious of how much physical activity you're getting; and you need to live your life to the full so that you can forget about food unless you're hungry. You owe it to yourself to eat the foods that make you feel so good that you can do these things with ease and grace.

Over to you

Here's something you can do immediately to put the ideas in this chapter into action.

What did you score in the food variety quiz in Diagnostic N°2d? If you're eating the same old 10 to 20 foods every week, it's highly likely that your diet is deficient in some vital nutrient, and your body therefore won't be working at optimum capacity. This will not only make you feel poorly, it can also make it unnecessarily difficult for you to lose weight, because it will rile your Famine Reaction, thereby making you hungry and desirous of quick-fix, kilojoule-rich, nutrient-poor foods.

If there are foods you don't eat, why is that? Is it because they really don't agree with you? If there are wholesome foods that you're actively avoiding for no other reason than habit or fear of gaining weight, for example, you may like to examine your beliefs more closely. Like Michelle, you could discover that the very foods you're avoiding turn out to be the 'missing link' you need to manage your weight more easefully and to feel your physical best.

The easiest way to increase the variety in your diet is to simply do the quiz in Diagnostic N°2d and then make a date with yourself to do the quiz again in a week's time. (If you'd like to download a free copy of the quiz to post on your fridge as a reminder, please see the back of this book for details of my website.) I'll bet you'll surprise yourself with your results, both in terms of eating foods you haven't eaten in a long time or have never tried, as well as in terms of how you feel. You may even notice, like Michelle, that the excess weight that your body seemed to be holding onto so tenaciously will now be easier to shift and easier to keep off.

Chapter 17

Step 2e. Is your diet too 'perfect' for your own good?

There is nothing either good or bad, but thinking makes it so.

William Shakespeare, English playwright and poet,
1564–1616

In a study designed to identify the psychological factors that predict success or failure in preventing weight regain after weight loss, Australian researcher Associate Professor Sue Byrne and her colleagues identified what they called 'dichotomous thinking' as a short cut to disaster.[110] Dichotomous thinking is the black-and-white mindset that makes you believe you won't reach your goal or maintain your weight unless you follow your diet and exercise regime to the letter; if you deviate in the slightest, your efforts will all be in vain, so the slightest slip will lead you to give up entirely. Dichotomous thinking is what leads millions of intelligent people to do things like drown their sorrows in a family-sized bucket of ice-cream because they broke their diet with a serve of white jasmine rice in a restaurant instead of sticking to carbs that are low on the glycemic index or avoiding carbs altogether. Or leads them to down half a loaf of bread, toasted and spread generously with butter and peanut butter, because they overshot their daily kilojoule allowance by a mere 10 per cent or because they had a couple of days of 'bad eating' after a month of vigilant efforts.

The problem with dichotomous thinking is that even though you haven't done anything that will put the slightest dint in your overall weight management progress, you *think* you've ruined everything and so you give up and then proceed to do things that really *will* set you back if you keep them up.

In this chapter, I'm going to show you that it *is* possible to manage your weight while eating foods of all colours, tastes and textures, and thereby help you to ditch the 'black or white', 'good or bad' mindset once and for all.

Does this apply to you?

One of the surest ways to ensure your attempt to lose weight will leave you feeling frustrated and heartbroken is to take the all-or-nothing approach that many conventional diets espouse. While many people can follow a diet's artificially imposed restrictions and cut out white bread or sugar or whatever for a few weeks or a few months, being a saint in the weight loss stakes is way too difficult a role to maintain. Moreover, the more saintly you try to be as you lose weight, the more drastically it tends to backfire. Here's a quick and easy diagnostic test to help you determine if your diet is too 'perfect' for your own good.

Dr Amanda's Diagnostic N°2e: Is your diet too 'perfect' for your own good?

Read through the following questions and choose the answer that best applies to you and your most recent weight loss attempt. You don't need a pen; just keep reading.

1. **In the few days before I start a new weight loss plan:**
A. I eat about the same as I normally would.
B. I eat a bit less than I normally would; I'm getting a head start on my diet.
C. I eat more than I normally would, eating things I wouldn't normally eat, in quantities I wouldn't normally eat. I'm

---

about to start the Diet To End All Diets and I don't know when, if ever, I'll be able to eat like this again.

2. When I finish trying to lose weight:

A. I eat about the same as I did while I was trying to lose weight, but enjoy slightly larger servings of everything.

B. I have what feels like a mini-splurge for a day or so, enjoying noticeably larger servings of everything, as well as a few treats, but then I get back to eating moderate portions.

C. I go on a rampage, frenetically eating all the things I wasn't allowed to eat while I was on the diet. I eat noticeably more than what I was habitually eating before I started the diet.

3. I'm standing outside a restaurant, ready for a nice meal, but after scouring the menu I realise there's absolutely nothing on it that my diet will allow.

A. I go to another restaurant that has safer options.

B. I order something that appeals and that has vegetables in it, and I eat as much as I need. I might even share a dessert with someone else, but I stop eating when I feel elegantly satisfied.

C. I either order nothing but a mineral water or a pot of tea and sip it dutifully as others tuck in, or I say 'Stuff the diet' and order whatever rich dish I fancy followed by dessert. I polish off everything and then feel overfull and awful about myself. Because I've blown it anyway, I buy myself a chocolate bar or two to eat on the way home. As soon as I can, I dive into bed to sleep it all off like a boa constrictor.

4. Someone offers me a chocolate that's impossible to resist.

A. I graciously accept and then put it in my bag to enjoy later when I feel a bit peckish.

B. I graciously accept, pop it in my mouth and savour a moment of sheer bliss. It was a delicious chocolate! Luckily it's not me holding the box or I'd probably eat all of them.

C. I fight a battle in my mind, groan audibly and then say begrudgingly, 'OK'. I pop it in my mouth. It tastes great, but I hardly notice because I'm drowning in a wave of negative thoughts such as 'Now I've done it. I've broken my diet. I'll never reach my goal. I'm useless.' I then go and scoff a mountain of 'illicit' foods because I've ruined my diet anyway and I think I might as well go for it.

5. I'm packing my suitcase for a much-anticipated holiday.

A. My comfortable walking shoes/swimsuit and goggles/gym kit are one of the first things I think to put in my bag. I'm looking forward to having more time to exercise so that I can come back feeling trim, taut and terrific.

B. I pack clothes that fit me comfortably and that have a waistband; they remind me not to go overboard with the holiday treats. If I can at least maintain my current weight while I'm on holiday, I'll be pleased.

C. As I throw my stretchy clothes with elastic waistbands into my suitcase, I'm munching my way through a packet of treats. I know I'm going to come back from my holidays a good few kilos heavier than I am now, so I've given up on my diet and have started my holiday overindulgences already. The diet starts when I get back.

6. I weigh myself and see I've gained back some of the weight I had previously lost.

A. I say, 'Oh well, all those Easter eggs really did catch up with me, after all,' and then get right back on track, eating in the way that I know will help me to lose the weight again.

B. I feel a bit grumpy for the whole day, and I may get a bit lax about the types or amounts of foods I eat, but within the week I'm back on track and feeling great.

C. I tell myself that there's no point in even trying to control my weight when my efforts are rewarded so dismally, so I cook myself up a batch of pancakes for breakfast and eat them all with butter and maple syrup, then proceed to eat chocolate and other fun foods until I feel physically uncomfortable and totally dreadful about myself.

Scoring

If you answered C to two or more of these questions, you're in danger of getting stumped by all-or-nothing thinking. Learning to incorporate more fun into your diet *while* you're losing weight will help you to lose weight and keep it off sustainably. It may seem ironic, but the tighter your grip on the reins of the weight loss wagon, the harder it is to stay on it. It's only when you loosen your grip that staying on becomes easier. You're less likely to fall off the wagon in the first place, and climbing back on is so much easier because all that white-knuckling hasn't weakened your hands.

Pat loosened the reins and two years later she's *still* on the wagon

Sixty-eight-year-old Pat has tended towards all-or-nothing thinking her whole life. This attitude has helped Pat enormously throughout her life. If she wasn't so steadfastly committed to achieving goals that are important to her, Pat doesn't think she would have done as good a job as she has in having a loving relationship with her spouse, raising three children (plus the four her husband brought with him!), maintaining a beautiful home on an acreage block, and holding down a demanding full-time job in a trustee company. When it came to taking care of her weight, however, Pat's dichotomous thinking style was a double-edged sword. Since her mid-twenties, Pat had followed a range of restrictive diets that became fashionable in the decades from the

1960s through to the 1990s. No doubt many people reading this book will be able to reel them off. While all-or-nothing thinking enabled Pat to stick staunchly to rigid kilojoule allowances or avoid long lists of forbidden foods until she had lost all the weight she wanted to lose, the slightest slip-up would often bring her completely undone. 'I remember once going on a diet with one of my daughters. It was the continual salads. Although I do like salad, as time went on I started hanging out for some lamb's fry. My daughter told me to have a vitamin B capsule – not the same, is it?' When Pat finally yielded and ate the lamb's fry she'd been longing for, she was so certain that she had completely mucked up (lamb's fry wasn't allowed on that diet) that she threw in the towel, went back to her normal way of eating and gained back all the weight she had lost, plus more.

Two years ago, weighing 96.2 kilos for her 1.6 metre tall frame, Pat heard me being interviewed on the radio about losing weight by listening to your body and eating normal foods (including vegetables and fruit). While Pat agreed with the logic and thought it sounded like an extremely do-able way of losing weight ('I can do this,' she said to herself), she was sceptical. The last time she had lost weight was more than 10 years ago, when she lost some 30 kilos over the course of a year by scrupulous attention to fats and kilojoules, only to start gaining it back again after just six months. Would eating in this more liberal way really result in weight loss? And if she could eat whatever she felt like – as long as she also ate enough vegetables and fruit every day – would eating lamb's fry and all the other foods that were no-nos according to all the diets she had ever been on send her off the rails again? 'To make sure I really believed in the concept, I bought and read your book *The Don't Go Hungry Diet*. I had to convince myself that if I did have "naughty things" it wasn't the end of the world – I really do mark myself hard,' she said. Pat also used a Success Diary for a couple of weeks.

By studying her body signals, Pat soon became proficient at eating only when hungry and stopping before she had eaten too much. 'I photocopied those two pages from your book where you explain what hunger feels like and how to know what you really feel like eating, and I stuck them on the wall near my desk at work and at home. Whenever I felt like eating something I'd go through your lists and try to figure out how I felt. Often I'd discover that I wasn't actually hungry at all,' Pat recalled. In addition to connecting with her body signals and following their lead, Pat dramatically improved her diet, largely thanks to getting organised and planning what she would eat. Before she started her weight loss adventure, Pat would usually eat something fatty and fast like a takeaway bacon and egg muffin on her way to work, and if she felt peckish mid-morning she would duck out of the office for something like a sausage roll, followed by a couple of chicken, salami or roast beef sandwiches at lunch time. Pat has always had more of a savoury than a sweet tooth, but because there were always biscuits available at work (with chocolate biscuits on Fridays), she would eat a handful on most weekday afternoons and then go home to a nutritious dinner of meat and vegetables with her family, or a takeaway if she decided not to cook. Simply by getting organised and packing more nutritious breakfasts to eat when she got to work and nutritious lunches based on salads or vegetables, Pat significantly increased her fruit and vegetable intake and decreased the number of kilojoule-rich, nutrient-poor takeaway foods she was eating. She also stopped eating biscuits at work, which wasn't a huge hardship, because she had never liked them that much anyway. 'With exercising, I commenced using a walking machine at home and tried to achieve 8000 steps in a day,' Pat told me in an email several months after she started her adventure. 'In the beginning I could only walk half a kilometre. It took me 6 minutes and 16 seconds and at the end of that I felt totally puffed out and terrible. But I do like a challenge and I soon got fitter. I have now hit the pavements and at night I top up to 12,000 steps on the walking machine if needed.' Pat's commitment to doing things well certainly helped her to achieve all of these feats. However, she also did something she had never previously allowed herself to do while trying to lose weight: she cut herself some slack and had a bit of fun. The highlight of Pat's working week is going to the pub for lunch on Fridays with the girls from work. Rather than telling them, 'I can't eat this or that, I'm dieting', she just continued to enjoy her Friday lunches as she had in her non-dieting periods. If there was grilled barramundi, chips, salad and some kind of dressing on the menu, then that's what she ate, always accompanied by a couple of glasses of wine. In the past, she would not have dreamed of allowing herself to have a pub lunch if she was trying to lose weight, but as Pat was being attentive to her body signals and checking that she didn't end up feeling oversatisfied, she knew that she was still on track. For her mother's 99th birthday, Pat made a rich cake laden with fruit, nuts and liquor, just the way she loves it, and every night for three weeks she savoured a finger-sized slice of it with a cup of tea after dinner. If she occasionally felt like going out for a Thai meal, she certainly didn't let the fact that she was trying to lose weight hold her back. While all of these carefully selected slices of paradise meant that Pat didn't lose weight as fast as she had in the past, within five months she had still lost an impressive 14 kilos. But the burning question was: would all-or-nothing thinking eventually resurface and get the better of Pat?

Time rolled on and I often wondered how Pat was getting on. Recently, two years after she started her weight loss adventure, I sent Pat an email asking how she was going. She must have made *huge* advances in overcoming her all-or-nothing attitude towards weight loss, because she emailed back and told me that she was now 65.8 kilos, a massive 30.4 kilos less than she weighed when she started. 'I have found that if I overindulge, it is now more easy than before to get back on track,' she wrote. 'My doctor is very impressed with my progress. He has taken me off my blood pressure and anti-inflammatory medicines. My cholesterol levels are good.' What wonderful news! Curious to know how she did it, so that I could share her secrets with you, I called Pat to learn more.

While Pat doesn't think she'll ever stop being all-or-nothing in her thinking, one of the things that helped her to tame this tendency enough to stay on track for two years was to constantly remind herself that one overindulgence wouldn't ruin everything. 'I kept telling myself that it took *years* to put on all this weight, and if I muck up at one meal or one day, it's not going to make me fat again because it took years of muck ups to get fat in the first place. On the other hand, if I let one muck up turn into a week of muck ups, I'll definitely be on the way up again.' As a result of these constant reminders, Pat now finds that when she does overindulge, she doesn't do so to the extent she would have in the past. For example, while she might occasionally eat until she feels oversatisfied when she goes out for a meal, she doesn't eat to the point of feeling uncomfortably stretched, as once she would have done. And if she's at a dinner and someone puts a slice of cake or a dessert in front of her, she might still eat it just because it's there, even if she doesn't particularly enjoy it, but then she gets straight back to her normal way of eating at the very next meal.

IT TAKES A LOT OF CONSISTENT OVEREATING AND INACTIVITY TO GET FAT

- How many years did it take you to reach your highest weight ever?
- How many times did you need to overindulge in order to reach that weight?
- And how inactive did you need to be to reach that pinnacle in your weight?

It took *much* more than one hamburger with chips, one piece of cake, one week of inactivity or even one month of festive follies to reach the highest weight you've ever been. That's why you never need to worry about occasional treats or periods of overindulgence or inactivity as you're losing weight, as long as you make a habit of getting back on track afterwards. It's literally *impossible* for occasional slip-ups to send you back to where you were before, because it takes much more than that to get fat.

Another thing that helped Pat to tame all-or-nothing thinking about her diet is that the way she is eating to lose weight has now become her normal way of eating, and she actually prefers it to how she was eating before. In other words, Pat enjoys being 'on the wagon' more than being off it. Achieving this change involved ignoring some of the rules about food that she'd learned in Diet Dungeon.

I was never much of a cereal eater, but I shopped around for the tastiest muesli I could find. A lot of diets I've followed would have said, 'Oh no, you can't have that; it's toasted', but every day I take a little bundle of my favourite toasted muesli with me to work, mixed with some bran and ground linseeds and almonds, and I much prefer eating that with fruit and milk over anything else I used to eat for breakfast.

In fact, the last time Pat had a takeaway bacon and egg muffin she noticed that it left such an unpleasant aftertaste and fatty coating in her mouth that she now rarely eats such things. Because Pat knows that she can eat any vegetable or fruit she feels like and still lose weight (unlike so many diets she had been on in the past, which prohibited long lists of natural foods), her cooking has become much more adventurous and tasty. 'I make a mean vegetable curry,' she told me over the phone, 'and I absolutely drool over my salads at lunchtime. I make a point of buying excellent olive oil, and it tastes divine drizzled over any vegetable.' Eating to manage her weight and to be healthy has now become a way of life for Pat. 'The trouble with most of the diets I tried before is that you cannot do them forever; there is a limit to the number of grapefruit you can eat even if you like them. The fact that I'm in charge and that I have flexibility and variety with food means that I can quite easily see myself eating like this forever. For the first time in my life, I *lived* while I was losing weight,' she told me.

Pat has certainly done a lot of living since she started her weight loss adventure. Last year she went on a one-month holiday to Canada with one of her daughters. She saw a lot of magnificent sights; she also enjoyed a lot of foods that were intriguingly different from what she usually eats in Australia. 'There was so much delicious seafood, and by the end of the holiday I didn't think I'd ever be able to look at another lobster. I also loved their pub meals; they had things like jacket potatoes with a range of delicious sauces.' Several times during the holidays Pat ate more than she needed, but it didn't catapult her into an eating rampage, as once it would have done. 'The next day I'd just wake up and get back into my fruit and muesli, and I kept up with my walking even though I wasn't eating perfectly. I have to admit that each time I went off a diet in the past I also stopped exercising. Has to be done, doesn't it!' Even when Pat came back home after her holiday and discovered that she'd gained 2 kilos, she wasn't fazed. She just climbed back on the wagon, lost the 2 kilos again, and then proceeded to lose even more weight.

Pat said that if she hadn't enjoyed so many indulgences as she lost weight she probably would have lost those 30 kilos much faster than the two years it has taken her. On the other hand, the time has flown by. 'Because I was living while I lost weight, it doesn't feel like it's been two years, it hasn't felt like a chore.' Additionally, if Pat *hadn't* enjoyed regular treats as she lost weight, I doubt very much that she'd still be on the wagon so long after climbing aboard.

> *Last week one of my girlfriends at work said to me, 'Pat, I've just got this feeling that this time the weight's not coming back again. I've got the feeling that this time you've really licked it.' And you know what? I feel so pleased and so proud of myself, and I feel more confident that this time the weight really is gone for good.*

Paradoxically, allowing all foods can put an abrupt end to bingeing. So why wait?

Pat is 68. I often wish that younger women could learn to do as she has done, letting go of rigid rules about what to eat, following their hunger signals, and gradually and peacefully reaching their optimum biological weight. Instead, almost all of the women I've helped have already spent decades of their lives in yoyo dieting – often at great financial and personal cost – before discovering that easing up on the rules they learned in Diet Dungeon is the fastest and most sustainable way to lose weight once and for all. Indeed, most of the people who kindly shared their success stories and experiences for this book are in their forties, fifties and sixties. This is one of the reasons why I love giving university lectures. Every time I walk into a lecture theatre to explain the physiology of weight management to young students in medicine, dietetics, nursing or human movement, I know that my knowledge will probably help them to assist their future patients and clients, but I secretly also hope that it will help them to improve their own lives. Some years ago I was giving a plenary lecture to some 400 first-year and second-year medical students. It was hard to know what impact I was having, because the lecture theatre was so large that I couldn't see anyone's face. Little did I know that out there in the sea of faces, a young life was about to change.

When she came to my lecture at 11 am that day, 19-year-old Sabrina was having a good morning. A good morning in Sabrina's books would start with as small a breakfast as she could get away with without too much nagging from her parents, usually some chopped-up fruit, a spoonful of yogurt and a tablespoon of oats – with the quantity of oats gradually decreasing as each day went by.

Sometimes I would be 'strong enough' to hold on and continue eating very little for the whole day, but normally at about 10 o'clock I would start feeling hungry – and I would make myself wait until I got home to have lunch because I was scared of the 'hidden bad foods', even in the healthy foods in the cafés at uni. But I'd get home at 3 and think, 'You know what? I'm strong enough, I can pull this off and not eat until dinner,' so it would start with a carrot, some celery. Then another carrot, maybe some capsicum. Then some cheese. Then I'd feel like something sweet, so I'd 'treat' myself to a biscuit, and then I'd eat the entire 250 gram packet! And the inevitable 'well I've blown it now' would sink in – and in roll the giant bowls of cashews (which in all honesty I don't even like!!!), bowls of ice-cream with chocolate topping, huge cheesy grilled sandwiches (with more butter on them than bread!). Sure enough, I'd go through this cycle of something salty, then need something sweet, and then go back to salty again. I would eventually manage to stop eating, but not until I felt so sick and thought my stomach would explode. And the guilt! The guilt would convince me that I could remedy the situation by trying to explain to my parents that I 'wasn't hungry' or 'wasn't feeling well' and couldn't eat dinner. But it never worked; I always managed to eat all of my dinner, too! The guilt was something dreadful. I felt bad at ending up back in this position when I knew how much I wanted to conquer binge eating. I felt bad about what I was doing to my poor body and digestive system – probably giving myself pancreatitis (I get terrible reactions to eating large quantities of fat. I break out in horrible pimples, have awful cramping, bloating, gas and diarrhoea). I hated myself for seemingly voluntarily doing that to myself all the time! And then there was the guilt about making myself fat, about not reaching my goal weight, the feelings of inadequacy and depression. Sometimes after these episodes I would feel ready to tackle my bingeing and my weight with my semi-starvation method of dieting again, always in the mornings. On other days I would just wander around uni from store to store, buying the unhealthiest things I could find. Chips, chocolate, ice-cream and more chocolate. I used to go on chocolate bar runs, where I would go from store to store and pick out a new chocolate bar at each one. Oddly enough, these days were normally dictated by what I had eaten for breakfast – if it was something light, I had the willpower and the reason to continue dieting, but if I had eaten toast – then the whole day started and ended with chocolate!

In addition to starving herself after binges, Sabrina would try to make up for overeating with gruelling amounts of exercise.

I used to sit down and calculate everything I'd eaten in my binge and the number of calories it contained – and then try to 'offset the guilt' with negative calories from exercise!!! I used to go on ridiculous walks. I'd take a backpack and just keep walking for hours until my legs spasmed and cramped and I had blisters and bruises all over my feet. Several times I walked for over five hours from my house to my old high school and back (about 20 kilometres), and one day I even walked home from uni (over 30 kilometres and 8 hours of walking!). That used to help keep my weight down a bit – but as you could imagine, no one could keep that up for long!!

Having been in this cycle of endless starving then bingeing for more than four years, Sabrina's internal anguish was now showing on the outside. At 75 kilos and 1.66 metres tall, she felt fat and uncomfortable. Listening to my lecture, however, gave Sabrina a glimpse of light at the end of the tunnel. 'I remember being totally dumbfounded and excited by what I was hearing – and I remember being very sadly disappointed that your book wasn't due to come out for another year.' Two-and-a-half years ago, Sabrina found my book *The Don't Go Hungry Diet* in a bookstore and decided to give it a go. Her weight by then just over 80 kilos, she was very afraid of gaining more weight if she simply ate nutritious foods according to her body signals instead of trying to be so restrictive about what and how much she ate, but understanding the physiology of weight management after reading my book and hearing my lecture helped her to take the leap of faith. 'There's no way I would have had the courage to start if I hadn't seen the solid medical basis behind your approach, which indicated that I might not actually gain weight in the process!' But even stronger than her fear of gaining more weight was Sabrina's fear of continuing to live the way she was.

At the time I sat down and had a talk with myself about my priorities. I had thought that the worst thing that could possibly happen to me if I gave up dieting as I knew it would be to gain weight. But when I actually thought about it, the only thing I hated more than the idea of gaining weight was the prospect of more of that guilt, that awful feeling that comes when I have completely over-eaten. And I think it was that realisation that really helped me to achieve my goal.

I started writing in your Success Diary in August, monitoring my eating patterns and my triggers for hunger and satiety. I confess that writing in the diary didn't work for me because I was still in that stupid mind frame of dieting; I was still eating a lot less than I needed to eat most of the time, and I kept having 'blank days' where I did not fill in the foods I ate and how I felt because a) I couldn't remember, or b) was too ashamed and wanted to start afresh. I guess I was just too reluctant and scared to start using your principles of eating normally and not having weight loss as a definite outcome. I still couldn't get used to the unknown! However, what writing in this diary did do was allow me to realise what I feel like when I am hungry, and how I feel when I am full. So even though my weight and eating patterns were still everywhere in those first few months, I learned some of the most important things about my body – things that I had never noticed before and had always managed to ignore.

At the start of December that year, something indescribable happened. I had stopped writing in the diary for a month or two and I slipped into another one of my bingeing phases where I really didn't care what I ate because I knew that in a few days or weeks I'd start on my 'new' diet. But I got lazy, I just kept moving along with my 'junk food period' and never started my diet – I guess I had had enough. I was so sick and tired of dieting because it wasn't working. Gradually I no longer got cravings for chocolate, junk food and pastries. I would still occasionally get a craving, and I'd just buy whatever I wanted, eat it straight away and get on with my day. I would eat larger breakfasts, lunches and dinners than I had ever had in my life; I would eat all the rice and pasta on my plate (I had previously had a carbohydrate phobia!), I would add cheese to my pasta when I wanted to, and I would have huge delicious toasted cheese, roasted vegetable and salad wraps with pesto sauce – things that are healthy but that I would never previously have let myself have! A part of me was paranoid that I was putting on weight again – but I had had enough, I had really given up. I ate my chips and chocolate and cake whenever I wanted them – but I honestly found that I didn't want them as much any more.

It was therefore amusing when I went back to university on the 10th of January and my research supervisor commented, 'Have you lost weight? You look great!' Sure enough, when I went home and stood on the scales I saw that I had lost 5 kilograms!!! From eating everything I wanted in sight! I was flabbergasted. So it was then that I realised that I could eat what I wanted and lose weight for good – and that what I had to do to stop those binge periods was to not diet anywhere near as hard as I used to, and to eat the cheese and bread or yogurt and muesli as soon as I found myself going down that spiral of wanting food again – which would previously have been a huge no-no! And I now do so, without guilt; I eat that bowl of whatever it is that I feel like eating and I continue on with my day.

So after losing those 5 kilograms I was intrigued. I knew that I really needed to lose a bit more weight, but I also now knew that I needed to take it easy. So over the next few weeks I reduced what I was eating, just a little bit – I still ate all that my body was craving, but I was careful to avoid eating too much of the chocolates or chips and things out of boredom, unless I was craving it. So over the next three weeks I lost 3 more kilograms. Isn't that amazing? Although I expected to lose weight slowly on account of all the dumb diets I've done over the years and their probable effects on my metabolism, I lost weight as fast as someone who had never messed around with their metabolism by dieting!!!!

Ten months after she started listening to her body, Sabrina had lost a total of 14 kilos and had reached a healthy 66 kilos, which she has now maintained for more than two years.

I always had plans to eventually get down to 60 kilograms. But to be honest, I've been at this weight for a while now and I'm actually quite happy here. Maybe one day I'll want to get my weight down further, but I fit into all the clothes in my wardrobe, I'm happy enough in a swimming costume, and I don't hate photos of myself any more. So I'm starting to think that maybe this is my body's weight for me.

With the passage of time Sabrina's new eating habits became more ingrained than her old erratic ones, and it now seems highly unlikely that she will go back to her pattern of starving then bingeing. Looking back over her progress, Sabrina sees the crucial role that eating more liberally played in her success.

It's so liberating to now be able to cook without feeling that I have to remove all sugar or oils, wine or cheese from recipes! I haven't had a binge in such a long time, and I've found a perfect balance between exercise, eating, uni study and social life (I never used to be able to 'diet' and

*'live' at the same time!). One big thing that was impor-
tant for getting my binges under control was to include
crushed linseeds and almonds with my breakfast cereal
every morning. It sounds silly, but I used to put nuts and
seeds in the 'bad food' pile and not let myself eat them
– which is probably why I used to have such massive
break-outs and intense cravings for fatty foods! But now
my 10 am Sesame Snap and regular lunchtime feeds at
the AMAZING salad bar they've recently opened at uni
have been a godsend! I'm proud to say that last night my
mum was cooking a lamb roast – and my first thought
was actually 'yummy!' If you gave me a lamb roast three
years ago, I would have been filled with the dread of one
who knows they are about to 'break their diet' and there
is nothing they can do about it . . .*

*I've been to counsellors in the past to try to get help
for my bingeing – and they showed me the model of the
four stages of change and told me that I needed to work
out what was my 'danger point' for relapses – but I never
could find it or tackle it! Now, frankly, I find it hilarious
that I managed to break the cycle of endless eating BY
eating. In recent months I've been seeing a psychologist
for depression and anxiety, and she was absolutely stunned
that I'd managed to kick binge eating away, and in as short
a period as a year. But of course, the approach of eating
my way out of bingeing made perfect sense to her; I 'broke
the psychological cycle' by removing my trigger factor (not
eating enough).*

In addition to giving up punishing restrictions about what and
how much to eat, Sabrina gave up her unsustainable exercise
habits. 'I made a pact with myself when I started this whole
journey of listening to my body that I would never make myself
eat/not eat/exercise whenever I didn't want to . . . those were my
terms!' she told me. Nowadays Sabrina is still active, but she
does it for pleasure or necessity, not for punishment.

I bargained with myself that if I'm going to expend energy for fitness, I may as well get some use or pleasure out of it! So incidental exercise has become my way of life. I walk to and from the station, I run between floors in the shopping centre to get the best bargains, I walk in the city to save money on bus fares, I swim in the (freezing!) pool at home, cook for hours in the kitchen until my feet ache, clean my room (an infinite job) or clean the house, and I even do silly dancing alone in the family room when I feel a burst of energy! Additionally, I've just started the soccer season again – which is guaranteed to be good for me (mentally, socially and physically), and is most definitely something I enjoy! When I feel energetic, I subconsciously realise that my body needs to move and I get up to do something. If I'm tired, I recognise that rest is important and that I shouldn't push myself.

Sabrina said goodbye to a heartbreaking relationship

Many people who struggle with their weight have told me, 'You're so lucky that you have gained control of your weight now, while you're so young.' Most seem to have huge regrets about having been overweight for most of their life. Call me lucky, but I actually don't have to do any work at all to stay at this weight – I literally don't think about what I eat any more, other than trying to eat a balanced diet so that my body runs well and won't get sick. No one actually believes me when I say that, they think I'm lying, hyperthyroid, or taking some strange diet pills I guess. It makes me sad when I see so many of my friends struggling with their weight, trying diet after diet – and I feel helpless as I don't know the best way to impart what I've learned onto them without it sounding silly or like just another fad. A few times I have suggested your book to friends, and while they read it – I think they just aren't at the right time to challenge themselves mentally like that, as they usually get super excited and try it for a while and treat it like another fad. Perhaps the only reason it worked for me at this time was because I was not broken-hearted about being overweight, I was broken-hearted about having such a stupid relationship with food – and that was what I wanted to change.

Thank you so much for your wonderful research and book. I never thought I would say goodbye to unwanted weight for ever, and say goodbye to binge eating forever, but I have.

How long have you been broken-hearted about your relationship with food: struggling to resist forbidden foods, white-knuckling it against genuine hunger, walking around with giant carbo-hydrate phobias or bingeing uncontrollably when it all gets too hard? If you don't want to face another 10, 20 or 50 years in Diet Dungeon obsessing about food or being unhappy about your weight, there's no better time than right now to start your journey to freedom. Yes, it may be scary, you may wonder if you're ever going to lose weight, and you may be tempted to go back to your old ways of rigid dieting. But if you trust your body and bravely leap into the unknown despite your fears, then – like Pat and Sabrina – you'll have the rest of your life to enjoy all the pleasures that life with a lean body and a healthy relationship with food can bring.

Let the Fat Brake work its magic

If the only way you've ever shed weight has been through rigid restriction, having a bit of fun as you lose weight may seem next to impossible. To lose weight and keep it off, there's no doubt that you need to keep fun foods and liquid kilojoules such as alcohol to a workable minimum; otherwise, you won't lose any weight at all. Neither Pat nor Sabrina achieved the success they did by eating whatever treat happened to come their way. Instead, they consciously decided to indulge in only those foods or beverages they were really craving, deliberately turning down almost all of the freeloading kilojoules that had no particular appeal other than just being there. But while you need to keep your most treasured treats to a workable minimum, it's really important to include them in your diet or you'll give up long before you reach the weight you're biologically meant to be. Instead of feeling like a pressure cooker about to explode from the build-up of excess steam, having some of the things you love allows you to let off some steam when you feel the urge rather than exploding and eating not just one or two but a whole packet of biscuits.

One of the reasons you don't need to worry about the effects of occasional indulgences on your weight is that consuming more kilojoules than you need activates your Fat Brake.[6, 28–32] If you're listening to your body and the reduced appetite your Fat Brake instigates, then your Fat Brake will help smooth out any bumps for you. In *The Don't Go Hungry Diet* I wrote about my friend Grace, 41, who lost 12 kilos in 18 months by listening to her body, and then another 5 kilos in the same way over the ensuing years. Grace has now maintained a stable weight of around 65 kilos for more than three years. Recently Grace sent me an email about her experiences of fun foods and her Fat Brake.

> *Today I was thinking about the wonders of the fat brake. Yesterday, I went to the grocery store and got these frozen apple turnovers that I hadn't gotten since I was a child. And you know they were so delicious, I had two of these buttery, flaky pastries, and I didn't feel any guilt.*
>
> *And today, Amanda, I couldn't have a pastry if I tried. It's amazing, my body has just said No to any high-fat foods. I ate very little today. It's just amazing how, if you listen to your body, it just takes care of you and you don't have to worry. How phenomenal the human body is.*

Of course, if you're eating kilojoule-rich, nutrient-poor foods every day and not getting the nutrients your body needs, your Fat Brake will get overwhelmed, you won't lose weight and you may even gain weight. But when you indulge in the foods you love from time to time, or when you occasionally overshoot the mark and eat more than you really need, your Fat Brake helps you to undo any excesses and keep excess weight off, just as Grace has done, just as Sabrina has done, and just as Pat is now learning to do.

Over to you

Here's something you can do immediately to put the ideas in this chapter into action.

As you lose weight, watch out for any signs of dangerous pressure build-up.

Pressure can build up for all sorts of reasons as you're losing weight. It can happen when you're consistently not eating enough to meet your physical needs. It can happen when you're not eating the types of foods that really satisfy your physical cravings. It can happen when you're doing unsustainable levels of physical activity, or it can happen when you're not allowing yourself any of the treats you truly love.

When pressure builds up to dangerous levels, you know it because you start feeling like a pressure cooker about to explode. You feel it in a desire to eat vast quantities of foods you otherwise try to avoid, or a desire to throw your arms up in despair and let your exercise routine go to the dogs.

Don't be a pressure cooker waiting to explode. Open that steam vent from time to time and gently let off some steam. Eat the types of foods you're really craving (including occasional treats), in the quantities your body really needs, and don't ever drive your body to painful levels of physical activity. You may not lose weight as quickly as you would if you used an all-or-nothing approach, but instead of blowing the lid off your weight loss efforts and seeing all your good intentions go up in smoke, years from now you'll probably still be simmering away nicely, with your weight sitting just where it's biologically meant to be.

Step 3: Move

Losing weight and keeping it off boils down to kilojoules in versus kilojoules out. If you burn a greater number kilojoules than you consume, you lose weight. If the number of kilojoules you burn is the same as the number of kilojoules you consume, you stay at the weight you are, neither losing nor gaining.

Eating only as much as your body needs and making healthy food choices, as covered in Step 1 and Step 2, will take you a long way towards consuming fewer kilojoules than you burn. But if you want to achieve *permanent* results, you'll need to maximise the number of kilojoules you burn off by optimising your level of physical activity. As well as burning more kilojoules, physical activity seems to lower the Set Point so that you can lose weight without too much opposition from your Famine Reaction.

If you're fed up with Diet Dungeon and you want to lose weight and keep it off once and for all, turn the page and let's take a look at this third essential step for permanent weight loss.

Chapter 18

Step 3. How to get the physical activity you need for permanent weight loss

My grandmother started walking five miles a day when she was sixty. She's ninety-three today and we don't know where the hell she is.

Ellen DeGeneres, American stand-up comedian, television host and actor

When it comes to the relationship between exercise and weight management, confusion abounds. We've all heard that physical activity is essential for permanent weight loss, and as a result many people are perplexed when they don't lose weight after extensive efforts to be more active. Research shows, however, that unless you're watching how many kilojoules you put into your body in the form of foods and beverages, then increasing the number of kilojoules you burn through exercise won't lead to significant weight loss,[111] especially in women.[60, 112] Sure, exercise can help you lose a kilo or so of fat while gaining lean body mass,[112, 113] the overall result being that your clothes may get a bit looser even if you don't lose much weight.[51] Exercise can also give you significant health benefits regardless of whether you lose weight.[114] Additionally, exercise can regulate your appetite and make it easier for you to tune into your hunger and satiety signals and eat accordingly.[64] Nonetheless, exercise per se can only take you so far in the weight loss game. It's only by watching how much and what you eat and drink that you can create enough of a kilojoule deficit to lose appreciable amounts of weight and fat, and what physical activity does is speed up the process and help the weight to stay away. It's for this reason that I always emphasise the importance of eating according to your physical needs and being mindful of your food and beverage choices either before or at the same time as you start looking at physical activity.

Physical activity is essential for permanent weight loss, but it can't do the job on its own
If you're taking on the challenge of additional physical activity and you want your efforts to result in notice-able losses of weight and centimetres, you *must* address the question of how much and what you're consuming either at the same time as, or before, you start being more active.

I've met many people who've worn themselves ragged in the belief that they can lose weight solely by exercising. When 46-year-old Jane enlisted my help to lose some 10 kilos via telephone coaching, I learned through her Success Diary and our telephone conversations that she was exercising rigorously for almost two hours a day, seven days a week, in an attempt to lose weight and keep it off. She would wake up at the crack of dawn to go for a one-hour brisk walk with her dogs before setting off for her work as a country veterinarian, which kept her fairly active for most of the day as she visited, examined and treated horses, cows, dogs and other animals. After work, Jane would go for a 50-minute run. She told me that meanwhile the paper-work related to her private veterinary business was getting out of hand and could benefit from more of her time, and she was troubled by a stress fracture in her foot, which was getting worse with all the walking and running she was doing. Jane's doctor had told her that her foot needed several weeks' rest in a plaster cast in order to heal properly, but she was putting it off because she didn't know how she was going to manage her weight if she couldn't walk and run. Indeed, whenever she has stopped exercising at this pace in the past, she has gained weight. In the first of the Success Diaries that Jane sent me, however, I noticed that there was at least one –1 or 0 on every page, meaning that at least once a day she was eating when she wasn't physically hungry, and she was also enjoying a glass of wine or two every night at dinner with her partner. The solution to Jane's predicament was clear to see. If she addressed these two factors that were leading her to consume an excessive number of kilojoules, she would be able to lose weight and keep it off without exercising so intensively. By reducing her alcohol intake in some weeks and by gradually eliminating the –1s and 0s in her Success Diary, Jane lost 2 kilos in three months. For most of that time Jane continued to exercise as much as she had when I first spoke with her, but I was delighted that she noticed she *didn't* gain weight when a bad cold meant that she couldn't get out for her daily walks and runs for almost a week. It may take a while for this new knowledge to fully sink in, but this experience has opened the way for Jane to question her long-held, but in fact mistaken, belief that the only way she can avoid gaining weight is to keep exercising at her accustomed pace – even though this is clearly unsustainable in the long term.

The combined benefits of physical activity and watching how much you eat and drink

If you play your cards right and eat according to your hunger and satiety signals as described in Step 1, and watch your food and beverage choices as described in Step 2, then increasing your level of physical activity will give you a distinct advantage in the weight loss game. In this chapter I'm going to give you a scientifically based guideline as to just how much physical activity you need for permanent weight loss. It's a great deal less than Jane's level of activity, but it's also more than what most people do.

The good news is that the benefits of physical activity for weight management and health are dose-dependent rather than all-or-nothing, meaning that even if you're not terribly active, doing a bit more than you're currently doing will give you a better result. You'll lose weight faster, you'll lose more weight or waistline than you would if you weren't as active, you'll have a better chance of keeping the weight off permanently, and you'll have a healthier, more youthful silhouette – plus you'll enjoy the numerous benefits of regular physical activity for your overall mental and physical wellbeing.

In this chapter I'm going to take you on a guided tour of these benefits of physical activity for weight management, drawing on recent scientific studies. Being an 'energy efficient' person myself (some might say lazy), it's rare that I do anything without strong evidence that it's going to give me good results, and that includes exercise. But when I read studies such as the ones I'm about to share with you, they motivate me to keep up my own efforts to be physically active. I trust that you'll find them motivating, too. In this chapter I'm also going to give you some specific examples of people, including myself, who've risen to the challenge of increasing their commitment to physical activity, with noticeable effects on weight management. If you're still umm-ing and ah-ing about being more physically active for the sake of your weight or your waistline and just can't seem to get started, these stories will soon have you saying, 'I'll have what she's having.'

Physical activity will increase your rate of weight loss

If you're watching what and how much you eat and drink, adding regular physical activity to the mix will help you to lose weight and body fat significantly faster than if you're inactive but still just as careful with your diet. This is the resounding conclusion of a recent review of more than 18 randomised controlled trials investigating the difference between dieting with or without the addition of exercise.[115] For instance, when people with a body mass index in the obese range did four to five sessions of walking per week, each session ranging from 45 minutes to an hour or a distance of 4.8 kilometres, they lost an average of 3 to 4 kilos *more* over the course of a year than people who followed exactly the same diet but didn't do the exercise. When you think about how mindful you need to be to lose 3 or 4 kilos, and when you think about how long it could realistically take to lose all the excess weight you want to lose (it's usually longer than most conventional diets would have you believe), wouldn't you love to lose a few extra bonus kilos simply by adding exercise to the list of things you're already being mindful of?

If you're already in a steady relationship with exercise, adding *more* exercise to your life will give you better results, not only in terms of faster weight loss but also in terms of metabolic health. This is an example of the benefits of exercise being dose-responsive rather than all-or-nothing. And before you start thinking that you're too old or too unfit to exercise, take a look at the following study from the University of Vermont in Canada.[116] The men and women who volunteered for this study were an average age of 64 and had an average weight of 94 kilos. All of them were undergoing rehabilitation after myocardial infarction (heart attack), coronary bypass surgery or chronic angina. The cardiac rehabilitation program included a weight loss component comprising diet plus three exercise sessions a week, each session being 25 to 40 minutes in duration, the preferred form of exercise being walking. At the end of five months the volunteers who followed this standard cardiac rehabilitation program had lost an average of 3.7 kilos – 2.8 kilos of which were fat – and 5 centimetres off their midriffs. However, only half the volunteers had been assigned to follow this standard program. The other half had been randomly assigned to pursue what turned out to be the fast track. While they followed exactly the same diet as the volunteers on the standard program, instead of exercising for 25 to 40 minutes three times a week, they exercised for 45 to 60 minutes five to seven times a week. In other words, their prescription for exercise was to 'walk often and walk far'.

At the end of five months they had lost an average of 8.2 kilos, an impressive 4.5 kilos *more* than the people in the standard program, and they had also lost an average of 3.1 kilos more fat and 2 centimetres more off their waistlines than the people in the standard program. In addition, their overall risk for subsequent cardiac problems – as assessed by a combination of factors such as blood pressure, blood lipid concentrations and insulin sensitivity – was significantly reduced compared to the people in the standard program.

Taken together, this study and the other studies mentioned in this section show that if you're already being careful about what and how much you eat and drink, adding physical activity – or greater levels of physical activity – to your life can turbocharge your weight loss and your metabolic health.

HOW MUCH PHYSICAL ACTIVITY IS REQUIRED TO ACCELERATE WEIGHT LOSS?

As a general rule, 22 minutes per day of moderate-intensity activity – such as walking at a pace that allows you to comfortably keep up a conversation – promotes a modest rate of weight loss, whereas 32 to 60 minutes per day of moderate-intensity activity can more than double this rate of weight loss.[60]

How much physical activity do *you* need to release the brakes on your own weight loss?

The figures above are based on an evaluation of many independent studies on exercise and weight loss, but it's important to note that they are just a guide to how much activity you're likely to need to lose weight. The best way to find out exactly how active you need to be is to experiment with increasing levels of physical activity until you start losing weight at a satisfying pace. When 45-year-old Felicity started the Don't Go Hungry Diet, she didn't lose any weight. Although I saw from her Success Diary that she was a natural at eating only when hungry and stopping before she felt overfull – as well as eating veggies every day – when we looked back over its pages it was clear that she wasn't eating enough fruit and that her alcohol intake was too high. On the exercise front, Felicity felt that she was doing just fine. With a three-year-old daughter to chase after, Felicity estimated that she was getting around 11,000 steps a day – 'no wonder I get tired,' she said to me in an email. But even when she started eating more fruit and reduced her alcohol intake to around two standard drinks per week instead of two standard drinks per day, Felicity's weight remained stubbornly fixed at 82 kilos. Where could the problem lie? Felicity had an inkling that exercise would be the solution to her predicament, because she bought a pedometer and discovered that she wasn't getting as much physical activity as she had thought: around 7000 steps per day. This knowledge empowered her to make the change that finally tipped her into the exhilarating realm of weight loss. Felicity's email tells the story.

From: Felicity
Sent: Tuesday 22ⁿᵈ July 4:16 PM
To: Dr Amanda Sainsbury-Salis
Subject: My weight loss

Hi Amanda,
  Success at last! After seven months on the Don't Go Hungry Diet I have finally beaten my plateau. I am now 79 kilos, 3 kilos down in the six weeks since I came back from my Queensland holiday. I owe my weight loss to exercise. The girls in my Mum's group started a walking group, and now we go for a 90-minute walk twice a week. It is quite hilly where we live and we get a really good workout.
  I always thought that my eating habits were not that bad, and that I had worked out my hunger signals but couldn't understand why I didn't lose weight. More exercise is what I needed, and three hours of strenuous exercise a week seems to have done it. Best of all I really enjoy going for walks with my Mother's group as

it enables me to have a good chat and release the tension that would usually be taken out on my husband and/or daughter, a win–win for all.

I really enjoy the fact that when I eat I don't have to think 'how fattening is that' or 'what is the least fattening thing to eat', I just eat what my body wants until it is satisfied. I find this great as I do dine out quite a bit and no longer is my only choice the 'warm chicken salad'.

Sincerely,

Felicity

Siobhan identified the obstacles to her weight loss

Another example of someone who found the level of exercise they needed to kick-start their weight loss is 48-year-old Siobhan. Siobhan's weight had been creeping up slowly over the years, and at 76 kilos and 1.69 metres tall she had a body mass index (BMI) of 26.6 kg/m^2, putting her fair and square in the 'overweight' range, a position she very much disliked. In the seven months after reading my book and following the Don't Go Hungry Diet, Siobhan lost and regained just one lonesome kilo. Being a nurse and knowing all about the pitfalls of restrictive diets, she was resolute in not giving in to the allure of a quick-fix diet. Determined to get rid of 6 pesky excess kilos before menopause rendered them even harder to lose – and determined to do it in a sustainable way – Siobhan got in her car and drove for seven hours from her home in Kalgoorlie to Perth, where I was giving a workshop on physical strategies for successful weight loss. She knew there must be a logical reason why she wasn't losing weight, but she couldn't see it at the time. 'At that time I felt I was doing enough exercise by attending the gym fairly regularly (three times a week usually) and walking 40 minutes a day on the other days,' she told me in an email some time after the workshop. 'I have always been pretty good at listening to my body signals and I rarely overeat. Perhaps that was why I never veered into the obese range, I usually managed to stay within the healthy weight range until I became perimenopausal.' At that workshop on a rainy winter's morning in Perth, Siobhan realised that there were probably only two things standing between her and her ideal weight. One was the amount of fun foods and alcohol she was enjoying, and the other was the amount of exercise she was doing. How can you tell if insufficient exercise is holding you back in the weight loss stakes? It's easy; all you do is crank up the frequency, duration or intensity of your current level of activity by a do-able increment, and see if you get a better result. That's what Siobhan did, and now she knows for sure why she wasn't losing weight.

From: Siobhan
Sent: Monday 4th May 9:56 PM
To: Dr Amanda Sainsbury-Salis
Subject: Hello from Siobhan in Kalgoorlie

Hi Amanda,

I attended your advanced workshop in Perth last year to fine-tune your methods that I had already been following. Well, I am pleased to report that while on vacation visiting my relatives in Ireland for six weeks in December and January I managed to start losing weight. Knowing that I was on holiday with few distractions, I was motivated to get serious about my weight! I started walking for an hour each day with my brother who set quite a fast pace (lots of huffing and puffing) and we walked up and down hills, through forests and fields, amounting to an average of 8000 steps per walk! Added to this, I limited alcohol to an occasional glass or two of wine on the weekend or for a social occasion and I followed your principles strictly. I avoided the little bites here and there and ate three good meals a day, usually with fruit and yogurt for snacks. I never skimped on dinner, eating my fill and often with a little pat of Kerrygold butter on my delicious Irish spuds! I lost the desire for desserts after dinner every night and saved them for special occasions. By the end of the six weeks when I set off on my journey back to Australia I had lost 4 kilos and was

THRILLED! My greatest challenge now would be to keep it off on my three-week journey back, which would see me stopping for a week each in Toronto, Alabama (where I just LOVE their southern barbeque), and San Francisco. How was I going to maintain my exercise routine and curb my usual desire to try everything different!!! Well, fortunately, a lot of friends and family that I stayed with had their own gym equipment such as treadmills, or they belonged to a gym where I could attend as a guest. Where this was not available, I walked where I could, and even did a workout on one friend's staircase for 40 minutes, varying my pace up and down to the sounds of my iPod!!! With all this exercise and sticking to your principles, I not only maintained my loss but lost another kilo too! And was able to satisfy my desire to eat barbeque and try out some different foods! Since returning to Australia I have lost another kilo and I now weigh 70 kilos (that's a total loss of 6 kilos), and I am finding it so much easier to keep a check on my weight with regular exercise and not too many fun foods! Back in Kalgoorlie I now go for vigorous 35-minute walks three or four times a week and I use a cross trainer at home as well as attending fun dance classes at the gym at least three times a week! Yes, the increased exercise was what I really needed to kick-start my efforts. I also really needed to cut back on 'fun foods' as you call them. Now, whenever I feel like popping a lolly, biscuit, or any other tasty little snack into my mouth, I pause and ask myself whether I really need it now. Thinking about what I ate helped me to lose this weight, and I would allow myself that treat at another more appropriate time like when in company, at book club, at morning tea or another special occasion. So thank you so much Amanda, first and foremost for undertaking all the study that brought you to where you are today, and for being generous enough to share it with us all in such a lovely way!

Cheers,

Siobhan

Twelve months after Siobhan sent me this email, I wrote and asked her how she was going with keeping the weight off. 'I am happy to report that I have pretty much maintained my weight loss,' she wrote back, 'although I do fluctuate between 70 and 72 kilos depending on my exercise level. It is very clear that exercise is the key to keeping my weight down. I should also add that I only have approximately three or four glasses of wine per week now, usually less if I am not socialising, and I guess that that makes a difference, too!'

What I want to show you with Felicity and Siobhan's stories is that if you're already eating only when physically hungry and being mindful about what you eat and drink but you're not losing weight or waistline at a satisfying pace, then finding ways to increase your overall level of physical activity could mean the difference between struggling on for months on end with nothing to show for it or flicking the switch that turbocharges you towards lasting success.

MAKE PHYSICAL ACTIVITY SOMETHING YOU ENJOY

If you don't enjoy physical activity, you won't keep doing it. That's why it's important to try lots of different ways of being active until you find activities you actually enjoy. I'll always remember a young woman who came to one of the first workshops I gave, over six years ago. I'd asked the group to split into pairs to discuss what forms of physical activity they might do, as well as the nitty-gritty logistics of when and how they might do it. Yalinda later told the group that as she was telling her partner that she was going to get up in the mornings and go walking, and then go for a walk around the block at lunchtime, she felt more and more deflated and bored; she actually loathed walking! However, out of the blue it occurred to her that she could start dancing again. As she told her workshop partner about the various dance classes she was going to enquire about and the things that were important to her in a dance class, she was suddenly filled with energy and enthusiasm. Yalinda had attended a lot of dance parties in her late teens and early twenties, and the idea of dancing again didn't feel like exercise at all, it just felt like fun. When Yalinda subsequently told the group about her idea to start dancing again, it was as if she'd plugged herself into a giant power point delivering life force. She sat up straight in her chair, her gestures became natural and enthused, she smiled as she talked, her eyes sparkled and she looked not a day over 21 even though she was in her thirties. I'll never forget that phenomenal transformation.

Last week I emailed Yalinda and asked her how she was going with the dancing. She must have found something she truly loved because she's *still* doing it! 'Thank you for remembering my personal details!' she wrote back. 'What a surprise, even my friends don't remember what I'm doing!! My dancing with Jazzercise is going great, thank you! When I first started I remember being a bit sore and achy and very tired, but I took it slowly and within a couple of months I passed that initial phase and actually started to look forward to my classes and really missed them if went on holiday or something. I've seen so many people come to their first Jazzercise class and push themselves so hard they don't enjoy it and don't come back. But I love it. It's so good to be in a regular dance class where our competitive natures keep us motivated and working hard,' she said.

When you find a form of physical activity that you love, then, like Yalinda and her dancing, you'll most likely stick with it for years. What activities would plug *you* into that giant power point delivering life force and make you want to get moving?

Physical activity can help to lower your Set Point

In Chapter 3 I discussed the concept of your ultimate Set Point or optimum biological weight, the weight below which you cannot go without unnatural restriction over what or how much you eat. Some people's optimum biological weight is just few kilos heavier than they'd ideally like it to be; for others it's 10 or more kilos heavier than their ideal. While being a few kilos more or a few sizes larger than you'd like to be is really no big deal in the grand scheme of things, what if you're trapped at a weight that not only puts you at a higher risk of disease but also makes you feel extremely physically uncomfortable? What if, despite your best efforts, you just can't get down to a comfortable weight or stay there? Whether you're a few sizes more than your ideal or you're carrying 50 or more kilos of excess weight, emerging research suggests that exercise is the key to kicking your Set Point down to a lower level. Let's take a closer look at exactly what this research shows.

When you lose weight, your metabolic rate slows down,[1, 4–7] which means that you are burning, or expending, less energy. Part of the reason for this is simply that it takes less energy to maintain and move a smaller versus a bigger body, just as it takes less petrol to power a smaller than a bigger car. However, the reductions in metabolic rate and energy expenditure that occur with weight loss are *greater* than those that can be explained by reduced body size alone, and that's because the Famine Reaction converts the 'small car' of your now smaller body into a *fuel-efficient* small car. This boost in metabolic efficiency is one of several ways in which your Famine Reaction protects you from wasting away in times of scarcity. Indeed, studies show that the degree to which metabolic rate drops during weight loss predicts the degree of subsequent weight regain.[117, 118] The Famine Reaction is activated whenever you consume fewer kilojoules and fewer nutrients than your body needs to maintain its fat stores and/or when you have less fat than your Set Point. Therefore, if your Famine Reaction is switched on (which is usually indicated by increased physical hunger or cravings for fattening foods), it's a sign that your weight is too far below your current Set Point for comfort. In several studies, this boost in metabolic efficiency, as well as other effects of the Famine Reaction, was deactivated when the reduced weight was maintained for periods of time ranging from one week to three months.[7, 8, 12, 13, 119] It's as if, by staying at the same lower weight and consuming more kilojoules during that time, the body comes to accept the lower weight as its new Set Point. This, in turn, is a signal to the Famine Reaction that it's no longer needed, with the result that energy metabolism returns to normal and the likelihood of weight being regained is reduced. It's important to note that the volunteers who participated in these studies demonstrating normalisation of energy efficiency after weight maintenance at a reduced body weight were doing moderate levels of physical activity, such as walking and occasional non-intensive recreational activities. In retrospect, this seems to have played an important part in deactivating the Famine Reaction, because in another study where physical activity was intentionally restricted so that weight loss was achieved solely through reduced food intake, the Famine Reaction was *not* deactivated when the reduced weight was maintained for over 14 days.[6] While these studies weren't specifically designed to test the effects of physical activity on the Famine Reaction in people (it just happened by chance that the different studies used different levels of physical activity), they highlight the possibility that physical activity plays a pivotal role in reducing the Set Point and deactivating the Famine Reaction. More recent research in animals suggests that this is indeed the case.[73, 120]

In a study designed to directly test the effects of exercise on the Set Point and the Famine Reaction, Dr Paul MacLean and his colleagues at the University of Colorado in Denver fed sedentary rats a high-fat diet for 16 weeks.[73] Some of the rats remained lean despite this dietary onslaught, whereas others ended up almost twice as heavy as their lean counterparts. As with humans,[104, 121] some rats are genetically predisposed to overeat when given unlimited access to a fatty diet, whereas others stay lean because they instinctively eat less when the food they have access to is very rich.[122] The researchers then selected the most obese rats in the group (that is, the ones with the greatest genetic propensity to gain weight) and switched them to a low-fat, reduced-kilojoule diet that resulted in them losing 10 to 15 per cent of their body weight within two weeks. All rats were sedentary during the weight loss phase, but after that the rats were divided into two groups. One group remained sedentary for the remainder of the experiment, and the other group was trained to run on a treadmill for half-an-hour a day, six days a week. For the following eight weeks, rats in both the sedentary and the exercise groups were fed a low-fat diet sufficient to maintain them at their reduced body weight. After this period of weight maintenance, the rats in both groups were allowed to eat low-fat food ad libitum, meaning that they could eat as much as their appetite decreed. Now, what happened during the ensuing eight weeks of ad libitum feeding is a wonderful illustration of the benefits of physical activity for weight management:

Within eight weeks of eating according to their hunger, the sedentary rats had regained all of the weight they'd lost while on the reduced-kilojoule diet, whereas the exercising rats regained significantly less weight, weighing approximately 10 per cent less, and having approximately 13 per cent less body fat, than the sedentary rats. Most inspiringly, the total body fat of the exercising rats was no different from that of lean rats that had never been obese in their entire lives!

Seeking to determine the reason for these differences in weight regain between sedentary and exercising rats, Dr MacLean's team meticulously measured kilojoule intake and kilojoule expenditure in both groups during the eight weeks of ad libitum feeding. Surprisingly, the exercising rats weren't burning any more kilojoules than the sedentary rats, showing that exercise doesn't affect body weight simply by increasing energy expenditure, as is often assumed. Rather, exercise blunted appetite. While the sedentary rats wolfed down up to 50 per cent more food per day than the lean rats until they had regained their heavyweight status, the exercising rats *didn't* eat any more than lean rats. Taken together, these findings show that exercise enabled these weight-reduced rats to assume a lower Set Point without their Famine Reaction intervening and stimulating their appetite.

Exercise helped Valerie kick down her Set Point and lose two dress sizes

In light of these emerging findings, if you feel stuck at an uncomfortable weight, then physical activity could well be your passport to a lower Set Point and a feeling of greater comfort in your skin. This principle seems to work in everyday life as well as in the lab. One such example is Valerie, a 58-year-old academic who used the principles in this book to go from a size 20 to a size 16 over the course of a year and has maintained her leaner silhouette for more than two years. Valerie told me that her weight came down in a stepwise fashion and that the main thing that enabled her to 'kick it down' to progressively lower levels was the times she spent visiting and caring for her elderly father, who lived in a coastal town several hundred kilometres distant from her. Free from the time constraints of lectures and student contact for a week or more at a time, Valerie had time to not only clock up around 10,000 steps in various activities per day, as she normally did when she was at work, but also to go for vigorous bike rides or long, invigorating beach walks three or four times a week. Perhaps this sounds like a lot of exercise to you. Valerie certainly acknowledged that she was not able to sustain this level of physical activity into the semester. But from the feeling of poise she got when she shimmied into one of her brand-new fitted tank tops and easily buttoned one of her smart jackets over the top before heading off to university to give a lecture to an audience of hundreds of students, she found it well worth the effort to have packed in as much exercise as she could during her semester break.

Grace achieved a seemingly impossible reduction in her Set Point with exercise

My friend Grace is another example of the ability of exercise to help reduce the Set Point. Having lost 12 kilos in 18 months by listening to her body, and then another 5 kilos in the same way over subsequent years, 41-year-old Grace had maintained a stable weight of around 65 kilos for more than three years.

At 1.64 metres tall, and lean in all the right places, Grace assumed that this was the weight she was meant to be, her optimum biological weight. It was at that point, however, that something happened and Grace dropped another kilo, and for over 18 months her weight has hovered around 64 kilos instead of 65. This may not sound like a lot of weight to lose, but when you're already at your optimum biological weight, it takes a miracle to kick your weight down to a lower Set Point that your body will happily defend. That 'miracle' is called physical activity. What happened was that Grace went on a month-long trip, visiting friends across England, Spain and France. With her love of walking and Indian dance, Grace already maintains an active lifestyle, but during her holidays in Europe she was even more active. For hours every day she was on her feet walking and visiting museums and monuments. If you've ever worn a pedometer during a trip to an interesting museum, you'll know what a huge number of steps you can notch up with this type of tourism, especially if you use public transport to get there and back. Moreover, as she was staying at the homes of several different friends during her time abroad, Grace got a fair whack of incidental strength training as she dragged and lifted her 23-plus kilos of luggage between multiple planes, buses, trains and taxis. The thing that makes me suspect that it was this boost in physical activity that caused Grace's Set Point to shift is the fact that she didn't make any particular efforts to restrict how much she ate over this time. She has been listening to her body signals and eating accordingly for over 15 years now, and she has so much respect for her mind, body and spirit that in all that time I've never seen her eat more than she needs, nor deny her true needs. Interestingly, Grace has maintained her lower weight of 64 kilos ever since she got back from that holiday over 18 months ago, even though, despite still leading an active life-style, she hasn't been quite as active as when she was away.

The bottom line is that, regardless of how much you weigh, if you want to be the weight you're biologically meant to be, then using – really energetically using – your body to live your life to the fullest right now will help you to get there. Later in this chapter I'm going to show you the levels of physical activity that you need to aim for: enough to get the benefits of physical activity for your health and your weight but not so much as to cause injury or be otherwise unsustainable.

WHAT IF YOU HAD TIME TO EXERCISE?

I know you don't have time to exercise, but what if you were one of those people who did? What would you do differently? Could you try it out, just for one week?

These are the questions I read in a magazine once, and they prompted me to take the challenge and imagine – just for one week – that I was one of those women who seem to have time to do things like go walking before work or go to enlivening sessions at the gym. (In case you haven't noticed, I don't have a natural affinity for structured exercise; almost all of the physical activity I've achieved in my life has been as a by-product of doing other things like commuting, working, dancing and bringing up children.)

Well, let me tell you that this little experiment not only had an impact on how much exercise I did, as you'll read later in this chapter, it also had a totally unexpected impact on my sense of self-worth. When you tell your colleague that you can't accept his invitation to be the honorary secretary of some committee or other, or you tell that friend who only ever talks about herself, 'Sorry, I can't do coffee today' (and then go and use the extra time you carved out to do something for your own health and wellbeing), it's inevitable that you'll notice interesting changes in how much you value yourself. I liked this effect so much that I extended the experiment beyond the one-week trial, and now I'm one of those women who seem to have time for exercise because I keep going back to structured exercises like swimming and fast walking. You might like to try it for yourself – just for one week – and see what happens.

Physical activity helps to abate the effects of genes on body weight

Unquestionably, your genes have an important influence on your weight. For example, recent research shows that people with certain variations in the DNA sequence of a gene called the fat mass and obesity-associated gene, which is estimated to occur in at least 15 per cent of the population, have a larger appetite and are significantly heavier than those who don't have those variations.[104, 123] Sounds unfair, doesn't it? But if you feel that your genes may be loading the dice against you, don't despair, because it has been shown that people with this genetic variation who are physically active weigh significantly less than people with this genetic variation who are sedentary.[104] In other words, you can counteract any genetic tendency to carry excess weight by making the effort to be physically active. Honestly, the more I learn about physical activity and the various ways in which it affects weight management, the more motivated I am to make sure I get my quota.

Physical activity will help you keep the weight off for good

Exercise not only helps you to get lean and healthy, it also helps you to keep the weight off once you've lost it. When it comes to keeping excess weight off for the long haul, scientific studies unanimously show that physical activity is essential. If you're not an aficionado of moving your body, this statement may make you want to groan and give up. The good news is, however, that even relatively small amounts of exercise will bring you significant benefits. To show you what I mean, I want to tell you about a study that I learned about at a recent conference.[124]

This study followed 200-odd women during the year after they'd lost an average of 12 kilos by diet plus exercise. The women were randomly divided into three groups. All three groups participated in a year-long weight management program consisting of monthly group meetings with discussion about healthy diet and exercise. In addition, the first group of women was scheduled to do two 40- to 50-minute sessions of aerobic training per week under the supervision of an exercise physiologist. The second group, in addition to their monthly meeting, was scheduled to do two 40-minute sessions of strength training per week, also under the supervision of an exercise physiologist. The strength training session included a circuit of 11 exercises such as squats and sit-ups. The third group was not scheduled to do any structured exercise, but at their monthly meetings they received general instructions about the importance of regular physical activity for weight management.

At the end of the year, the differences among the three groups were clearly apparent. While this was to be expected, nobody suspected just how great the differences would be, nor how little time it would take for them to become apparent. Over the course of the year, some women in the study were found to have gained an additional 50 per cent of fat around their midriff (intra-abdominal adipose tissue). This fat sits around organs such as the liver and pancreas and contributes to metabolic diseases such as cardiovascular disease and diabetes. On the other hand, some women in the study did not gain *any* intra-abdominal adipose tissue in the year after they'd lost weight.

Which women do you think they were? As you'd expect, they were, quite simply, those who stuck with their program and exercised consistently, even if they missed a few sessions here and there. It didn't matter whether they did aerobic or strength training, all the women who did at least five of the eight training sessions they'd been assigned per month (an average of 48 to 60 minutes of supervised aerobic or strength training per week) avoided regaining belly fat. The amount of exercise they did is equivalent to, say, going to the gym and doing a 30-minute strength-training circuit twice a week. Or doing two 15-minute bursts of strength-training sessions at home involving exercises such as sit-ups or lifting hand-held weights plus swimming lengths of the pool for 30 minutes a week. Or going for a vigorous walk or a run-walk for an hour every week. In other words, moderate amounts of physical activity.

While 48 to 60 minutes of exercise per week was shown in this study to prevent people who had lost weight through diet and exercise from regaining the most dangerous fat, intra-abdominal fat, it usually takes more than this level of physical activity to keep weight off overall. Indeed, the women in the study who exercised and avoided regaining belly fat did regain a bit of weight over the year-long study (3 to 4 kilos on average), but this was significantly less than the amount regained by the women who didn't exercise (6 to 7 kilos on average). Once again, this shows that some exercise is better than none. The key question is then: exactly how much exercise would have prevented these women from regaining any weight at all?

How much is enough to keep weight off?

If you've lost weight and you want to keep it off, the verdict from current research is that you need to work up to doing an average of about 60 to 90 minutes of moderate-intensity activity per day.[60-62] Moderate-intensity activity is something like walking at a pace that allows you to comfortably keep up a conversation. If you use a pedometer, it's easy to see how much activity you're getting compared to the amounts recommended for preventing weight regain, because 60 to 90 minutes of moderate-intensity activity is equivalent to about 8000 to 12,000 steps.

THE PEDOMETER EFFECT

Using a pedometer can make you do things you didn't expect you would. Andy, 47, calls this mysterious force 'the pedometer effect', and it pushes her to do things like top up her step count at the end of the day by asking her husband to join her in a quick walk around the neighbourhood, or go for a walk first thing in the morning if she knows it will be the only chance she'll have to be active that day. She gets great satisfaction from looking at her pedometer at the end of the day and seeing a number higher than 8000. With the pedometer effect on your side, clocking up those daily 8000 to 12,000 steps can feel a lot more do-able.

While 60 to 90 minutes per day may sound like an awful lot of time to commit to something like walking, if you're doing more vigorous forms of exercise such as fast walking, dancing, swimming or cycling, the amount of time you need to spend being active in order to prevent weight regain is less. For example, whereas it might take you 90 minutes to clock up 12,000 steps by walking, you could achieve the same amount of activity in 40 minutes with a vigorous bike ride.

PEDOMETER STEP EQUIVALENTS
Your pedometer won't count steps reliably for any activities besides walking or running, but if you search 'pedometer step equivalents' on the internet, you'll find plenty of sites telling you how many steps various activities are equivalent to.

The other concept emerging from this research is that the total number of kilojoules expended through physical activity seems to be more important for preventing weight regain (or losing weight in the first place) than the type of activity you do. This means that whether you get your physical activity predominantly thorough a structured 60-minute session in the gym every day, or whether you get it in short bursts of activity accumulated over the course of the day, such as walking to and from the bus stop, taking the stairs instead of the lift, going for a short walk at lunch time and cleaning your home, it's all good.

Many people gasp in dismay when they see how much physical activity is recommended for preventing weight regain. If you're finding it difficult to scrape together 3000 steps a day, these numbers can sound demoralising. However, it's important to note that these numbers are only an *estimation* of how much physical activity is required to prevent weight regain in most people. It's also important to note that the amount of activity required to prevent weight regain is different for different people, depending on factors such as your genetic propensity to gain weight, your sex, size, age and health. Indeed, in studies of so-called Big-time

Losers – volunteers on an international registry of more than 5000 people who have lost more than 13.6 kilos and kept it off for more than a year – it has emerged that while the overwhelming majority do some form of regular physical activity – the equivalent of about one hour of brisk walking every day – some of them don't.[58] As such, these recommendations are not an all-or-nothing proclamation that doing 90 minutes of exercise per day will guarantee that your excess weight won't come back but that if you do 59 or fewer minutes of exercise per day you will instantly forfeit your chances of long-term success. This is not so. As you have seen from various case studies in this chapter, it's a question of trying out different levels of physical activity for yourself and watching how your weight and size respond until you find a level of physical activity that's right for you.

Approximate levels of physical activity required to prevent weight regain

To avoid regaining weight, you need to accumulate a total of about 60 to 90 minutes of moderate-intensity activity per day, such as walking at a pace that allows you to comfortably keep up a conversation, or 8000 to 12,000 steps per day.

Puff the magic dragon

One of the outstanding questions in research into the amount of physical activity required to prevent weight regain is whether vigorous activities that make you huff and puff, and whether strength training that makes you push against resistance, offer additional benefits for weight management over and above the number of kilojoules they burn. Emerging evidence suggests that they do. For instance, it was shown in a recent study that a group of Big-time Losers who had lost over 30.6 kilos and kept it off for an average of 14 years did 59 minutes of physical activity per day on average, with an average of 24 minutes of that time being spent doing higher intensity activities such as aerobic dance, jogging or, in the case of people taking part in that international study who live in snowy climates, cross-country skiing.[62]

There is some evidence that vigorous activity may blunt appetite and result in the body burning fat more efficiently.[61] For instance, one study compared the amount of food the same group of volunteers spontaneously ate after a bout of high-intensity exercise and after a bout of low-intensity exercise.[125] Even though both exercise sessions burned the same number of kilojoules, the volunteers ate less after the high-intensity exercise. New research also suggests that strength training may be important for weight management, mainly by preventing loss of lean body mass and the subsequent reductions in metabolic rate that contribute to weight regain.[60] For instance, a recent report showed that losing weight through dietary changes – with or without the addition of aerobic exercise – resulted in a significant reduction in lean body mass (including muscle mass), a decline in muscle strength and a drop in the resting metabolic rate.[63] Significantly, when three supervised 40-minute sessions of resistance (strength) training per week were added to this weight loss regimen, these adverse effects of weight loss did not occur.[63]

The greater the frequency, duration and intensity of your physical activity, the greater the benefits will be for your weight and your health

Before changing your physical activity habits, check with your doctor or health care provider that it is safe for you to do so. Additionally, when you do different types of physical activities from the ones you normally do – especially activities like strength training – it's best to do them under the supervision of a suitably qualified exercise physiologist or personal trainer, at least initially, to learn how to do them correctly and to reduce the risk of injuries.

While research into the usefulness of vigorous activity and strength training for weight management continues, what is already clear is that these two forms of physical activity bestow significantly greater benefits than moderate activity in terms of promoting mental health and preventing certain cancers, diabetes, heart disease and other disorders.[60, 126]

Once you've got the all clear from your doctor or health care provider, if you enjoy the feeling that comes from pushing your body that little bit further, pounding it out in a vigorous exercise session or feeling your muscles strain under resistance, go for it!

Exercise helped Tiffany to lose 28 kilos and keep it off for more than two years

If you know someone who has lost a significant amount of weight and kept it off for a significant amount of time, you'll probably notice that they lead a pretty active lifestyle. Last year I gave a series of lectures on the science of weight management to a group of practising and future weight loss consultants. At the end of my last lecture, a young woman came up to thank me for my lectures and tell me how they had made so many things click into place for her. Tiffany, 32 years old and 1.7 metres tall, told me that three-and-a-half years ago she had weighed 113 kilos; now she was 28 kilos lighter, and she had kept that weight off for more than two years. 'What an achievement!' I exclaimed. 'How did you do it?' Tiffany told me that she'd done it in *exactly* the way I'd talked about in my lectures. 'I listened to my body,' she said jubilantly. 'I knew instinctively back then that it was wrong to be so hungry that I couldn't sleep at night. I realised that if I was doing everything I could to lose weight and be healthy, then hunger was a sign that I was just expecting too much from my body and pushing myself too hard. So if I was hungry at night or whenever, I'd just go and eat whatever healthy food I needed to fill myself up.' Tiffany told me that the thing she appreciated most about my lectures was that she now understood the theory behind everything she had experienced in her own successful weight loss adventure. As such, she now felt confident that she would be able to help others to achieve similar success. 'To be able to pass what I've experienced in my own life and what I've learned from you on to other people is massive,' she said with a beam. 'I know the difference that this way of losing weight has made to my life. To be able to pass that on to another and know that it could impact their life so positively is just an awesome experience.' I wanted to ask Tiffany more about her experiences so that I could share them with you, but there were other students waiting to ask me questions and I had a train to catch, so I asked her if she'd have time to meet me for coffee some day.

Over a hot chocolate several weeks later, I soon learned that eating when she was hungry was only part of the story. Here are the three ingredients that Tiffany considers to be fundamental to her successful weight loss.

First, Tiffany recorded what she ate and drank in a food diary. 'I did this religiously for about eight months, then periodically thereafter,' she told me. Tiffany is a living example of what scientific studies have shown: that people who keep a written record of what they consume lose more weight and keep it off for longer than people who don't.[59, 127] (By the way, have you started your Success Diary yet? You won't need to use it forever, but it's the best way to ensure your success right from the outset.) Nowadays, Tiffany no longer keeps a food diary, because she has completely changed her eating habits and she no longer needs it.

The second secret to which Tiffany attributes her success is learning the art of patience. 'Because I was so big, I wanted my excess weight to be gone overnight. And it doesn't happen overnight. In the past I'd lose a lot of weight in about three months and then put it all back on again and more. This time I was focused on changing my lifestyle. I kept telling myself, "This is how it is. I'm doing everything well. I'm eating well, I'm recording what I eat, I'm exercising. If I just cruise along with it, it will work." I had to have faith that I would lose the weight, and I had to trust myself that I could keep going,' she told me. Tiffany's faith bore fruit. Within 12 months she had lost 25 kilos, and six months later she had lost a further 3 kilos and had reached her optimum biological weight.

The final thing to which Tiffany attributes her successful weight loss is – you guessed it – exercise. In fact, this is where Tiffany's winning journey began. One day, still reeling from the shock of seeing herself in a video taken at a recent family gathering, Tiffany saw an advertisement in her local paper for a new gym in her neighbourhood. She jumped at the opportunity to try it out, and before long she had joined the gym and was en route to success. Although Tiffany, a single mum, didn't get much support in her weight loss journey from her immediate family, at the gym there were several people who gave her 'that little bit of extra oomph'; her trainer, the gym staff and other gym members would all cheer her on and encourage her to keep going. The gym has become an important part of Tiffany's life. She goes there six days a week for a vigorous workout consisting of resistance and cardio training. On most days she does a one-hour workout, and two days a week she does a two-hour workout. On average, therefore, Tiffany gets 70 minutes of moderate to vigorous physical activity per day, in line with the 60 to 90 minutes of moderate physical activity recommended for permanent weight reduction. 'Exercise is critical,' Tiffany says of her success. 'It keeps my appetite in sync, and it keeps me energetic and enthusiastic about being healthy. I love going to the gym,' she says. I can see how much pride Tiffany takes in being fit and healthy. As she sipped her hot chocolate and told me about her experiences, Tiffany looked like a porcelain doll with her soft curves and a baby pink tank top, but I've learned not to be fooled by appearances. With a look of steely determination, she told me that she can do about 6 kilometres on the treadmill in 40 minutes!

It has now been more than two years since Tiffany lost all that weight, and her continued commitment to exercise undoubtedly helps her to keep it off. 'In my whole adult life, I've never been the same weight for this long. Never. I was always either losing weight or gaining it back, and the longest I've ever kept weight off in the past was one year maximum. Now, I know the weight's gone forever,' she said jubilantly.

ALL-WEATHER ACTION

One of the most common obstacles to regular physical activity is the weather. If you feel it's too hot, too humid, too sunny, too dark, too cold, too windy or too rainy to get outside and do the physical activity you enjoy, what *can* you do instead? There are so many ways to be active even when the weather is against you. There's 'mall walking' (a walk through the long, winding corridors of a shopping centre), ice-skating, squash, following an exercise DVD in the comfort of your own home, bowling, or visiting a museum, plus, of course, going to an indoor pool, gym or dance class. When 65-year-old Beth – whom I introduced in Chapter 7 – decided to lose weight, she not only had to overcome muscle weakness brought about by Hashimoto's Thyroiditis, with which she was diagnosed 10 years earlier, and years of fatigue and inactivity, she also had to find sustainable ways to beat the weather. However, having lost 9 kilos in 10 months and kept it off for over 10 months, she has found her ideal solution.

For me the secret has been in finding a way to walk which was enjoyable and which I could do at any time of day or night, in any weather. I used to enjoy walking around the lake near my house at 6 am on warm summer mornings, but come Easter I'd give up because it was raining, too cold or too dark. So I knew when I started your program that I'd have to find a way to walk which wasn't unpleasant in any way, or I wouldn't keep it up. I started iPod walking when I was staying at my daughter's house looking after my grand-daughter, when it was too hot to walk outside. So we made a walking track inside her house through all the rooms and she joined me in my perambulations. We then discovered that the walk to and from school also was more enjoyable if we wore our iPods. I also found it imperative to have really comfortable (not necessar-

ily expensive) walking shoes, as any hint of discomfort results in a tendency to give up. Now I do most of my walking inside, and often half of it at night time. I really enjoy it and when I stop walking for a while and get back into it, I wonder why I didn't start again sooner – old habits die hard. The one problem is finding enough time, as I take almost two hours to walk 12,000 steps and I really need to do 12,000 daily to lose weight (about 5000 will keep my weight stable).

Dangerous curves ahead

Another benefit of physical activity – besides helping you to lose weight faster, reach your optimum biological weight and maintain your leaner physique – is that it can noticeably improve the appearance of your body. Studies show that physical activity results in greater fat or centimetre losses from around the waist than from around the hips, particularly with more intense forms of physical activity such as those that improve your strength and your cardiovascular fitness.[76, 78] This is probably because belly fat is more metabolically active than hip and thigh fat and is therefore more likely to be burned off when you consume fewer kilojoules than you need, and also because exercise can increase the size of muscles such as the gluteus maximus in your hip and thigh region. The result of these changes is that exercise can decrease your waist-to-hip ratio (your waist circumference divided by your hip circumference, as described in Chapter 3), resulting in not only a reduced risk for metabolic diseases such as diabetes and heart disease but also a more youthful physique. For men, this means less paunch and more six-pack, and for women it means less muffin top and more of the hourglass silhouette that has been idealised throughout the centuries (although nowadays the measurements that are in vogue are less ample than they tended to be in earlier times!). Another way to see the direct effects of physical activity on body shape is to see what happens when you stop. When a group of young female dancers ceased their regular training for two months, they didn't gain any weight but they showed significant increases in their waist circumference as well as their waist-to-hip ratio.[128] For many people, myself included, the effects of physical activity on appearance are very motivating, because the benefit of being active – or the consequence of *not* being active – can be seen in such a short time frame.

Knowing the many benefits of physical activity from the scientific literature, and having seen how my clients who exercised achieved better results than those who didn't, I decided some years ago that 'when I grow up I'm going to be one of those women who exercise'. Don't get me wrong; I'm no couch potato. Ever since I started my permanent weight loss adventure in my early twenties I've been in the habit of getting decent doses of daily activity: mostly around 8000 steps per day, sometimes around 12,000 steps or more per day, but sometimes only around 3000 steps or fewer per day. Mostly, I have achieved these levels of physical activity while doing things such as walking or catching public transport instead of driving whenever possible, shopping, dancing and sometimes going for a stroll. This 'incidental' activity – along with my husband, two young children, a medical research team and writing books – fits snugly and sustainably into my life and has helped me to lose 28 kilos and keep it off for what is now more than 13 years. However, I often wondered what kind of body I might have if I stepped up the pace and did some dedicated strength or aerobic training as well as my incidental activity. This question flitted sporadically through my mind for several years, until recently something happened and I finally decided that it was time to take action: I turned 40.

While this major milestone birthday put the seal on my decision to be more active, there was just one small problem: *when* was I going to make this heightened investment in myself? Was I going to go to the gym on weekends and book my children in for yet another session of child-care? No way. Was I going to nick out to the gym in my lunch break at work? Um, what lunch break? Was I going to join a local Pilates class on Thursdays when I stay home to catch up on things? Unfortunately, finding a class that was within walking distance from my home and that fell on a Thursday, in between my various appointments, deliveries and tax returns, plus the mad rush to go to the shops and then prepare dinner before my husband came home with the kids, proved impossible. I started to despair about my plans to improve my fitness. What could I change in my life in order to make it happen?

But wait . . .

What about my family's regular Sunday afternoon visits to the aquatic centre? Instead of just splashing around with my husband and children in the warm pool for the whole time we were there, I could ask Hubby to watch the kids for half an hour while I ploughed through some laps.

Brilliant!

Pulling against the water's resistance, I envisaged my arms firming up and my waist getting smaller, and I saw myself feeling fabulous in anything I chose to wear. My whole body feels addictively invigorated after my half-hour Sunday swim, and if I ever have to miss it for any reason I feel very disappointed. While my Sunday swim was a good start, I wondered what kind of body I might have if exerted myself like that every day. What else could I change in my life to bring it on?

Thinking I'd found the perfect solution, I ordered a Pilates DVD over the internet. In the comfort and convenience of my own home I'd be able to strengthen and shape my whole body. The kids would have a ball. But I was wrong. Not only did I find the 50-minute workout excruciatingly difficult and tedious, the kids got bored after five minutes and started climbing on me while I was trying to do killer crunches. The DVD is now languishing somewhere at the back of the wall unit.

Just as I was about to give up my dream of having a better body at 40 than I've ever had in my life, I had one of those life-changing 'Aha!' moments. It came from a book I was reading at the time: *Fit & Firm Forever* by award-winning journalist Paula Goodyer. In Paula's book I learned that you can shape, tone and strengthen your whole body simply by adding several sets of crunches, push-ups and other strength-building exercises to your weekly activities. This was a revelation for me.

Somehow I'd assumed that the only way I'd be able to get results from strength training would be with complicated gym equipment or supervised routines. Never in my wildest dreams had I imaged that such simple exercises as push-ups could give me results. This was something I could envisage fitting compactly and sustainably into my life.

Afraid of doing something wrong and damaging my body, and coaxed by Paula's intelligent book, I then did something that was previously unimaginable for me: I went and had a few sessions with a personal trainer. This was a fantastic investment. After explaining to Matthew exactly what I wanted (to shape and tone my body at home, without any complicated equipment and whenever I found a scrap of time), he showed me how to do a series of simple strength-building exercises without hurting myself, aided by just a few pairs of hand weights that I bought from a sports shop. He then designed a program specifically suited to my abilities. Matthew's personalised program blew me away with its ingenuity. Because there were only three different exercises to do on each of the five days in the program, and because those three exercises were different and worked different muscle groups on each day, and because it only took me 10 minutes to do all the prescribed reps and sets, and because I could do them in a little private corner of my bedroom at any time, the whole program was so incredibly do-able that I actually did it (most of the time).

Fuelled by mounting confidence in my physicality, I then did something else that was exhilaratingly unlike me. On my precious, busy Thursdays at home alone, I started driving to the pool and racing the clock to swim a kilometre. Exercise was starting to give me a real high. Triumphantly, I wrote to the author of the book that had helped me get going and told her of the strange and wonderful effects her book was having on me. She wrote back with an even stranger recommendation.

From: Paula Goodyer
Sent: Thursday 9th April 10:04 AM
To: Dr Amanda Sainsbury-Salis
Subject: strength training

Dear Amanda,

Good for you for starting strength training. It really helps to sculpt your body, building muscle tone, definition and a curvier silhouette.

By the way, just wondered if you'd considered doing a bit of jogging (or maybe you already are). A lot of people think it means running for long distances but (as long as your knees are OK) if you can work up gradually to just 20 minutes it boosts the intensity of a workout – and makes a short workout more effective when time is short. I started it when I had young kids because I could dash out and do it while my partner was at home. A 51-year-old friend who always said she 'couldn't run' has amazed me by taking it up – again, not running huge distances, but for about 20 minutes and then slowing down for a walk.

Have a good Easter!
Best wishes,
Paula

My initial reaction to Paula's email was to think it must have been intended for someone else. Me? Run? She obviously didn't know that when I was at school I was the cleverest kid at getting out of sport. Besides, it can't be good for the knees. However, when I looked into the emerging research on knees and running, it seemed that provided you don't have any existing problems with your knees, short bursts of occasional running may actually help prevent problems later on.[129] Moreover, the idea that running could save me time held massive appeal.

Ten days later, and who's that running in her local park?

Although I could only run three-quarters of a length of the park before stopping, I was delighted that I could actually run at all. In the ensuing month I worked up to running four lengths of the park before taking a walking break. I can't say I loved running, but I was rather smitten by the buzz it gave me afterwards. One Wednesday my husband and children were at home sick, so I stayed with them. By 5 pm, after pottering around our apartment all day, I actually craved the feeling that running gave me. I pulled on my runners and ducked out. In 35 minutes flat I got in a 15-minute walk up and down stairs and inclines to and from the park and a 20-minute run-walk on lovely soft grass, totting up in the process 4500 steps on my pedometer and a priceless feeling of being fully alive. To help me maintain my motivation, knowing full well that most of the time I'd rather stroll to a café for a latte than go for a run, I decided to participate in a 4 kilometre fun run to raise money for the research institute where I work. Now that was motivating! Knowing that my family, friends and colleagues had paid money to sponsor my run, and knowing that many of them would be running with me on the day, I had no choice but to keep training.

Ignore the nay-sayers

Something that struck me on my journey to better form and fitness was the number of discouraging messages I received from people around me. Before I found Matthew, I spoke with two other personal trainers, both of whom told me that unless I committed to a certain duration of additional physical activity per week, an amount that I knew was totally unrealistic for me, I'd be 'wasting my time'. An active friend whose partner runs for an hour every day, upon learning that I'd taken up running, informed me that unless I ran continuously for more than 20 minutes I wouldn't get any benefit from it. If I didn't know better, having read many research publications showing that the benefits of exercise for weight management and health are dose-dependent rather than all-or-nothing (that is, the more you do, the more benefits you get), I might have given up.

The fact of the matter is that in just two months after increasing my level of activity from predominantly incidental activity to incidental activity plus a 30-minute swim, a 35-minute run-walk and four to five 10-minute bursts of strength training per week, I saw noticeable changes. The strength-training program Matthew wrote for me became too easy and I had to ask him to revamp it so that I could keep growing stronger. Whereas before I would struggle to swim 650 metres in half an hour, within two months I could swim a kilometre in the same time. Additionally, while I was still the same 65 kilos that I was before I started exercising, my clothes glided on more easily and my stuffing seemed to have shifted, so much so that sometimes I had to do a double take before recognising my body.

Were those really *my* arms in the mirror? Surely my arms used to have more wobbly bits on them?

And whose reflection was that in the shop window? Surely my curves weren't as 'dangerous' as that before?

And was that really *my* shadow cast upon the wall? I seemed to recall that my bum was slung lower than that before?

While part of me suspected that I was just imagining these changes, they must have been real, because I started receiving exhilarating compliments. Someone at work said to me, 'What have you been doing? You look fantastic!' That felt great. However, the most obvious effects of exercise on my body became apparent several months after I started. It was mid-winter, I'd been on holidays to see Mum and Dad in Perth with my husband and children, I'd stopped exercising for a week, a week without exercise turned into six weeks without exercise, and before I knew it my body had morphed back to how it was before! There was no doubt about it; all my extra efforts to be fit and strong really *had* benefited my body. This realisation prompted me to pull my hand weights and runners out from under my bed, dust them off and get going again.

It has now been more than a year since I resolved to get fitter and firmer by adding structured aerobic and strength-training exercise to my life, in addition to the incidental activity I was already doing, and I'm happy to report that I'm hooked. Sometimes I go for a week or a month without being as active as I usually am, but I keep coming back to exercise. Every time I 'fall off the wagon' and stop exercising, I learn more sustainable ways to stay on the wagon. For example, while I'd often come up with excuses for not going run-walking, and while I'd often need to write 'go for a run-walk!' in my diary, along with a long list of other things I needed to do but didn't particularly want to do, when I quit running and started fast walking in the hilliest part of my neighbourhood instead, the excuses stopped and I no longer needed to write it into my to-do list. Unlike running, I actually enjoy the process of fast walking (and swimming), not just the feeling it gives me afterwards, so it's no hardship to just do it. As another example, I learned to spice up my strength-training sessions at home by adding a wide variety of different exercises to the mix, using different techniques such as resistance bands, hand weights and sometimes just my own body weight, listening to music while I exercised, and only choosing to do exercises that I like doing, not the ones that make me think, 'Oh great, not this one again!' I also discovered that many gyms will allow you to participate in group fitness classes or use their equipment on a casual basis (without paying for ongoing membership), at a cost per visit that's similar to what it would cost you to go to the movies and buy a choc-top. So now I occasionally do a casual class in a gym, and this gives me additional variety and increases my motivation.

Before I started exercising, I used to spend hours devouring Trinny and Susannah's tips for disguising bingo wings, bra bulges and a voluptuous belly, as presented in their famous books and their television series on *What Not to Wear*. Now that I'm in a long-term sustainable relationship with the kind of exercise that demands more from my body than incidental activity does, I've got less to disguise and more to simply enjoy about my body.

If you're not already in a steady relationship with physical activity, particularly the kind that builds your cardiovascular fitness and strengthens your muscles, what kind of body might *you* be hiding from yourself and from the world?

Build up to it gradually

If you're new to the idea of moving your body, the levels of physical activity recommended for preventing weight regain may seem daunting. It's important to keep in mind, however, that you don't need to reach that level of physical activity immediately. It *is* possible to lose weight without much physical activity, it's just that exercise will speed things along or make it easier. Even relatively modest increments in physical activity will help in the beginning. For example, studies have shown that people who used pedometers and increased the number of steps they walked by 2100 or more per day lost approximately 1 kilo more than people who didn't.[60] While this is a modest increase in weight loss, it points to the benefits of even modest increases in physical activity, at least in the beginning. However, keeping weight off in the long term is critically dependent upon greater levels of activity. So, if you're starting your weight loss adventure from a completely sedentary position, a good aim is to gradually increase your level of physical activity towards the level recommended to prevent weight regain some time between now and when you reach your ideal biological weight. And unless you're trying to reach your ideal biological weight with a quick-fix diet that leaves you feeling hungry, this means you've got some time up your sleeve.

Do you remember Maree from Chapter 9 who came to one of my workshops and lost 12 kilos in 12 months and has maintained her svelte size 12 for the past eight months (and counting)? Maree is an excellent example of someone who has gradually built up her level of physical activity to the level recommended for permanent weight loss. When she started her weight loss adventure, 44-year-old Maree was so unfit that even changing a light bulb was a feat of endurance. 'I would stand on the step ladder and would have to put my arms down to rest several times before I was able to get the light fitting off to change the bulb,' she told me over the phone. It's easy to see how this could have happened; Maree's past was chequered with discouraging sporting experiences. 'In school I was never any good at sports and I was always the last to be chosen for the netball team. When I'd drop the ball, everyone would go "ohhhh" in disappointment,' she told me. Maree had tried to do some exercise training with videos and DVDs in the privacy of her own home, but even then she felt intimidated. 'Why is it that exercise videos always feature award-winning fitness instructors showing off?' she lamented. 'If you can't do the exercise as well as they can do it, you get the demoralising soft option such as "if you can't manage this one, just walk on the spot". Why doesn't somebody make an exercise DVD for overweight or obese people that's tailored to their level, instead of making them feel even worse about all the things they can't do?' On top of her acquired exercise phobia, Maree was still recovering from chronic fatigue syndrome and so was unable to do any activity over and above attending to the bare necessities of life.

In spite of these constraints, over the 12 months in which Maree lost all her excess weight she worked up to effective volumes of physical activity and became so fit that she's now the strongest woman in her gym class. 'I am the best boxer in my class, and none of the other girls can catch my punches. I have to get a man to hold the pads and catch my punches if I want to go all the way and use all the strength in my back and arms. Having never been good at anything physical, this feels fantastic,' she said. The thing that Maree found most surprising about her increased physical fitness was how much easier her day-to-day activities became. 'Last week I needed to change a light bulb and I was shocked at how easy it was this time. I got the fitting off, the bulb changed and the fitting reattached without having to rest my arms once, it was effortless!' she said. 'And picking up the soap in the shower is now so easy,' she continued. 'I never used to think it was hard to pick up the soap, but now that I see how easily I do it I realise that it was hard to do when I was overweight and unfit.' Having lost 12 kilos, Maree has noticed a dramatic change in her body, which she now describes as having 'no flabby bits from losing weight too quickly'. A major contributor to Maree's lack of flab is all the exercise she has done in the past year. Instead of having bingo-wings to hide, Maree is now happy to display her arms in the shortest of sleeves. 'Last week a friend commented on how thin and shapely my arms are now,' she told me. If Maree can work her way up to such an admirable level of physical fitness from struggling to change a light bulb or pick up the soap in the shower, then you can improve your fitness, too. The trick, as Maree discovered, is to start small and work your way up gradually.

The first thing Maree did in her journey to an active lifestyle was to measure how much activity she was already getting. At my workshop, Maree felt encouraged by my reassurance that bursts of activity accumulated over the day – whether in the form of running errands and doing the laundry or going for a couple of walks on the way to work and back again – would indeed help get the weight off and keep it off. She bought a pedometer and aimed for around 12,000 steps every day. It wasn't an effortless feat, but Maree doesn't have a car and so it wasn't an overly onerous task, either. 'I use walking as a form of transport. I walk to the station (40 minutes) instead of catching the bus, or I walk to the shops (20 minutes) instead of taking the bus. This level of activity is something I can sustain in the long term,' she told me. If you try using a pedometer yourself, you'll see what a head start it will give you in your journey to a more active lifestyle.

Having made a large amount of incidental activity a sustainable part of her life, Maree gained confidence and went on to incorporate more structured and vigorous forms of physical activity into her daily step counts. Maree tells of the radical changes she implemented and how she managed them.

My flatmate at the time was thin, attractive and blond. She started swimming and that motivated me to try. I've always been a reasonable swimmer. So I started going to the pool a couple of times a week and swam for 30 minutes. I really enjoyed it. Then I decided that I would like to take advanced swimming lessons to improve my style, it was really fun and I learned a lot more than I had expected. Every week after the lesson I would see a group of overweight people training in the park. It caught my attention because they didn't have an 'I'm hating this!' look on their faces; they seemed to almost be having fun. So, after a couple of weeks of watching them I started to think that maybe I should join the group and give it a go. After I finished my swimming lessons I started the personal training. At first I was going to go just once a week. That quickly increased to three times a week, I was so shocked by how much I enjoyed it as I've never enjoyed exercise before. The trainer is great and really understands each person's ability and encourages just the right amount for each individual. I have also started having one-on-one training as well as joining the group. I can now run 4 kilometres, which is incredible, and I absolutely love boxing (hitting pads not people). Exercising in the park is perfect for me as I love the outdoor setting. The other great thing is that with each training session I can actually notice an increase in fitness – such quick tangible results are a great encouragement.

As Maree says, 'Weight loss and regaining your vitality is a process, you start as a beginner doing easy things, then gain confidence and try a little more and so on.' My question to you is this: what easy things could you do today to get the ball rolling and start being more active? Whether it's slinging a pedometer on your body and finding out what level you're starting from, doing a few exercises in a chair, going for a gentle stroll, or leaving your car at home and using public transport, I promise that if you keep doing these kinds of do-able things, before long they'll become so much easier to do, you'll gain confidence and you'll be looking out for your next challenge. If you persist in gradually increasing your level of physical activity, it will only be a matter of time before you reach the levels recommended for permanent weight loss and you'll know exactly what it takes to stay at the weight nature intended you to be.

THE BEAUTY OF NEW AGE ACCELERATION PEDOMETERS

Last year I was giving a workshop when one of the participants pulled a pedometer out of her bra and checked her step count. The other people at the workshop were just as intrigued as I was: what an original place to wear a pedometer! It turns out that the pedometer she was wearing was actually an acceleration pedometer, one of the new generation of pedometers that uses acceleration sensors to count steps at any angle, whether you're carrying it in your bag or in your pocket, or wearing it around your neck.

For several months I coveted a pedometer I could wear in my bra. With my clip-on-the-hip pedometer, using it is dependent on what I wear. If I wear a tailored dress one day, I can't wear my pedometer, because it looks lumpy under my clothes. Then I lose my momentum and I forget to wear it the next day, and the one after that . . .

When I bought my own acceleration pedometer a few months later, I fell instantly in love with it. Every day it tucks discreetly into my bra regardless of what I'm wearing. Because I *can* wear it every day, I *do* wear it every day. It always amazes me the difference that seeing my daily step counts makes to my activity levels and my attitude towards activity. The first summer that I had my new pedometer I needed to do quite a bit more running around with our children than usual, what with working during the long school holidays, commuting, and doing the morning and afternoon drop-offs and pick-ups from vacation care and day care. As I've said previously, I'm an 'energy-efficient' person, and so burning kilojoules is not something that comes naturally to me. But when I saw how much this enforced incidental activity added to my step counts every day, I actually started to relish that activity. Several afternoons that summer I even found myself walking up the road under the hot sun to buy lunch rather than going upstairs to buy it in my workplace, just so that I could increase my step count. How bizarre (for me) but wonderful.

Watch out for the Famine Reaction's effects on your energy levels

So far in this chapter we've covered numerous benefits of physical activity in relatively high doses. But what happens when your commitment to eating well and being active results in weight loss or fat loss to the point that your Famine Reaction awakens and starts impinging on your progress? In its efforts to protect you from wasting away, your Famine Reaction can make you feel incredibly lethargic,[1, 4] like you're dragging your whole body through mud. In this situation, do you march on with your usual level of physical activity regardless, or do you listen to your body and do what it tells you to do? Someone who has tried both approaches and lived to tell the tale is 63-year-old Harriet.

I probably would never have met Harriet, who lives alone on a 30-acre property in a remote area of Western Australia, but for the fact that she ordered a set of bathroom scales from my website and I called her to arrange a special delivery. As we talked through the business of couriers and logistics, Harriet mentioned in passing how much she enjoyed my book *The Don't Go Hungry Diet*, and naturally I asked her how she was going with her weight. I'm certainly glad I did, because Harriet's story is a graphic example of what happens when you ignore your body signals as opposed to what happens when you respect them. As Harriet's story shows, the effects go well beyond weight loss.

For more than 30 years, Harriet's weight had yoyoed between 75 kilos and 65 kilos. Every time she'd reach 65 kilos, just a few kilos heavier than her goal, she'd hit a wall of resistance that she now recognises as a Famine Reaction. Without any clear under-standing of what was happening, Harriet would plough on with the actions that had helped her to lose the first 10 kilos: banish-ing processed carbs and upping her intake of veggies and fruit, plus walking vigorously for approximately 90 minutes a day on her sprawling property. As a result of trying to fight her body's survival instincts, however, hunger and fatigue would eventually overcome her and she'd give up on her diet and exercise regime and end up in bed, completely flattened by exhaustion. Every time it happened, Harriet had thought that she must be a lazy person with no tenacity, and her negative self-talk made it even harder to get out of bed and get on with life. This, combined with the fact that Harriet also struggled with periods of depression, meant that many times in the past she had spent weeks in bed – only getting up for the bare necessities of life – and she had often needed to take antidepressants to get her back on her feet.

One spring, Harriet decided that it was time to get her weight back down again. By improving her food choices and once again doing her vigorous daily walks, she lost 10 kilos as efficiently as she always did, bringing her weight down to 65 kilos by early December. It was at this point that the all-too-familiar mental and physical fatigue set in, and Harriet longed to crawl into bed and stay there. In the past, Harriet would have resisted this desire – or beat herself up if she succumbed to it. But having read my book eight months previously, she was now well versed in the Famine Reaction and its intractable ways. Could it be that her desire to crawl into bed was *not* because she was useless and lazy, as she'd always told herself, but because a simple physi-ological defence mechanism was slowing her down? Harriet was not totally convinced that the Famine Reaction could explain her plight, but she realised she had all the classic signs. Therefore, instead of giving up and throwing herself into another indefi-nite period of inactivity, as she would have done in the past, Harriet decided to take heed of her fatigue and take it easy for a while. Although these two scenarios may seem identical, there's a huge difference in the effects they had on Harriet's mental well-being. The first made her feel awful about herself, and the latter gave Harriet a sense of control. Harriet told me on the phone that it had taken a giant leap of faith to achieve this change in her mindset, but she was soon reaping the benefits. Instead of lying in bed eating and feeling bad, Harriet nurtured herself by reading and knitting in bed and pottering around her home, trusting that she would soon feel rested enough to get back to her usual routine. After just 12 days, Harriet felt energetic enough to leave the house and walk one kilometre on an errand. By the week before Christmas, Harriet's energy levels had returned to normal and she was back to her long, energetic walks and her normal activities, and all without the aid of a single antidepressant. Throughout Christmas and New Year Harriet maintained her weight at 65 kilos, and by Easter she had dropped to 62.5 kilos, a number she hadn't seen in more than 30 years of yoyo dieting. Now that she can fit easily into her favourite size 12 clothes – they are even a bit loose around her waist – Harriet is focused on maintaining her current weight and being toned and strong. When I asked her how she felt about maintaining this new lighter weight, she said to me, 'I now feel in my soul that my weight will never go up again.'

Although Harriet's Famine-induced fatigue was extreme, no doubt exacerbated by her propensity for depression, the important message in her story is that following your body's cues can give you a much better result than repeatedly trying to fight against them. So, if you're trying to lose weight and you hit a patch where you feel really tired for whatever reason, then giving yourself a suitable rest, rather than soldiering on with your usual level of activity, can be the fastest way to get back on track. A suitable rest can be anything from going for a slow amble around your neighbourhood instead of going for your usual power walk, or taking your goggles to a rock pool by the beach and checking out the life forms clinging to the rocks instead of ploughing through laps in an Olympic-sized swimming pool, or taking a break from exercise altogether for a day or so and contenting yourself with however much incidental activity you happen to clock up. Regardless of whether any feeling of fatigue lasts for one day or one month, if you continue to eat according to your hunger signals as described in this book despite any temporary drop in physical activity, there's no reason why you won't be able to at least maintain your weight while you're taking it easy.

The dangers of dichotomous thinking

In Chapter 17 I discussed the concept of dichotomous thinking – the black-and-white or all-or-nothing mindset that makes countless intelligent people give up on their diet and eat anything or everything if they deviate from their chosen path by even a fraction of a hair. Dichotomous thinking is also a frequent flyer in the exercise arena. Maybe you've succumbed to it yourself? Have you ever decided to give your walk a complete miss because you only had time for a 20-minute quickie instead of your usual 50-minute affair? Maybe this happened a few times in a row, and before you knew it you'd lost the habit of going walking at all and were back to a completely sedentary lifestyle. Have you ever flopped on the sofa in defeat, munching your way through a block of cooking chocolate (and a subsequent week-long binge), because your car broke down and you couldn't get to the Pilates class you'd psyched yourself up for? These are both examples of the dangers of dichotomous thinking, and they stem from the assumption that the intensity or duration of the activity you had planned is the *only* way to achieve success, and if you can't do it in its entirety you won't get any benefit and so you may as well give up. It's easy to see how this kind of thinking about physical activity has weaselled its way into our minds. Often when I read something about exercise in the popular press, and even when I was looking for a personal trainer, I hear things such as 'you need at least 20 minutes of aerobic activity in order to get a training effect', or 'unless you do at least 40 minutes of strength training in a single session, you're wasting your time'. Is it any wonder that dichotomous thinking pervades so many people's view about exercise? But I've said it once and I'll say it again: scientific research has shown that the benefits of physical activity are dose-dependent, not all-or-nothing, meaning that the more physical activity you do (the 'dose'), the greater the benefits, and the benefits start becoming apparent even after relatively small doses. If you're usually as active as the public health authorities recommend for permanent weight loss but you sometimes can't be as active as usual owing to family commitments or whatever, then even something like clocking up 3000 steps during a snail's-pace shopping expedition with your elderly mother on those occasions will bring more benefits to your weight and waistline than vegging out at home. *Any* form of movement will. So if for whatever reason your exercise routine is disrupted, what can you do instead that still involves *some* physical activity?

Do you remember when you were a child and the summer school holidays seemed to last forever? It wasn't an illusion; summer school holidays really *do* last forever. In Chapter 7 I mentioned that my children and I were staying with my mother in Perth for the school holidays while my husband was away on business. Well . . . thousands of words later I'm *still* here as I write this! Without the routine of school, daycare and my husband's help, the exercise routine I'd established in Sydney has gone to dust. If I hadn't known from my reading of the scientific literature about the benefits of accumulating smaller bursts of activity throughout the day, building up to a total of around 8000 to 12,000 steps per day, and if I hadn't experienced those benefits in my own life, I might well have given up on physical activity altogether these holidays. Instead, I do what I can with the resources I have. No more invigorating laps of the pool during the interminable school holidays . . . my kids still need to be within arm's reach of me or in constant visual contact with me in the water. But thankfully they can both swim in deep water, so I throw them into the diving pool and tread water while keeping watch over their exploits. I haven't looked to see how many steps I'd be getting if I exerted the same amount of effort on dry land, but I do know that by the end of our swim I'm totally knackered. Not only will this kind of activity 'have to do' until school goes back, it actually does very well; all my clothes remain comfortably loose, especially around my waist.

Again, any kind of physical activity is better than none. Another example of this principle in action is my friend Holly from high school, who I introduced in Chapter 11 and who has lost 13 kilos and kept it off over the past two-and-a-half years. Physical activity has been an important part of Holly's success, but with two toddlers she has had to snatch it from wherever she could.

Once I had my second child I was determined to lose weight, but with the motivation and all the responsibilities of motherhood I vowed never to do it in an extreme way again. I booked both of my small children into the creche at my local gym and they loved it. After six months the kids were not always so keen to be in the creche or even to sit in the pram when I went walking with them, so I started looking for other ways and opportunities to be active. I didn't always go to the gym, sometimes I went for a walk on my own when my husband came home, and sometimes I couldn't get out at all so I had to chase bikes, trolleys and prams up and down the driveway. I also sacked my cleaner and started cleaning myself.

So, if you can't be as physically active as usual in a structured way, what *can* you do? I promise that doing whatever activity you can manage will do you much more good than giving up and doing nothing . . . especially if giving up entails doing nothing for a long time and eating whatever the hell you want to boot. And remember, even if you do go through temporary periods where you can't manage much or any physical activity for whatever reason, listening to your body and eating only when you feel physically hungry will help you to avoid gaining weight until you can start moving again.

Dr Amanda's Diagnostic N°3

What's your current level of physical activity? The best way to know your current daily average is to write down in your Success Diary what physical activities you do during the day – even if it's just a 10-minute walk at the shopping centre or 15 minutes on your bike on the weekend. If most of the activities you do involve being on your feet (such as walking or running), an easy way to get an estimate of your overall activity levels is to use a pedometer.

Interpreting your results

Unless you're already moving with moderate intensity for a total of 60 to 90 minutes a day (approximately 8000 to 12,000 steps per day), including some vigorous activity several times a week and some strength training, then increasing the frequency, duration or intensity of your current level of activity will boost your ability to lose weight and keep it off, not to mention the benefits it will bring to your physical and mental wellbeing. The good news is that even modest increases in the frequency, duration or intensity of your activity compared to what you usually do will give you better results. Read on for further ideas on how to do this.

Ideas for increasing your activity levels if you're starting from zero

If you're not currently doing much physical activity at all, a good place to start is to get a pedometer and simply count how many steps you're currently averaging. Many people are surprised to learn that they're moving more than they thought they were, just through the incidental activities of daily living, and this encourages them to strive for the levels of physical activity recommended for permanent weight loss.

Once you know your starting activity levels, aim to increase your step counts in increments of about 1500 steps per day (or about 15 minutes of moderate-intensity activity such as walking). For instance, if your average step count is around 2000 per day, aim to increase this to around 3500. Once you're comfortably doing around 3500 steps per day, aim to increase your average step count to around 5000 steps per day, and so on. There are countless ways in which to increase your step counts. Maybe you could make a walking track around your home and walk to the tune of your iPod like Beth did, or give up your cleaner like Holly did and use housework as a golden opportunity to ratchet up your step counts.

If your feet or knees don't take kindly to walking, there are many other ways to increase your level of physical activity that will help you to lose weight. Notable examples include swimming, water aerobics, strength training – on land or in water using foam aqua dumbbells – and sitting in a chair and waving your arms vigorously. Whatever your starting level of activity, aim to increase it gradually in increments of about 15 minutes of moderate-intensity activity, aiming ultimately for the recommended 60 to 90 minutes of moderate-intensity activity per day, or 8000 to 12,000 steps.

If the shoe fits . . .
If you get a significant proportion of your physical activity while on your feet (e.g. by walking), it's essential to wear well-fitted walking or running shoes. A podiatrist will be able to tell you exactly what you need to look for when buying shoes, taking into account your specific needs. The right shoes for your feet (with orthotic inserts if necessary) will not only help prevent injury to your feet, legs, hips or back, they will also do wonders to alleviate any niggling discomfort you may experience as a result of being active.

Ideas for increasing your activity level if you're already reasonably active

If you're already getting a fair number of steps or their equivalent every day, is there anything you could do to beef it up to around the 12,000 mark? Perhaps you could leave your car at home and use public transport or your own feet, offer to walk to the shops if someone you know needs something around the home or office, or add an extra exercise session to your week, giving yourself the time you need to 'walk often and walk far' like the participants in that research study mentioned early in this chapter who got such first-class outcomes for their weight, waistline and cardiovascular health.

If you're already headed towards a steady 12,000 or so steps per day on average and you're serious about attaining and maintaining your optimum biological weight, is there anything you could sustainably do to increase the *intensity* with which you obtain those steps? Remember, research shows that the greater the frequency, duration and intensity of your physical activity, the greater the benefits will be for your weight and your health. Could you convert your regular walk to a run-walk or a run, or walk faster, in a hillier area or on softer ground at the beach, or buy a pair of Nordic walking canes, to really intensify your walk? What about that old bike in your garage; could you get it serviced and go for a fast spin around your neighbourhood? Or go for a swim and see how many laps you can do in a fixed time, constantly striving to beat the clock? And when you move, how many activities can you do that make you push against resistance, thereby increasing the strength of your muscles? You don't have to go to the gym to increase your strength; you can do it incidentally by putting more oomph into the activities of everyday life, being mindful of your back. Perhaps you know a child who'd be thrilled to be taken on a nice long piggyback ride? Or someone who could do with a hand to move house? In a more structured way, perhaps you could add a few sets of push-ups, sit-ups, lunges and other simple resistance exercises to your life, join a gym and do some supervised strength-training sessions, or learn how to use a set of foam dumbbells in the pool and pull against their buoyancy? There are countless ways in which to get the physical activity you need for permanent weight loss, and all you need to do is find activities you enjoy and just start doing them.

Over to you
Here's something you can do immediately to put the ideas in this chapter into action.

Provided that you're eating according to your hunger signals and choosing foods that help rather than hinder weight loss, any increase in your current level of physical activity towards the levels recommended for permanent weight loss, as outlined in this chapter, will help you to lose weight faster, lose more weight, prevent weight or fat regain, whittle your waist and give you a trimmer, more youthful body. Remember, in working up towards the recommended levels of physical activity, the more active you are, the greater the benefits will be, so *any* increase in the frequency, duration or intensity of your activity compared to what you usually do will help you to lose weight and keep it off, not to mention the benefits of activity for your health generally. My question to you is: what could you reasonably and sustainably do?

The trick is to keep trying different activities until you find the ones you enjoy so much that the excuses fall by the wayside and you keep going back to them. It doesn't matter what those activities are; you just need to enjoy them. I promise that if you start being more active than you currently are, then within a month you'll start noticing the benefits and you'll be on your way to being hooked. Once you're hooked on physical activity and the benefits it brings you, you're home and hosed, because you won't want to go back to the way you were before.

Making it sustainable for life

Chapter 19

The restorative power of a weight loss holiday

Adopt the pace of nature; her secret is patience.
Ralph Waldo Emerson, American essayist, philosopher
and poet, 1803–1882

One of the mistakes that many people make in their efforts to lose weight is *trying to lose weight all the time.* Although you'll never see your knuckles go white while losing weight by connecting with your body as described in this book, shedding excess weight in this way still requires considerable focus and attention. Occasionally you may find that a kilo will drop off here or there because you've been too busy to eat, or you've been sick or sad or particularly active, for example. For the most part, however, you'll be acutely aware of the efforts you've made to lose every kilo you've lost. You'll certainly have had a good reason for wanting to lose those kilos. You'll undoubtedly have taken control of your environment so that you had nutritious foods readily available and you didn't eat too many heavily processed foods just because they're there. You'll probably also have become more proactive and done things you enjoy doing or that give you satisfaction so that you didn't think about eating unless you were comfortably and physically hungry. None of these things require you to use brute force to resist your body's hunger signals, but they don't happen without desire, focus and organisation.

Because of the degree of mindfulness it takes to lose weight, it's important to know that you may sometimes need to take a break from trying to lose weight in order to conserve your energy. After all, losing weight and keeping it off is not a sprint; it's a marathon you need to sustain for the rest of your life. Sometimes your body may also need to take a break from losing weight – for example, when your weight dips so far below your current Set Point that your Famine Reaction comes into play and makes your weight loss stall. Not knowing this, many people who are trying to lose weight burn out way too early. Fuelled by conventional weight loss thinking that encourages continuous adherence, they focus on losing weight week after week, month after month. This leaves most people in a state of physical and mental exhaustion, where the prospect of losing more weight ends up in the 'too hard basket'.

If you've ever petered out while trying to lose weight in the past, you may like to try losing weight in shorter, more manageable chunks. The idea is to focus on losing weight when it feels right for you to do so, and then, when you feel like taking a break from all that vigilance, to switch your focus from trying to push your weight downwards to maintaining your new lower weight. In other words, you take a weight loss holiday. A weight loss holiday can be pre-booked, where you decide in advance when you're going to take a holiday; it can be sprung on you in surprise, such as when you've got every intention of losing more weight over the Easter holidays but you end up eating more chocolate bunnies than you anticipated; or it can be obligatory, when your Famine Reaction decides for you that it's time to take some annual leave and your weight loss naturally stalls. The beauty of a weight loss holiday is that unlike conventional holidays, which often end before you're ready to come back to earth, you can stay on a weight loss holiday for as long as you like. And what a restful holiday destination! While preventing weight regain is never easy, it's considerably easier than the degree of mindfulness it takes to lose weight in the first place. You can afford slightly more overindulgence: those times when you occasionally eat when you're not hungry, or when you occasionally eat more than you really need. What's more, you can afford to enjoy slightly more fun foods or alcohol while on a weight loss holiday without putting yourself off track. By taking a breather from time to time, you can refresh yourself and get ready for your next burst of weight loss. Just as real holidays help you to work more effectively, weight loss holidays help you to lose weight more effectively. Let's take a look at the science underpinning this principle.

The science behind taking a weight loss holiday

When it comes to losing weight, emerging evidence suggests that going about it in intermittent bursts is the way of the future. As I summarised in Chapter 2, where I covered the science of weight loss, our bodies are equipped with an incredibly resilient mechanism – the Famine Reaction – that's designed to protect us from losing too much weight too quickly. Whenever your weight dips too far below your current Set Point (for example, if you eat fewer kilojoules than you need to maintain your body's fat stores, or if you have liposuction to remove a few kilos of fat that you couldn't shift by diet and exercise), your Famine Reaction rouses and tries to slow your progress. It does this with such antics as making you hungrier[1-3] and more lethargic,[1,4] slowing your metabolic rate,[1, 4-7] and shifting your hormones so that your body tends to accumulate belly fat.[8, 41-49] My number one research mission for the past two decades has been to understand the Famine Reaction and to find ways to weaken it so that more people can attain and maintain an optimum healthy weight. The reason I have such enormous respect for this commander-in-chief is that whenever we try experimental approaches to weaken it by attacking certain branches of its army, we often see temporary increases in weight loss, but the Famine Reaction just goes and calls for back-up troops and ultimately wards off the attack. Thus far, the Famine Reaction has always won.

You see this resilience of the Famine Reaction clearly among people taking weight loss medications. At present there are very few prescription medications available that act on the brain to weaken the Famine Reaction. They do this by increasing the amount of noradrenaline and dopamine or serotonin in the brain, thereby reducing appetite, stimulating satiety and boosting the metabolic rate. However, it's usually only a matter of weeks before the Famine Reaction gets wise to the effects of the drug and figures out ways to overcome it. When 44-year-old Jacinta decided to lose weight, weighing 98.8 kilos for her 1.7 metre frame, she and her doctor decided that she would try Reductil. (Reductil, or sibutramine hydrochloride, has since been taken off the market.) Her exhaustive attempts to lose weight over the past 16 years – including home-delivered meals, joining a gym, fibre capsules, the cabbage soup diet, five different diet clubs, a low-carb, high-protein diet, meal replacement shakes, visualisation, hypnosis tapes and Xenical, as well as just trying to 'be good and eat very small portions and as little fat as possible' – had at best seen her lose up to 13 kilos, but each time, without fail, Jacinta's weight would eventually climb back to her Set Point of around 98 kilos. Reductil offered her a possible way out of Diet Dungeon.

> I had the prescription made up and I started taking it. I had such high hopes that this would work for me, and to tell you the truth, I think it did serve a purpose at first. It got me started. I went on the internet and looked up all the horrible side effects. They were awful, but I was desperate. I had the headaches, sleeplessness, terribly dry mouth and constipation – but happily, very little appetite. It was such an effort to eat a full meal. IT WAS A DREAM COME TRUE!

Jacinta was elated to lose 7 kilos within six weeks of taking Reductil. Of course she was watching what she ate and exercising as well (weight loss medications can only be truly effective when combined with diet and physical activity), but Reductil gave her efforts a discernible boost. That's why she was stunned at what happened next. It stopped working.

I couldn't believe it! I had read on some of the Reductil forums that other people had also said it stopped working for them and that was OK, they admitted that they just had to try harder to resist their hunger. It was madness – pay $114 a month for this drug and still have to try and resist my hunger??

Frustrating? Yes. But that's just the resilience of the Famine Reaction at work. You may be interested to know that Jacinta stopped taking Reductil and then went on to lose a further 10.5 kilos in three-and-a-half months using the principles outlined in this book. And that brings me to the effectiveness of *food* and the weight loss holiday for outsmarting the Famine Reaction.

In one study, people who lost weight in two-week to seven-week bursts of diet and exercise interspersed with prescribed breaks of two to six weeks in duration, during which time they ate more but nonetheless maintained their reduced weight by ongoing attentiveness, lost *just as much weight* after four months (8.2 kilos on average) as people who were instructed to follow the same diet and exercise regime continuously for the entire four months.[130] It seems that just as the Famine Reaction was gearing up for a war on famine, along came a weight loss holiday and the adequate food supplies it brings, and the Famine Reaction was left standing in the field, wondering where the hell the famine went. Then, just as it instructs the guys in the appetite, metabolic rate and other departments to lower their defences, along comes another burst of vigilant diet and exercise. Because the Famine Reaction's defences are down, these efforts are met with satisfyingly efficient weight losses. For example, after two groups of volunteers had both followed the conventional diet for six weeks, one group took a break for seven weeks while the other group stayed on the conventional diet for the whole time (13 weeks). In the month following this 13-week period, the volunteers who took the seven-week weight loss holiday lost an average of 3 kilos, whereas people who endured the long, slow grind of the conventional diet for all that time lost absolutely nothing in that month.[130] In light of these findings, it seems that taking regular weight loss holidays can improve your weight losses relative to the amount of effort you put into them, possibly by weakening your Famine Reaction's defences. In fact, if you're losing weight by connecting with your body as outlined in this book, you'll achieve these benefits automatically, as you'll see below.

Some weight loss holidays are enforced, so you might as well enjoy them

When you're losing weight by connecting with your body, your Famine Reaction will naturally thrust a weight loss holiday upon you from time to time, whether you want it or not. This will most likely occur for the first time once you've skimmed off the initial 'easy' kilos that were in excess of your current Set Point, when your weight starts dipping to new lows. When this happens, your Famine Reaction will rouse and start pushing you to eat more than you were eating before, and this will often mean you stop losing weight, even if you continue eating to the precise tune of your hunger and being active. Sometimes your weight loss will stall like this for a month or more while your body comes to terms with your new weight and accepts it as its latest Set Point. That's where accepting the pace of nature will bring you much better results than trying to deny your body's need for a break.

In Chapter 4, I introduced you to Lauren, 58, who has lost 35 kilos since she started listening to her body five years ago. Every time she lost approximately 10 kilos, Lauren's body would take a weight loss holiday and there was nothing she could do to get her weight moving downwards (short of denying her hunger and starving herself). Even though she was continuing to do all the things that had helped her to lose all those kilos – eating only when hungry and stopping when she felt nicely satisfied, eating mainly unprocessed foods with adequate vegetables and fruit, and walking for about an hour every day or doing 30-minute to 60-minute strength and cardio training sessions with her personal trainer or at home – her weight would stay stuck on the same number for up to two months. In the past, Lauren would have rebelled against her Famine Reaction by eating less than she really needed and pushing herself to do uncomfortable levels of exercise. However, having seen this brute-force strategy backfire unfailingly during her 40 years' experience of yoyo dieting, and now being wise to the Famine Reaction's wilful ways, Lauren knew that she just had to accept her body's enforced weight loss holiday. 'I've learned that the key is to not stress about it,' she told me over the phone. 'I know it's just my body getting used to the new weight, and it will take as long as it takes. I have to let it go and let it run its course.' And the Famine Reaction always ran its course. Lauren can't say exactly how she knew when the Famine Reaction had subsided, but she got a sense that it was safe to start trying to lose some more weight. 'It's hard to explain,' she said, 'but something told me that I've got to try a bit harder. So I'd cut back a bit on how much I was eating and I'd exercise a bit more, and the weight would start coming down again.' By being patient with her body as it took the weight loss holidays it needed, Lauren is now reaping handsome dividends. She has absolute confidence in her body's ability to help her attain and maintain her optimum biological weight. 'I just know that I will *never* weigh 134 kilos again,' she said. 'My goal is to eventually get down to around 75 kilos by just working slowly at it. And I'll get there.'

Some weight loss holidays are accidental, so you might as well enjoy those, too

In addition to the weight loss holidays that your Famine Reaction will probably enforce upon you, sometimes you may have every intention of losing weight and your body may be perfectly amenable to it, but circumstances make it too difficult for you to do the things you need to do to actually lose weight. That's when accepting these accidental weight loss holidays – rather than berating yourself because you didn't achieve your immediate goal – will give you a mental break, too. And as with all holidays, you'll probably find yourself feeling re-energised when you 'come back' from your break, and this will help power you onwards towards your ultimate goal.

Every 12 to 18 months in the past five years, Lauren has been on an overseas trip with her husband or friends. 'Although I always try to be moderate and do the best I can when I'm away, it's more difficult to stay on track,' she told me. For example, two years ago she visited her family in England and Wales. 'My family are big eaters and they eat a lot of processed foods and things from packets, and they served that to me.' The result was that even though Lauren continued with her hour-long daily walks while she was away, and even though she pretty much ate only when hungry and avoided feeling overfull, inadequate fruit and vegetable intake meant that she ended up eating far more kilojoules than she needed. At the end of five weeks with her family she had gained about 5 kilos. Usually she gains less than that when she goes on a trip. 'Last year I went on an Alaskan cruise and there was food available 24 hours a day. That made it a bit harder to eat only as much as I needed, although I have to say that my husband and our friends and I saw so many people piling their plates up at the buffet table, it really put me off going too far overboard.' After the cruise, Lauren and her travelling team went on a three-week bus tour of Canada and saw some amazing sights. 'The trip of a lifetime, really,' she said. There, again, it was not as easy to eat in the way she needs to eat in order to lose weight, although she still maintained her daily routine of hour-long walks plus she did plenty of strolling around museums and monuments. Mealtimes sometimes fell when she wasn't actually hungry, but she had to eat anyway to protect herself from getting dangerously hungry. And when she *was* hungry, sometimes the best available food choice was a hamburger and an orange juice. In addition, Lauren ate out in restaurants, and shared a few more desserts and enjoyed a few more gin and tonics than she normally does when she's at home. However, instead of fretting about these small kilojoule excesses, as she might have done in the past, she gave herself a mental break. 'This is going to be a lifetime commitment,' she told me over the phone. 'I need to balance looking after my health with living and doing what I want to do. You have to say to yourself, "This is just the way it is. It's just a temporary thing," and you have to realise that you can't be 100 per cent in control all the time.'

Although Lauren gained 2 to 3 kilos after her Alaskan–Canadian tour, a weight gain typical of most of her overseas trips, accidental weight loss holidays such as this one energise her to keep pursuing her goal.

By the time I return from a trip I'm usually excited about getting back on track. Eating too many sugary or cheap starchy foods doesn't agree with me any more; they actually upset my stomach and sometimes give me diarrhoea, so now I prefer eating my own whole fresh foods. And when I'm away I really miss my strength training; it makes me feel so strong and fit. So one of the first things I do when I get back from holidays is call my personal trainer and book myself in for a few one-hour sessions with her. That always helps me; it motivates me to keep working out on my own at home on days when I can't get out for a walk.

As a result of these changes, Lauren invariably reverses any holiday-induced blips in her weight rapidly, and then goes on to lose even more weight. 'My body really responds very quickly now when I get back to basics and start using my Fat Brake again,' she said.

HOW TO EAT WELL WHEN IT MEANS EATING DIFFERENTLY FROM THE PEOPLE AROUND YOU

Have you ever struggled to stick to healthy food choices or to eat according to your body signals when you're with other people? Whenever Leanne, 46, visits her parents, they always offer her fried takeaway foods and profuse quantities of home-baked biscuits and slices. Although it's blatantly obvious that Leanne struggles with her weight – she is only

1.56 metres tall and weighs over 98 kilos – it creates such a ruckus to explain to her parents that she's not hungry or that she's trying to eat healthily that she usually just shuts up and eats.

Sometimes people take it almost as a personal insult if you refuse their food, and they'll tell you how delicious it is and keep trying to persuade you to eat it. That's where briefly explaining your particular needs and doing your own catering can prove invaluable. Next month Lauren will set off again to visit her family in Europe and England. Not wanting to gain 5 kilos, as she did the last time she was with them, but not wanting her family to feel she is criticising the food they eat, she has emailed in advance to say that she can't eat too many sugary or starchy foods such as cakes or dumplings with gravy because they upset her stomach, so while she is with them she'll largely be catering for herself and eating her own foods. She figures that this way she will avoid hurting anyone's feelings, and it may even help her family to get a taste for healthier foods while she's with them.

The before and after benefits of the pre-booked weight loss holiday

So far we've looked at two types of weight loss holidays: those that are enforced by your Famine Reaction and those that happen accidentally or spontaneously, when you go through a period of eating or drinking more than you originally intended. And that brings me to the third kind of weight loss holiday – the *pre-booked* weight loss holiday – where you decide in advance that you'll try to lose weight for a predetermined period, after which time you'll take a break. This is my favourite type of weight loss holiday, because it not only energises you after the holiday, it can also energise you in the countdown leading up to it. Have you ever noticed that when you've got a holiday to look forward to, you can get far more done than if you didn't have a holiday on the horizon? Like a horse bolting back to the stables after a long walk, you suddenly find the second wind you need to finish up projects or chores, attack the important tasks you've been accumulating in your 'too hard basket', and spritz over your workplace so that it will look inviting when you get back. And so it is with the pre-booked weight loss holiday. Whereas eating strictly only when hungry or drinking fewer than four standard alcoholic drinks per week may seem too hard, when you know that you only need to do it until your pre-booked weight loss holiday, you'll be amazed at what you can do.

My salvation in short bursts

When I first started losing weight by connecting with my body, I didn't find it easy. Having just come out of six years of bingeing and yoyo dieting, my eating wasn't as healthful or as in tune with my body's needs as it is now. I wanted fun foods such as chocolates, sticky buns and fatty, salty corn chips far more often than I do today, and several times a week I ate when I wasn't hungry. Although this eating pattern didn't make me put on weight – probably because I had naturally stopped eating until I felt stuffed once I gave up conventional dieting, and also because, having taken up flamenco dancing, I had a more active lifestyle – it didn't allow me to lose weight, either. I learned, however, that if I cut my fun food consumption back to about 25 grams of chocolate per day (two Swiss chocolate truffles I bought when I was out and about – no question of my keeping a stash at home), that if I was mindful about eating only when hungry, and that if I was active in the form of walking or dancing *every* day, my weight would shift downwards. I wanted my weight to shift downwards, but I also loved to eat. I solved this conundrum by deciding that I'd only try to lose weight for defined periods of time; 5 to 14 days, or until my Famine Reaction struck, whichever came sooner. After that I'd take a pre-booked weight loss holiday, reverting back to my normal, comfortable way of eating for weight maintenance for as long as I wanted. Sometimes my Famine Reaction would strike before the end of my short burst, in which case I'd immediately declare a weight loss holiday. But in most cases I don't think I lost enough weight during my short burst to have initiated a Famine Reaction; I just wanted to give myself a break.

This strategy turned out to be my salvation. In my old diet club days, I would start yet another rigidly counted diet and fully expect to stick to it until I reached my goal weight, but the sheer prospect of spending an undefined period of time in that straightjacket for foodies made me want to pig out immediately. In contrast, knowing that I'd only be cutting back modestly for a maximum of 5 to 14 days with my short-burst strategy, I found it much easier to do what I needed to do in order to lose weight. To help me stay on track until my pre-booked weight loss holiday, I made a paper chain out of pieces of gaily patterned wrapping paper in my favourite colours, each piece 5 centimetres wide by 12 centimetres long. Every day that I did what I knew I needed to do to lose weight – enjoying my daily treat of 25 grams of chocolate, making sure I was hungry before eating anything, and doing something active every day – I folded up one of my pieces of paper into a flat link and added it to my zigzagging and growing paper chain just before going to bed. It's amazing what a positive influence that flat paper chain had on me. I'd hold it and admire it, congratulating myself on the number of successful days I'd already clocked up, counting down the days until my pre-booked weight loss holiday and wondering how much weight I'd have lost when I weighed in again after my short burst of concerted effort. These factors were so motivating that at most there would be one day out of five when I didn't score a link on my paper chain. It was such a helpful technique that I used it until my paper chain was several metres long – that's how many successful days it had helped me to achieve. If I hadn't learned through my medical research and personal experiences that it was OK to lose weight in short bursts, I might still be stuck in Diet Dungeon today, miserably counting kilojoules and obsessing about food, and all the while feeling unattractive and matronly in my heavy-duty bras and plus-sized clothes that looked more like curtains.

It all gets easier with time

While I distinctly remember going through highly conscious short bursts of effort to lose those first 8 kilos of excess weight, the short bursts that got me from 85 kilos to 75 took a lot less effort. By then, doing what I needed to do to lose weight and keep it off came so much more naturally to me. At the time I was weighing in once a month at the lightest part of my menstrual cycle, and all it took to help ensure that a nice loss of one or more kilos would show up on the scales from one weigh-in to the next was a bit more mindfulness about my eating and exercise habits for about five days before my weigh-in. After my monthly weigh-in I'd still take a pre-booked weight loss holiday and be a little more liberal in my interpretation of hunger and how many treats I ate, but I must have been pretty in tune with my body's needs, because it's unlikely that I lost that one or more kilos in the five or so days of watchfulness before weighing in.

One of the things I loved about taking pre-booked weight loss holidays was that occasional overindulgences between weigh-ins just didn't set me back like they used to. One Easter, all of my colleagues from the lab and I were invited to dinner at another colleague's house just across the Franco–Swiss border. We dined around an oversized rustic wooden table in Isabelle's giant, barn-style lounge-dining room. I remember feeling a bit overwhelmed by the event; all my colleagues at the time were at least 10 years older than I was and seemed to live in another world, with conversations about parents and partners, children and schools, houses and cars. I had nothing to contribute to these conversations. What I did have, however, was a giant bowl filled with Swiss chocolate Easter eggs right in front of me on the dinner table. Isabelle always did things lavishly and aesthetically. Most people interpreted Isabelle's Easter eggs as a table decoration and politely ate two or three, but I got stuck into them. I ate Easter eggs before dinner, I ate Easter eggs in between the entrée and the main meal, I ate Easter eggs after dinner, and I ate Easter eggs straight after dessert and then during coffee as well. I can't remember how many Easter eggs I ate that night, but

Isabelle kept filling up the bowl and by the time I got home I felt awfully sick and bloated. However, because my weigh-ins rolled around just once a month, and because I knew that occasional splurges wouldn't make me gain weight as long as I had time to be scrupulously careful about my habits for a burst of about five days before my weigh-in, I wasn't worried. Once again, I didn't gain weight.

Another thing I appreciated about weight loss holidays was that I could give myself an extension whenever I wanted. Whenever I was faced with an overwhelming temptation like that memorable Easter egg fest during one of my short bursts of intentional weight loss, I'd weigh up the desirability of what I wanted to eat versus how much I wanted to lose weight at that time. If the food won, I'd say, 'Nah, I'm not really trying to lose weight right now, I'm having a break.' Because I'd honed the art of weight maintenance during weight loss holidays thanks to my Fat Brake, it really didn't matter how much 'annual leave' I took.

Bursts of concerted effort and regular weight loss holidays helped me lose the last 10 kilos

The closer you get to your body's ideal weight, the harder it will be to lose weight, because your Famine Reaction will be that much more discerning about how much weight it lets you lose and when. Almost all of the weight I lost between 75 kilos and my natural weight of 65 kilos was achieved with deliberate, conscious effort. Thank goodness I had weight loss holidays to look forward to between bursts of concentrated effort; otherwise, I wouldn't have had the tenacity I needed to keep going. Those weight loss holidays undoubtedly also helped my body to accept progressively lower Set Points.

My weight got stuck on a plateau of 75 kilos for several months, but a week-long ski camp was an ideal opportunity to kick it down to the next level with another short burst of deliberate effort. Although sometimes I ate a bit more than I really needed during the day (I didn't want to get caught unawares by ravenous hunger and fall flat on my face in the snow), I was particularly careful about eating in tune with my body signals at dinnertime and about keeping desserts and chocolate to a minimum. When I got home after that holiday, I weighed 73.5 kilos and felt fantastic. The jump from 69 to 68 kilos also remains vividly in my memory. I'd been stuck at 69 kilos for more than four months, and it took a 'short burst' of a whole month of scrupulous attentiveness to get my weight down to 68 kilos. I went out and bought an expensive pair of designer jeans to celebrate, and declared another weight loss holiday. Even if I hadn't wanted to take a pre-booked weight loss holiday at that time, my Famine Reaction would probably have thrust a compulsory one upon me in any case, while my body accepted my new weight as its current Set Point. It was months before I felt I had the courage to undertake another 'short burst' to get from 68 to 67 kilos, which also took a whole month of strong focus and desire. And then I got stuck at a new Set Point of 66.8 kilos for about a year. If I hadn't broken up with the boyfriend I'd been living with for more than two years and cried so much that I couldn't eat like I usually did, I might never have lost those last 2 kilos.

Fun foods, alcohol and the 'short burst' approach to weight loss

To lose weight by connecting with your body, you need to cut your intake of fun foods and alcohol right back, enjoying occasional small doses of only those treats you'd hunt and kill for if they weren't immediately available to you. This can be problematic for people like myself who have strong attachments to gustatory pleasures such as chocolate, ice-cream and sticky date pudding. That's where losing weight in short bursts can be so much more do-able than trying to be constantly vigilant. For 53-year-old Bernice, the short burst approach to weight loss was one of the key things that helped her to lose the 5 kilos she hadn't been able to shift in more than 15 years.

In her work as senior sales consultant for a company producing earthmoving equipment, Bernice frequently travelled overseas, where she wined and dined customers and made multi-million-dollar sales. When at home in Australia, one of her favourite ways to relax and enjoy life was to go out for a nice meal with her husband and have a glass or two of wine with her dinner. Although her alcohol intake was moderate (never more than about 10 standard alcoholic drinks per week, well below the maximum levels recommended for good health, as outlined in Chapter 15), it was too high to allow her to lose weight. Bernice already knew this from past experience, so when she decided to lose weight by connecting with her body she cut her alcohol intake back to around three or four standard drinks per week. She lost 1.5 kilos in her first fortnight of using a Success Diary and was thrilled. Within a total of 16 weeks she had lost 5.3 kilos and had reached her optimum biological weight of 62 kilos, which she has now maintained for more than 18 months. Bernice's success came in a series of short bursts of effort of about 7 to 14 days each, with pre-booked weight loss holidays between bursts.

Knowing that it wasn't feasible to cut her alcohol intake right back when she had a spate of particularly heavy trips and sales meetings coming up, Bernice would wait until she had a 'clear run' ahead of her, with adequate time at home or with her family overseas in which to unwind and focus on her goals, before trying to get her weight down by another half a kilo or a kilo. During her 'burst week', she would focus on enjoying refreshing glasses of sparkling mineral water and the sensation of her trousers getting looser whenever she was in situations where she would normally enjoy an alcoholic drink, and she would also focus on getting in a good vigorous run or a bike ride almost very day of the week. During her pre-booked weight loss holidays, she would keep up her exercise by running or using her hotel's gym if it was too dark or treacherous to exercise outside, and she would follow her body's directives about what and how much to eat. It's thanks to these habits that Bernice was able to maintain her weight (to within half a kilo) during each weight loss holiday, despite the fact that she would enjoy a fair few more cocktails, beers or glasses of wine than when she was in a 'burst' week. Here is what Bernice said about losing weight in this way.

What I loved the most about your weight loss program is that it was so simple and so totally different to all the weight loss programs I have tried over the past 20+ years. I did not have to count points, weigh food or only eat specific foods.

I travel a lot and dine out a lot with clients so eating specific foods, weighing food and counting points does not work for me.

Amanda, you have helped me to see my weight loss journey as exciting and positive. You helped me to fine-tune how to go about changing my eating and exercise habits so I could lose weight almost effortlessly. I am still quite stunned at how easy it has all been. I have been trying to lose this weight for more than 15 years. Also I know without any doubt that the weight I have lost is permanently lost, as I have permanently changed my habits.

I have had several people (including my husband) say I look 10 years younger. Not only do I look 10 years younger but I feel it too.

Thank you Amanda, and I am so glad I 'found' you.
Bernice
PS: I threw out all the trousers in my wardrobe that are now too big for me. There is no going back!

You may wonder how losing 5 kilos could possibly make a person look 10 years younger. That's precisely what I wondered. But when Bernice sent me her before and after photos, I knew exactly what she meant: *She literally looks 10 years younger.*

If you want to look and feel younger but find it hard to cut back on your favourite pleasures, why not try cutting back in short bursts and then taking a weight loss holiday and focusing on maintaining your weight until you're ready for another burst. Instead of spending another 15 years yoyoing in and out of Diet Dungeon and feeling frustrated, you could be enjoying *la dolce vita* as Bernice is now doing.

CHANGE YOUR THINKING: BE TENACIOUS IN BURSTS

Many people mistakenly believe that unless they're losing weight all the time, they're failing. In fact, it's highly unlikely that your weight will go down in linear weekly losses until you reach your ideal weight. Rather, your weight loss adventure will probably consist of a series of stepwise weight losses interspersed with periods of weight maintenance that are due to either the Famine Reaction or accidental or pre-booked weight loss holidays. Accepting these periods as inevitable rather than struggling against them can give you the confidence you need to keep going until you reach your optimum biological weight.

In Chapters 9 and 18 I introduced you to Maree, 44, who lost 12 kilos in 12 months and has kept it off for more than 8 months using the principles outlined in this book. Maree says that one of the things that helped her to conquer her excess weight – at a time when she was also recovering from chronic fatigue syndrome at that – was knowing that it's OK not to be losing weight all the time. In the first month of her weight loss adventure Maree lost 4 kilos, but then her weight got stuck on the same number for several months, what with her Famine Reaction's antics, Christmas and a period when she felt particularly tired. 'But instead of hitting that first plateau and panicking because my weight loss had stopped, then overeating and packing it on again, I was able to have confidence and just keep going,' she told me. Maree lost weight in fits and starts – 3 kilos here, a kilo or two there. Accepting that her journey was not a linear one has made all the difference to her success.

How long should each short burst be?

If you're losing weight in intermittent bursts of focused attention interspersed with regular weight loss holidays, each burst of effort needs to be long enough to produce a measurable and motivating result in terms of weight loss or loss of waistline centimetres (as opposed to being a random dip due to normal fluctuations), while also being short enough to feel do-able. This will most likely change over the course of your weight loss adventure, with longer efforts usually being required the closer you get to your optimum biological weight.

An easy way to know if it's time to end a burst of effort and take a weight loss holiday is when your motivation wanes and you start wanting to eat things like three slices of fruitcake swimming in custard and cream. In Chapter 12 I introduced you to Brooke, now 53, who lost over 7.5 kilos and reached her optimum biological weight of 67.5 to 69.5 kilos, which she has now maintained for more than 18 months. Brooke's journey from 77 kilos to her current weight was not the continuous grind her diet club encouraged but an adventure that included at least two lengthy weight loss holidays.

I took 'pit stops' along the way and allowed my weight to settle. First it settled at around 73 kilos, then it settled at around 71 kilos, and now it is very firmly settled at around 69.5 kilos or under. When I stopped to let my weight settle it was either because I felt that I had been trying to lose weight for a while and wanted 'a rest' from it, or quite simply because I temporarily lost the motivation to do so. Taking a break for a few months was the perfect way to avoid the dreaded plateau as well as those awful eating binges that seem to so readily happen when I try to lose weight for a lengthy period of time.

Each of Brooke's bursts of focused effort lasted for several months. If you're interested in the short burst approach to weight loss, then as a starting guideline you might like to try losing weight in short bursts of approximately 14 days and see how you go. The reason for this recommendation is that when research volunteers sign up to participate in weight loss trials, they usually have no trouble following the program for two weeks, but after that time small deviations from the program start to appear. The important thing to note is that if you can maintain your weight losses between each burst of focused effort, it doesn't really matter how long (or short) your more intensive efforts are. And that brings me to the all-important topic of weight maintenance.

How to maintain your weight during weight loss holidays

When it comes to weight loss holidays, the secret of success lies in ensuring that you are maintaining your weight between each period of weight loss. If you know how to maintain your weight, it doesn't matter how long each weight loss holiday lasts; whether you are actively moving towards, or maintaining, a lower weight, you are still headed in the direction of permanent weight loss.

You may wonder what you need to do to maintain your weight. That's easy. Take a look at a recent period where you were trying to lose weight but you didn't succeed – not because you were having a Famine Reaction and your body was adapting to a new Set Point, but because you didn't manage to do what you know you need to do in order to shift some of the excess. Maybe you were trying to eat only when hungry, but your routine was disrupted with a weekend away and you ended up having a few more non-hungry meals or snacks than you planned. Maybe you were trying to enjoy your favourite martini only on Friday and Saturday nights, but long-lost friends unexpectedly flew into town and you ended up having a fair few drinks with them during the week as well. Maybe you intended to eat almost all healthy foods except for an occasional small treat, but you had a disagreement with your partner and ended up comforting yourself with quick-fix takeaway dinners two nights in a row. Whatever you did during that period, that's exactly the kind of thing you need to do in order to maintain your weight. You weren't losing weight, but you weren't gaining, either. If you kept a Success Diary during that time, you'll know *exactly* how you did it.

Throughout this book you've seen many examples of people who were trying to do what they needed to do to lose weight but nonetheless didn't lose any. While this outcome is often disappointing, it still offers an invaluable lesson in weight maintenance. Carmen discovered that although drinking six to eight glasses of wine per week was too much to allow her to lose weight, it didn't stop her from maintaining her weight. What an empowering discovery; she now knows that whenever she wants to lose weight, 'all' she needs to do is keep doing the things that enabled her to maintain her weight while enjoying her wine but to cut back to around two to four glasses of wine per week. And in between periods of actively trying to lose weight (such as when she takes an accidental or a pre-booked weight loss holiday), as well as once she reaches her optimum biological weight, there's no reason why she can't go back to enjoying her six to eight glasses of wine per week if she wants to. Indeed, she recently came back from a skiing holiday in France where she enjoyed wine, cheese and croissants and didn't gain any weight.

As you can see, weight maintenance still requires effort. You can't just consume any old foods or beverages whenever you feel like putting something in your mouth, and you can't just give up on doing some kind of regular physical activity. However, these things are *much* easier than the super vigilance it requires to actually lose weight. The more experiences you have of maintaining your weight throughout the many adventures that life will throw your way, the more confident you'll become about never going back to your highest ever weight, and Diet Dungeon will seem but a distant memory.

Monitor your size regularly during your weight loss holiday

It's vitally important that you keep weighing or measuring yourself regularly throughout your permanent weight loss adventure, *especially* during periods of weight maintenance. Margo, 59, is exceptionally good at losing weight. Throughout her life she has lost over 30 kilos in less than a year at least four times. But when it comes to weight maintenance, she really struggles. It's usually only a matter of months before she has gained back all the weight she lost. Margo can't say exactly how long it took her to gain the weight back each time, because once she tips the scales at 5 kilos or more above her slimmed-down weight she feels so certain she has failed that she goes back to her old patterns of eating and can no longer bear to look at the scales. These two factors – all-or-nothing thinking and not weighing herself consistently – probably contribute to her downfall. If Margo looked those creeping kilos square in the face and did something about them before they became seemingly unmanageable, she would stand to feel so much more in control of her weight and would be much more likely to keep the weight off once she has lost it. Have you ever noticed that even the biggest, scariest tiger of a task often turns out to be a meek little pussy cat once you stop procrastinating and start doing it? So it is with tackling small weight gains. In fact, in the previously mentioned one-year study of some 2500 'Big-time Losers' who have lost over 13.6 kilos and kept it off for more than a year, it was found that almost all of them were weighing themselves regularly at home at the start of the study, but a year later there were marked differences.[50] Those who over the course of the year weighed themselves as often as, or more often than, they had at the start of the study maintained their weight to within 1.8 kilos of their starting weight, but those who reported weighing themselves less frequently than they had at the start of the study gained significantly more weight: an average of 4 kilos. While it's not exactly clear what comes first (do these people gain weight because they stop weighing themselves as frequently, or do they stop weighing themselves as frequently because they know they are gaining weight), it's probably a combination of both factors. The authors of the study hypothesised that consistent self-weighing can help prevent weight regain by nipping small gains in the bud before they become overwhelming.

So, whatever frequency of weighing and measuring works best for you while you're losing weight – whether it's once a month, once a fortnight, once a week or once a day, as discussed in Chapter 4 – take care to keep it up during weight loss holidays as well as once you reach your optimum biological weight.

Additionally, keep using your hands and your clothes as a guide to how you're going, so that you can quickly adjust your approach when necessary. Lauren weighs and measures herself once a month, so whenever she goes on an overseas trip for four or five weeks, she weighs herself before she leaves and then again when she gets back. While she's away, her clothes let her know how she's going. If her waistbands start feeling a teensy bit too tight or her buttons start straining, she knows it's time to be a bit more discerning about how often she shares a restaurant dessert or enjoys a gin and tonic before dinner. Lauren's regular self-monitoring undoubtedly contributes to the fact that the most she has gained on any accidental weight loss holiday has been 5 kilos, and usually she gains only 2 to 3 kilos. What's more, she is quick to get on top of those excess kilos when she gets back to her regular life.

Weight maintenance guides you for subsequent weight loss

When you know what you need to do in order to maintain your weight, you learn a valuable lesson in how to lose weight. Whenever your weight stays the same (plus or minus a kilo) for several weeks or more, it means that the number of kilojoules you're consuming is the same as the number of kilojoules your body is burning. If you're not having a Famine Reaction at the time (you'll know that you're not having a Famine Reaction if, for example, you're just starting your weight loss adventure after a period of overeating, or if you're just getting back into losing weight after a long weight loss holiday), then either cutting back a bit on your kilojoule intake or increasing your energy expenditure a bit, or both, will result in an energy deficit and will therefore lead to weight loss. It's an immutable law of nature. Often all it takes is a little bit of fine-tuning in order to get the ball rolling.

Lesley, 39, knew that there was a thinner Lesley inside. Since her late teens she'd consistently weighed around 58 kilos, but when she took on a stressful position as a human resources manager three years ago, her weight climbed to an uncomfortable high of 70 kilos. As she hadn't gained any more weight in the past six months – largely thanks to working out vigorously in the gym at work for 45 minutes five days a week and being careful with her food choices – she was in energy balance. In other words, her kilojoule intake matched her kilojoule output. Any reduction in how many kilojoules she ate, or any increase in how many kilojoules she burned, would necessarily result in weight loss. But Lesley couldn't see how it would be possible for her to achieve that. She couldn't possibly cram any more exercise into her already jam-packed schedule, and she was already eating only nutritious whole foods and only when hungry. On inspection of her Success Diary, however, Lesley noticed that she was drinking two flat white coffees every weekday morning and afternoon, usually when she wasn't physically hungry, making for at least seven –1s or 0s in her Hunger column every week. If she gave them up or had a cup of tea instead, she would most likely create enough of a kilojoule deficit to lose weight, but Lesley wasn't prepared to do that. Her coffee breaks and the comfort of that consistent flat white taste and texture gave her a much-needed 'sanity break' from the otherwise constant demands of her long and hectic working days. Lesley found the ideal solution. By eating a bit less at breakfast and lunch, she realised that she would get comfortably hungry (at a level of –2 or –3) in time for her coveted coffee break. After two weeks of implementing this modest change, she had lost 0.7 kilos and was on her way.

If you're currently maintaining a consistent body weight and you're not having a Famine Reaction, even a modest decrease in how many kilojoules you consume, or a slight increase in how many kilojoules you burn, even if it's just a 15-minute increment, will help you to lose weight. So, if your weight or measurements have been stuck on the same numbers for longer than you care for, what small changes could you make to get your weight heading downwards?

Once you learn how to maintain your weight, accidental weight losses can be an added bonus

One of the great things about learning to maintain your weight is that whenever you lose a chunk of excess weight accidentally, because of such things as minor illnesses or going through a period of sadness, you may not regain it and you'll be that much closer to your ideal biological weight. Annie, a 34-year-old woman from Auckland, New Zealand, is so good at maintaining her weight that she accidentally lost 6.1 kilos in less than seven months and reached a svelte 57.4 kilos for her 1.61 metre frame, a weight she has been for most of her adult life and the weight at which she feels best.

From: Annie
Sent: Saturday 28th February 10:34 AM
To: Dr Amanda Sainsbury-Salis
Subject: Re: Hello and thank you

Hi Amanda,

It's been about a year since I read your book and first wrote to you and I thought I'd let you know how it's all been going. It's been going great!

I started revising my eating straightaway after buying your book, and I have to tell you that ALL my stress about food literally melted away overnight – and it has never come back. It took several months before I started losing weight though. In fact it wasn't until early June last year (so about five months) that I noticed any change at all. But during those months I didn't care! I was eating lovely food, as much as I wanted, and I wasn't gaining weight. Win!

In early June I took a 10-day trip to Thailand. I slept very badly while I was there, and learned that when I'm past a certain point of tiredness I stop feeling hungry. The only thing I could really do was ensuring that when I ate, I ate good food – no great hardship in Thailand! When I came home I found that I'd lost about a kilo. I caught up on all that missed sleep and resumed eating as normal. I didn't regain the weight.

Six weeks later I had another bout of sleeplessness, accompanied by lack of appetite. I lost another kilo. I got my sleep and appetite back on track, and didn't regain the weight. This has happened several more times since then, and each time I lose roughly the same amount and it never comes back. The upshot is that at last weigh-in I'd lost 6.1 kilos over the six to seven months. My starting point was 63.5 kilos so that's almost 10% of my bodyweight. 10%!!! How cool is that!

Amanda, not only do I have my body back in a form that I recognise, but I'm happier than I can remember being for many years. Food is no longer a constant nagging worry at the back of my mind, like a distant fingernail eternally scraping down a blackboard. I eat what I want, when I want. At exam time this includes several large chocolate bars. So thank you, really thank you, from the bottom of my heart.

I hope everything is going well for you too.

Best,

Annie

You'll have noticed that each of Annie's accidental weight losses was relatively small, about a kilo, and that they took her back towards a weight she recognised as right for her. These are important points. Had her accidental weight losses been too fast, or had they taken her too far below her current Set Point, they would have activated a raging Famine Reaction that would have made it extremely difficult to prevent regain.

In Chapter 15 I told you about the emergency cholecystectomy I had to remove my gallbladder and gallstones. Two things about that operation remain particularly strongly imprinted in my mind. The first is the excruciating pain I felt after the operation, which involved a 14 centimetre incision in my abdomen and a lot of poking around in my ducts to ensure there were no little chips of gallstone remaining that would wreak subsequent havoc. I was in so much pain after the operation that I scarcely ate anything in the first five days, and during the remainder of my 12-day hospital stay I was a little tentative about eating with my normal level of gusto. The other thing I vividly remember is that when I got home and weighed myself, I had lost 3 kilos. For more than three months I had been stuck on a Set Point of 73 kilos and my weight just wouldn't budge no matter what I did, and now I had lost 3 kilos in a matter of just 12 days. Some of the weight loss would have been due to loss of body water and lean body mass on account of my almost total inactivity in hospital, but some of it would have been due to fat loss. I felt wonderful, but I'd obviously gone too far below my current Set Point too fast, because the weight came back again in less than two months, even though I was already fully proficient at maintaining my weight. The moral of the story is that if you lose weight accidentally and you put it back on again, you shouldn't feel bad about yourself. But if you do keep it off, what a bonus!

How long do you need to spend on each weight loss holiday?

When you take a weight loss holiday, you need to stay on holiday for at least as long as it takes to deactivate your Famine Reaction. Research suggests that this can take anything from one to 12 weeks, possibly longer if you've been struggling with a lot of excess weight for many years.[7, 8, 12–14, 17] However, if you're listening to your body and following its cues about what and how much to eat, you won't need to worry about whether your Famine Reaction has been deactivated; the beast won't let you cross the bridge to ongoing weight loss until it is totally convinced the famine has vanished. If you try to lose more weight by eating less than you really need but your Famine Reaction is still on high alert, the teensiest weight reduction will be met with a hunger that pushes you to eat until you regain that weight. In other words, you'll be having an enforced weight loss holiday.

Because of the Famine Reaction's effects on your appetite and cravings, you'll probably be able to sense when the Famine Reaction has dissipated and it's safe for you to lose some more weight. Every time Lauren came out of one of those periods when her weight had refused to go down (the enforced weight loss holiday), she had a sense that it was time to start trying a bit harder. My own experience is that whenever I'd been on a weight loss holiday for a while, especially the ones I took at the end of my journey, when it took month-long bursts to push my weight down, I got a sense that being another kilo or so lighter would be nicer than the woodfired pizzas I was sometimes enjoying when I wasn't physically hungry, or the chocolates I was savouring a little too liberally. Before then, the prospect of losing more weight had felt too onerous. Maybe it had been my Famine Reaction grumbling, making sure that I didn't try to cross the bridge to further weight loss.

When you take an accidental or a pre-booked weight loss holiday, you may end up taking more annual leave than your body needs in order to appease the Famine Reaction. During my 28 kilo weight loss adventure, I took many lengthy weight loss holidays. I used to convince myself that I was taming my Famine Reaction, but in reality it probably didn't need that much taming, I was just indulging my Labrador-like tendencies to want to eat as much as possible. But what does it matter if you take a longer weight loss holiday than your body actually needs? Holidays are not just for the benefit of your body; they're for your mind as well. There's no point in trying to lose weight when there are too many things competing for your energy. For Bernice, this meant slotting in each short burst of weight loss at a time when she had a 'clear run' ahead of her, a week or two when she had few or no overseas trips or sales meetings to interfere with her need to keep alcohol intake to a minimum. If you're going through any kind of challenging period where it's a struggle just to attend to the basic necessities of your life – let alone organising your kitchen and being mindful of your hunger signals – then it's probably best to wait a bit longer before attempting to lose some more weight. The only right time to come back from holidays is when your body is fully rested *and* you feel wholly ready to get back to work.

Over to you
Here's something you can do immediately to put the ideas in this chapter into action.

Remember that there is absolutely no reason why you have to be trying to lose weight all the time in order to reach your optimum biological weight. In fact, interim periods of weight maintenance as you progress towards your body's healthiest weight may even improve your chances of success by helping to physically wash out any trace of the Famine Reaction and to re-energise you mentally for the mindfulness it takes to lose weight.

If you're in a situation where it seems too difficult to lose weight, whether it's because the Famine Reaction has forced a weight loss holiday on you, an accidental weight loss holiday has been sprung on you, or you just want to take a pre-booked rest from trying to lose weight, try focusing on maintaining your weight instead. Weight maintenance is never easy, but it's a darned sight easier than the degree of vigilance you need to actually lose weight. Through trial and error, you'll soon learn exactly what it takes to maintain your weight. If you do those things consistently, then every kilo you lose will be a kilo gone for good.

Write and tell me how you're going

The mediocre teacher tells. The good teacher explains.
The superior teacher demonstrates. The great teacher
inspires.
William Arthur Ward, American writer, 1921–1994

This brings me to the end of the real-life success stories I have brought together in this book. I've had the privilege of getting to know the intimate details of many people's relationship with food and their body, and I trust that through their stories and experiences, as well as the scientific studies cited in this book, you've seen that it *is* possible to lose weight and keep it off by listening to that ultimate teacher, *your own body*. Most of all, I hope that this work has inspired you to start listening to your body – starting with that all-important stepping stone, your Success Diary – and to use the 10 diagnostic tests in this book to identify which specific strategies you need to use to lose weight and keep it off without wasting another precious day of your life in Diet Dungeon.

I know as well as anyone does what it's like to be constantly worried about your weight and obsessing about what, when and how much to eat. I spent six years in that miserable state, until I learned through my medical research that there *is* a way to lose weight once and for all without reconciling myself to a lifetime of servitude in Diet Dungeon. If you've had enough of counting kilojoules, of low-fat, tasteless diet foods, of eating separate meals to your family and friends, of paltry little diet portions that leave you feeling unsatisfied, or of getting on the scales and panicking because you either haven't lost weight or have regained the weight you lost, why not put all that behind you and let your body show you an easier way to lose excess weight and keep it off? The three simple steps in this book are based on years of medical research into successful weight management. They will enable you to lose weight and keep it off by working with your body, not against it. Others who have followed these simple steps have lost weight and are keeping it off, and you can, too.

One of my biggest joys is to hear from my readers. If you'd like to tell me about your Don't Go Hungry Weight Loss Adventure, please drop me a line via my website or postal address, below. It will make my day to hear how my six years in Diet Dungeon and a career in scientific research have helped you to change your life for the better. With your permission, your story could feature in one of my newsletters or my next book and inspire others to reach their true potential.

Have fun, and I look forward to hearing from you.

Sincerely,

Amanda.

Dr Amanda Sainsbury-Salis, PhD

To contact Dr Amanda
Website: http://www.DrAmandaOnline.com
Mail: Dr Amanda Sainsbury-Salis
           PO Box 544
           Kogarah NSW 1485
           Australia

Acknowledgments

Writing a book is an adventure. To begin with, it is a toy and an amusement; then it becomes a mistress, and then it becomes a master, and then a tyrant. The last phase is that just as you are about to be reconciled to your servitude, you kill the monster, and fling him out to the public.

Sir Winston Churchill, British orator, author and
prime minister during World War II, 1874–1965

True to Sir Winston Churchill's words, writing this book has certainly been an adventure. What I thought would be a quick and straightforward project turned out to be much bigger than I ever imagined. However, the feeling of fulfilment it gives me to bring this message to my readers is worth every hair-tearing moment. I could never have achieved this feat without the help of the following people.

I will forever be grateful to my husband for encouraging me to write this book in the first place – for no other reason than that he knew I felt called to do so. Even though writing this book has meant sacrificing a lot of family times together, he has stood behind me and cheered me on. Thank you, Honey; I'm looking forward to having our weekends for us again.

To all the people who shared their experiences in this book so that others could learn from them and be inspired by them, thank you for helping me bring my message to life. Many people have told me that the real-life examples in my first book gave them the courage to let go of rigid dieting and follow their body signals to arrive at a healthier weight and a peaceful relationship with food, and now your stories have the potential to inspire more people to do the same.

I am grateful to all the people who contacted me and told me about their weight management adventures after reading *The Don't Go Hungry Diet* or attending my live workshops. Your questions, comments, challenges and successes have been instrumental in shaping this book.

A huge thank you goes to Annette (Carter) Sayers, editor, for scrupulously editing this book and ensuring consistency throughout, and for helping me to bring my message to my readers in a clear, easy-to-read form.

I am extremely grateful to Mel Cox at Random House Australia, who championed this book right from the start and so generously helped me to get a better understanding of publishing. Without your encouragement, this book might have taken many more years to come to fruition.

To my Mum, Bev Sainsbury; my sisters, Sally and Belinda Sainsbury (and Tim Hughes and Christian O'Connor); as well as to Kathryn Dixon, thank you for babysitting so that I could continue writing during the school holidays. It was wonderful knowing that my children were laughing, learning and getting lots of love and hugs in your care.

Special thanks go to Associate Professor John Dixon, Head of the Obesity Research Unit in the Department of General Practice at Monash University, and National Health and Medical Research Council Senior Research Fellow in the Human Neurotransmitters Laboratory, Baker IDI Heart and Diabetes Institute, for invaluable discussions about gastric surgery and the associated risks and benefits.

Thank you to Allan Borushek, author of CalorieKing.com.au, the free online website from which all kilojoule counts in this book were obtained.

The food variety quiz in Diagnostic N°2d is reproduced from 'Food variety as nutritional therapy', Dr Gayle S. Savige, Dr Bridget Hsu-Gage and Professor Mark L. Wahlqvist, *Current*

Therapeutics, in March 1997, with permission from Adis, a Wolters Kluwer business (©Adis Data Information 1997). All rights reserved. An electronic version of this quiz can be found on Professor Wahlqvist's website: http://www.healthyeating-club.org

I gratefully acknowledge the warm welcome of my favourite writing cafés: Dome Café in Claremont, WA; Home Style Food Bar in Claremont, WA; Michel's Patisserie in Kogarah, NSW, and Gloria Jean's Coffees in Kogarah, NSW. There's nothing like one of their wonderfully smooth caffé lattes and the clatter of background noise for bringing logic and form to a sea of ideas.

Finally, I'm grateful to my penpal Nartana for her persistent encouragement throughout the creation of this book, and for reminding me of the world's need for the message within it.

References

1. Sainsbury A, Zhang L. Role of the arcuate nucleus of the hypothalamus in regulation of body weight during energy deficit. *Molecular and Cellular Endocrinology* 2010; 316(2): 109–119.

2. Doucet E, Imbeault P, St-Pierre S, Almeras N, Mauriege P, Richard D *et al*. Appetite after weight loss by energy restriction and a low-fat diet-exercise follow-up. *International Journal of Obesity and Related Metabolic Disorders* 2000; 24(7): 906–914.

3. Westerterp-Plantenga MS, Saris WH, Hukshorn CJ, Campfield LA. Effects of weekly administration of pegylated recombinant human OB protein on appetite profile and energy metabolism in obese men. *American Journal of Clinical Nutrition* 2001; 74(4): 426–434.

4. Martin CK, Heilbronn LK, de Jonge L, DeLany JP, Volaufova J, Anton SD *et al*. Effect of calorie restriction on resting metabolic rate and spontaneous physical activity. *Obesity* 2007; 15(12): 2964–2973.

5. Rosenbaum M, Nicolson M, Hirsch J, Murphy E, Chu F, Leibel RL. Effects of weight change on plasma leptin concentrations and energy expenditure. *Journal of Clinical Endocrinology and Metabolism* 1997; 82(11): 3647–3654.

6. Leibel RL, Rosenbaum M, Hirsch J. Changes in energy expenditure resulting from altered body weight. *New England Journal of Medicine* 1995; 332(10): 621–628.

7. Weinsier RL, Nagy TR, Hunter GR, Darnell BE, Hensrud DD, Weiss HL. Do adaptive changes in metabolic rate favor weight regain in weight-reduced individuals? An examination of the set-point theory. *American Journal of Clinical Nutrition* 2000; 72(5): 1088–1094.

8. Friedl KE, Moore RJ, Hoyt RW, Marchitelli LJ, Martinez-Lopez LE, Askew EW. Endocrine markers of semistarvation in healthy lean men in a multistressor environment. *Journal of Applied Physiology* 2000; 88(5): 1820–1830.

9. Niskanen L, Laaksonen DE, Punnonen K, Mustajoki P, Kaukua J, Rissanen A. Changes in sex hormone-binding globulin and testosterone during weight loss and weight maintenance in abdominally obese men with the metabolic syndrome. *Diabetes Obesity & Metabolism* 2004; 6(3): 208–215.

10. Beck B, Jhanwar-Uniyal M, Burlet A, Chapleur-Chateau M, Leibowitz SF, Burlet C. Rapid and localized alterations of neuropeptide Y in discrete hypothalamic nuclei with feeding status. *Brain Research* 1990; 528(2): 245–249.

11. Swart I, Jahng JW, Overton JM, Houpt TA. Hypothalamic NPY, AGRP, and POMC mRNA responses to leptin and refeeding in mice. *American Journal of Physiology* 2002; 283(5): R1020–R1026.

12. Westerterp-Plantenga MS, Lejeune MP, Nijs I, van Ooijen M, Kovacs EM. High protein intake sustains weight maintenance after body weight loss in humans. *International Journal of Obesity and Related Metabolic Disorders* 2004; 28(1): 57–64.

13. Hunter GR, Byrne NM. Physical activity and muscle function but not resting energy expenditure impact on weight gain. *The Journal of Strength & Conditioning Research* 2005; 19(1): 225–230.

14. Belza A, Toubro S, Stender S, Astrup A. Effect of diet-induced energy deficit and body fat reduction on high-sensitive CRP and other inflammatory markers in obese subjects. *International Journal of Obesity (London)* 2009; 33(4): 456–464.

15. Buscemi S, Verga S, Maneri R, Blunda G, Galluzzo A. Influences of obesity and weight loss on thyroid hormones. A 3–3.5-year follow-up study on obese subjects with surgical bilio-pancreatic by-pass. *Journal of Endocrinological Investigation* 1997; 20(5): 276–281.

16. Filozof CM, Murua C, Sanchez MP, Brailovsky C, Perman M, Gonzalez CD *et al.* Low plasma leptin concentration and low rates of fat oxidation in weight-stable post-obese subjects. *Obesity Research* 2000; 8(3): 205–210.

17. Larson DE, Ferraro RT, Robertson DS, Ravussin E. Energy metabolism in weight-stable post-obese individuals. *American Journal of Clinical Nutrition* 1995; 62(4): 735–739.

18. Weinsier RL, Hunter GR, Zuckerman PA, Redden DT, Darnell BE, Larson DE *et al.* Energy expenditure and free-living physical activity in black and white women: comparison before and after weight loss. *American Journal of Clinical Nutrition* 2000; 71(5): 1138–1146.

19. Szymanski LA, Tabaac BJ, Schneider JE. Signals that link energy to reproduction: gastric fill, bulk intake, or caloric intake? *Physiology & Behaviour* 2009; 96(4–5): 540–547.

20. de Rijke CE, Hillebrand JJ, Verhagen LA, Roeling TA, Adan RA. Hypothalamic neuropeptide expression following chronic food restriction in sedentary and wheel-running rats. *Journal of Molecular Endocrinology* 2005; 35(2): 381–390.

21. Sweeney ME, Hill JO, Heller PA, Baney R, DiGirolamo M. Severe vs moderate energy restriction with and without exercise in the treatment of obesity: efficiency of weight loss. *American Journal of Clinical Nutrition* 1993; 57(2): 127–134.

22. Brooks RC, Simpson SJ, Raubenheimer D. The price of protein: combining evolutionary and economic analysis to understand excessive energy consumption. *Obesity Reviews* 2010, in press.

23. Beard J, Borel M, Peterson FJ. Changes in iron status during weight loss with very-low-energy diets. *American Journal of Clinical Nutrition* 1997; 66(1): 104–110.

24. Dulloo AG, Jacquet J. Low-protein overfeeding: a tool to unmask susceptibility to obesity in humans. *International Journal of Obesity* 1999; 23(11): 1118–1121.

25. Frank A, Anke M, Danielsson R. Experimental copper and chromium deficiency and additional molybdenum supplementation in goats. I. Feed consumption and weight development. *Science of the Total Environment* 2000; 249(1–3): 133–142.

26. Selvais PL, Labuche C, Nguyen XN, Ketelslegers JM, Denef JF, Maiter DM. Cyclic feeding behaviour and changes in hypothalamic galanin and neuropeptide Y gene expression induced by zinc deficiency in the rat. *Journal of Neuroendocrinology* 1997; 9(1): 55–62.

27. Specter SE, Hamilton JS, Stern JS, Horwitz BA. Chronic protein restriction does not alter energetic efficiency or brown adipose tissue thermogenic capacity in genetically obese (fa/fa) Zucker rats. *Journal of Nutrition* 1995; 125(8): 2183–2193.

28. Wijers SL, Saris WH, van Marken Lichtenbelt WD. Recent advances in adaptive thermogenesis: potential implications for the treatment of obesity. *Obesity Reviews* 2009; 10(2): 218–226.

29. Stock MJ. Gluttony and thermogenesis revisited. *International Journal of Obesity and Related Metabolic Disorders* 1999; 23(11): 1105–1117.

30. Roberts SB, Young VR, Fuss P, Fiatarone MA, Richard B, Rasmussen H *et al.* Energy expenditure and subsequent nutrient intakes in overfed young men. *American Journal of Physiology* 1990; 259 (3 Pt 2): R461–R469.

31. Levine JA, Eberhardt NL, Jensen MD. Role of nonexercise activity thermogenesis in resistance to fat gain in humans. *Science* 1999; 283(5399): 212–214.

32. Rising R, Alger S, Boyce V, Seagle H, Ferraro R, Fontvieille AM *et al.* Food intake measured by an automated food-selection system: relationship to energy expenditure. *American Journal of Clinical Nutrition* 1992; 55(2): 343–349.

33. World Health Organization. Obesity: preventing and managing the global epidemic. Report of a WHO consultation. *Word Health Organization Technical Report Service* 2000; 894(3): 1–253.

34. Alibhai SM, Greenwood C, Payette H. An approach to the management of unintentional weight loss in elderly people. *Canadian Medical Association Journal* 2005; 172(6): 773–780.

35. Chapman IM. Obesity in old age. *Frontiers of Hormone Research* 2008; 36: 97–106.

36. Shahar A, Shahar D, Kahar Y, Nitzan-Kalusky D. [Low-weight and weight loss as predictors of morbidity and mortality in old age]. *Harefuah* 2005; 144(6): 443–8, 452.

37. Hocking SL, Chisholm DJ, James DE. Studies of regional adipose transplantation reveal a unique and beneficial interaction between subcutaneous adipose tissue and the intra-abdominal compartment. *Diabetologia* 2008; 51(5): 900–902.

38. Lovejoy JC, Sainsbury A. Sex differences in obesity and the regulation of energy homeostasis. *Obesity Reviews* 2009; 10(2): 154–167.

39. Lear SA, James PT, Ko GT, Kumanyika S. Appropriateness of waist circumference and waist-to-hip ratio cutoffs for different ethnic groups. *European Journal of Clinical Nutrition* 2010; 64(1): 42–61.

40. Linder J, McLaren L, Siou GL, Csizmadi I, Robson PJ. The epidemiology of weight perception: perceived versus self-reported actual weight status among Albertan adults. *Canadian Journal of Public Health* 2010; 101(1): 56–60.

41. Panter-Brick C, Lotstein DS, Ellison PT. Seasonality of reproductive function and weight loss in rural Nepali women. *Human Reproduction* 1993; 8(5): 684–690.

42. Hukshorn CJ, Menheere PP, Westerterp-Plantenga MS, Saris WH. The effect of pegylated human recombinant leptin (PEG-OB) on neuroendocrine adaptations to semi-starvation in overweight men. *European Journal of Endocrinology* 2003; 148(6): 649–655.

43. Johnstone AM, Faber P, Andrew R, Gibney ER, Elia M, Lobley G et al. Influence of short-term dietary weight loss on cortisol secretion and metabolism in obese men. *European Journal of Endocrinology* 2004; 150(2): 185–194.

44. Poehlman ET. Menopause, energy expenditure, and body composition. *Acta Obstetricia et Gynecologica Scandinavica* 2002; 81(7): 603–611.

45. Blouin K, Despres JP, Couillard C, Tremblay A, Prud'homme D, Bouchard C et al. Contribution of age and declining androgen levels to features of the metabolic syndrome in men. *Metabolism* 2005; 54(8): 1034–1040.

46. Kamel HK, Maas D, Duthie EH, Jr. Role of hormones in the pathogenesis and management of sarcopenia. *Drugs & Aging* 2002; 19(11): 865–877.

47. Rosen CJ, Ackert-Bicknell CL, Adamo ML, Shultz KL, Rubin J, Donahue LR et al. Congenic mice with low serum IGF-I have increased body fat, reduced bone mineral density, and an altered osteoblast differentiation program. *Bone* 2004; 35(5): 1046–1058.

48. Natsui K, Tanaka K, Suda M, Yasoda A, Sakuma Y, Ozasa A et al. High-dose glucocorticoid treatment induces rapid loss of trabecular bone mineral density and lean body mass. *Osteoporosis International* 2006; 17(1): 105–108.

49. Curtis JR, Westfall AO, Allison J, Bijlsma JW, Freeman A, George V *et al*. Population-based assessment of adverse events associated with long-term glucocorticoid use. *Arthritis and Rheumatism* 2006; 55(3): 420–426.

50. Butryn ML, Phelan S, Hill JO, Wing RR. Consistent self-monitoring of weight: a key component of successful weight loss maintenance. *Obesity (Silver Spring)* 2007; 15(12): 3091–3096.

51. Church TS, Martin CK, Thompson AM, Earnest CP, Mikus CR, Blair SN. Changes in weight, waist circumference and compensatory responses with different doses of exercise among sedentary, overweight postmenopausal women. *PLoS One* 2009; 4(2): e4515.

52. Wojtaszewski JF, Nielsen JN, Richter EA. Invited review: effect of acute exercise on insulin signaling and action in humans. *Journal of Applied Physiology* 2002; 93(1): 384–392.

53. Everson G, Kelsberg G, Nashelsky J, Mott T. Clinical inquiries. How effective is gastric bypass for weight loss? *The Journal of Family Practice* 2004; 53(11): 914–918.

54. Picot J, Jones J, Colquitt JL, Gospodarevskaya E, Loveman E, Baxter L *et al*. The clinical effectiveness and cost-effectiveness of bariatric (weight loss) surgery for obesity: a systematic review and economic evaluation. *Health Technology Assessment* 2009; 13(41): 1–190, 215–357, iii–iv.

55. Boneva-Asiova Z, Boyanov MA. Body composition analysis by leg-to-leg bioelectrical impedance and dual-energy X-ray absorptiometry in non-obese and obese individuals. *Diabetes, Obesity and Metabolism* 2008; 10(11): 1012–1018.

56. Watson PE, Robinson MF. Variations in Body-Weight of Young Women during the Menstrual Cycle. *British Journal of Nutrition* 1965; 19: 237–248.

57. Klem ML, Wing RR, Lang W, McGuire MT, Hill JO. Does weight loss maintenance become easier over time? *Obesity Research* 2000; 8(6): 438–444.

58. Wing RR, Phelan S. Long-term weight loss maintenance. *American Journal of Clinical Nutrition* 2005; 82(1 Suppl): 222S–225S.

59. Streit KJ, Stevens NH, Stevens VJ, Rossner J. Food records: a predictor and modifier of weight change in a long-term weight loss program. *Journal of the American Dietetic Association* 1991; 91(2): 213–216.

60. Donnelly JE, Blair SN, Jakicic JM, Manore MM, Rankin JW, Smith BK. American College of Sports Medicine Position Stand. Appropriate physical activity intervention strategies for weight loss and prevention of weight regain for adults. *Medicine & Science in Sports & Exercise* 2009; 41(2): 459–471.

61. Saris WH, Blair SN, van Baak MA, Eaton SB, Davies PS, Di Pietro L *et al.* How much physical activity is enough to prevent unhealthy weight gain? Outcome of the IASO 1st Stock Conference and consensus statement. *Obesity Reviews* 2003; 4(2): 101–114.

62. Phelan S, Roberts M, Lang W, Wing RR. Empirical evaluation of physical activity recommendations for weight control in women. *Medicine & Science in Sports & Exercise* 2007; 39(10): 1832–1836.

63. Hunter GR, Byrne NM, Sirikul B, Fernandez JR, Zuckerman PA, Darnell BE *et al.* Resistance training conserves fat-free mass and resting energy expenditure following weight loss. *Obesity (Silver Spring)* 2008; 16(5): 1045–1051.

64. Martins C, Morgan L, Truby H. A review of the effects of exercise on appetite regulation: an obesity perspective. *International Journal of Obesity (London)* 2008; 32(9): 1337–1347.

65. Maurer J, Taren DL, Teixeira PJ, Thomson CA, Lohman TG, Going SB *et al.* The psychosocial and behavioral characteristics related to energy misreporting. *Nutrition Reviews* 2006; 64 (2 Pt 1): 53–66.

66. Weihrauch MR, Diehl V. Artificial sweeteners – do they bear a carcinogenic risk? *Annals of Oncology* 2004; 15(10): 1460–1465.

67. Ha EJ, Caine-Bish N, Holloman C, Lowry-Gordon K. Evaluation of effectiveness of class-based nutrition intervention on changes in soft drink and milk consumption among young adults. *Nutrition Journal* 2009; 8: 50.

68. Palmer M, Capra S, Baines S. To snack or not to snack: results from an eating frequency weight loss study. *Nutrition and Dietetics* 2008; 65, supp 2: A14.

69. Marmonier C, Chapelot D, Fantino M, Louis-Sylvestre J. Snacks consumed in a nonhungry state have poor satiating efficiency: influence of snack composition on substrate utilization and hunger. *American Journal of Clinical Nutrition* 2002; 76(3): 518–528.

70. Johnson PM, Kenny PJ. Dopamine D2 receptors in addiction-like reward dysfunction and compulsive eating in obese rats. *Nature Neuroscience* 2010; 13(5): 635–641.

71. Saris WH, van Erp-Baart MA, Brouns F, Westerterp KR, ten Hoor F. Study on food intake and energy expenditure during extreme sustained exercise: the Tour de France. *International Journal of Sports Medicine* 1989; 10 Suppl 1: S26–S31.

72. Burke L. Fasting and recovery from exercise. *British Journal of Sports Medicine* 2010; 44(7): 502–508.

73. MacLean PS, Higgins JA, Wyatt HR, Melanson EL, Johnson GC, Jackman MR *et al*. Regular exercise attenuates the metabolic drive to regain weight after long-term weight loss. *American Journal of Physiology* 2009; 297(3): R793–R802.

74. Simkin-Silverman LR, Wing RR, Boraz MA, Kuller LH. Lifestyle intervention can prevent weight gain during menopause: results from a 5-year randomized clinical trial. *Annals of Behavioral Medicine* 2003; 26(3): 212–220.

75. Lovejoy JC, Champagne CM, de Jonge L, Xie H, Smith SR. Increased visceral fat and decreased energy expenditure during the menopausal transition. *International Journal of Obesity (London)* 2008; 32(6): 949–958.

76. Sternfeld B, Bhat AK, Wang H, Sharp T, Quesenberry CP, Jr. Menopause, physical activity, and body composition/fat distribution in midlife women. *Medicine & Science in Sports & Exercise* 2005; 37(7): 1195–1202.

77. Sternfeld B, Wang H, Quesenberry CP, Jr., Abrams B, Everson-Rose SA, Greendale GA *et al*. Physical activity and changes in weight and waist circumference in midlife women: findings from the Study of Women's Health Across the Nation. *American Journal of Epidemiology* 2004; 160(9): 912–922.

78. You T, Murphy KM, Lyles MF, Demons JL, Lenchik L, Nicklas BJ. Addition of aerobic exercise to dietary weight loss preferentially reduces abdominal adipocyte size. *International Journal of Obesity (London)* 2006; 30(8): 1211–1216.

79. Silva JE. The thermogenic effect of thyroid hormone and its clinical implications. *Annals of Internal Medicine* 2003; 139(3): 205–213.

80. Empson M, Flood V, Ma G, Eastman CJ, Mitchell P. Prevalence of thyroid disease in an older Australian population. *Internal Medicine Journal* 2007; 37(7): 448–455.

81. Zimmermann MB. Iodine deficiency. *Endocrine Reviews* 2009; 30(4): 376–408.

82. Li M, Eastman CJ, Waite KV, Ma G, Zacharin MR, Topliss DJ *et al*. Are Australian children iodine deficient? Results of the Australian National Iodine Nutrition Study. *Medical Journal of Australia* 2006; 184(4): 165–169.

83. Iossa S, Lionetti L, Mollica MP, Crescenzo R, Barletta A, Liverini G. Fat balance and serum leptin concentrations in normal, hypothyroid, and hyperthyroid rats. *International Journal of Obesity and Related Metabolic Disorders* 2001; 25(3): 417–425.

84. Rosenbaum M, Hirsch J, Murphy E, Leibel RL. Effects of changes in body weight on carbohydrate metabolism, catecholamine excretion, and thyroid function. *American Journal of Clinical Nutrition* 2000; 71(6): 1421–1432.

85. Wansink B, Painter JE, North J. Bottomless bowls: why visual cues of portion size may influence intake. *Obesity Research* 2005; 13(1): 93–100.

86. Kokkinos A, le Roux CW, Alexiadou K, Tentolouris N, Vincent RP, Kyriaki D *et al*. Eating slowly increases the postprandial response of the anorexigenic gut hormones, peptide YY and glucagon-like peptide-1. *Journal of Clinical Endocrinology & Metabolism* 2010; 95(1): 333–337.

87. Ames BN. Increasing longevity by tuning up metabolism. To maximize human health and lifespan, scientists must abandon outdated models of micronutrients. *EMBO Report* 2005; 6 Spec No: S20–S24.

88. Ames BN, Wakimoto P. Are vitamin and mineral deficiencies a major cancer risk? *Nature Reviews Cancer* 2002; 2(9): 694–704.

89. National Health & Medical Research Council. *Dietary Guidelines for Australian Adults*, Commonwealth of Australia: Canberra, 2003.

90. Savige GS, Hsu-Gage B, Wahlqvist ML. Food variety as nutritional therapy. *Current Therapeutics* 1997; March: 57–67.

91. Lin S, Thomas TC, Storlien LH, Huang XF. Development of high fat diet-induced obesity and leptin resistance in C57Bl/6J mice. *International Journal of Obesity and Related Metabolic Disorders* 2000; 24(5): 639–646.

92. Lin S, Storlien LH, Huang X. Leptin receptor, NPY, POMC mRNA expression in the diet-induced obese mouse brain. *Brain Research* 2000; 875(1–2): 89–95.

93. El-Haschimi K, Pierroz DD, Hileman SM, Bjorbaek C, Flier JS. Two defects contribute to hypothalamic leptin resistance in mice with diet-induced obesity. *Journal of Clinical Investigation* 2000; 105(12): 1827–1832.

94. Enriori PJ, Evans AE, Sinnayah P, Jobst EE, Tonelli-Lemos L, Billes SK *et al.* Diet-induced obesity causes severe but reversible leptin resistance in arcuate melanocortin neurons. *Cell Metabolism* 2007; 5(3): 181–194.

95. Rolls BJ, Drewnowski A, Ledikwe JH. Changing the energy density of the diet as a strategy for weight management. *Journal of the American Dietetic Association* 2005; 105(5 Suppl 1): S98–103.

96. Bell EA, Castellanos VH, Pelkman CL, Thorwart ML, Rolls BJ. Energy density of foods affects energy intake in normal-weight women. *American Journal of Clinical Nutrition* 1998; 67(3): 412–420.

97. Karhunen LJ, Juvonen KR, Huotari A, Purhonen AK, Herzig KH. Effect of protein, fat, carbohydrate and fibre on gastrointestinal peptide release in humans. *Regulatory Peptides* 2008; 149(1–3): 70–78.

98. Schroder KE. Effects of fruit consumption on body mass index and weight loss in a sample of overweight and obese dieters enrolled in a weight-loss intervention trial. *Nutrition* 2009.

99. Alinia S, Hels O, Tetens I. The potential association between fruit intake and body weight – a review. *Obesity Reviews* 2009; 10(6): 639–647.

100. National Health & Medical Research Council. *Australian Guidelines to Reduce Health Risks from Drinking Alcohol*, Commonwealth of Australia: Canberra, 2009.

101. Mourao DM, Bressan J, Campbell WW, Mattes RD. Effects of food form on appetite and energy intake in lean and obese young adults. *International Journal of Obesity (London)* 2007; 31(11): 1688–1695.

102. Yeomans MR. Effects of alcohol on food and energy intake in human subjects: evidence for passive and active over-consumption of energy. *British Journal of Nutrition* 2004; 92 Suppl 1: S31–S34.

103. Gee C. Does alcohol stimulate appetite and energy intake? *British Journal of Community Nursing* 2006; 11(7): 298–302.

104. Loos RJ. Recent progress in the genetics of common obesity. *British Journal of Clinical Pharmacology* 2009; 68(6): 811–829.

105. Loos RJ, Bouchard C. FTO: the first gene contributing to common forms of human obesity. *Obesity Reviews* 2008; 9(3): 246–250.

106. Hukshorn CJ, Westerterp-Plantenga MS, Saris WH. Pegylated human recombinant leptin (PEG-OB) causes additional weight loss in severely energy-restricted, overweight men. *American Journal of Clinical Nutrition* 2003; 77(4): 771–776.

107. Farooqi IS, O'Rahilly S. Mutations in ligands and receptors of the leptin-melanocortin pathway that lead to obesity. *Nature Clinical Practice Endocrinology & Metabolism* 2008; 4(10): 569–577.

108. Sainsbury A, Schwarzer C, Couzens M, Jenkins A, Oakes SR, Ormandy CJ *et al.* Y4 receptor knockout rescues fertility in ob/ob mice. *Genes and Development* 2002; 16(9): 1077–1088.

109. Hill AJ. The psychology of food craving. *Proceedings of the Nutrition Society* 2007; 66(2): 277–285.

110. Byrne SM, Cooper Z, Fairburn CG. Psychological predictors of weight regain in obesity. *Behaviour Research and Therapy* 2004; 42(11): 1341–1356.

111. Sodlerlund A, Fischer A, Johansson T. Physical activity, diet and behaviour modification in the treatment of overweight and obese adults: a systematic review. *Perspectives in Public Health* 2009; 129(3): 132–142.

112. Westerterp KR, Meijer GA, Janssen EM, Saris WH, Ten Hoor F. Long-term effect of physical activity on energy balance and body composition. *British Journal of Nutrition* 1992; 68(1): 21–30.

113. Westerterp KR, Meijer GA, Schoffelen P, Janssen EM. Body mass, body composition and sleeping metabolic rate before, during and after endurance training. *European Journal of Applied Physiology and Occupational Physiology* 1994; 69(3): 203–208.

114. Ross R, Bradshaw AJ. The future of obesity reduction: beyond weight loss. *Nature Reviews Endocrinology* 2009; 5(6): 319–325.

115. Wu T, Gao X, Chen M, van Dam RM. Long-term effectiveness of diet-plus-exercise interventions vs. diet-only interventions for weight loss: a meta-analysis. *Obesity Reviews* 2009; 10(3): 313–323.

116. Ades PA, Savage PD, Toth MJ, Harvey-Berino J, Schneider DJ, Bunn JY *et al.* High-calorie-expenditure exercise: a new approach to cardiac rehabilitation for overweight coronary patients. *Circulation* 2009; 119(20): 2671–2678.

117. Pasman WJ, Saris WH, Westerterp-Plantenga MS. Predictors of weight maintenance. *Obesity Research* 1999; 7(1): 43–50.

118. Goran MI. Energy metabolism and obesity. *Medical Clinics of North America* 2000; 84(2): 347–362.

119. Weinsier R, Hunter G, Schutz Y. Metabolic response to weight loss. *American Journal of Clinical Nutrition* 2001; 73(3): 655–658.

120. Levin BE, Dunn-Meynell AA. Chronic exercise lowers the defended body weight gain and adiposity in diet-induced obese rats. *American Journal of Physiology* 2004; 286(4): R771–R778.

121. O'Rahilly S. Human genetics illuminates the paths to metabolic disease. *Nature* 2009; 462(7271): 307–314.

122. Levin BE. Why some of us get fat and what we can do about it. *Journal of Physiology* 2007; 583(Pt 2): 425–430.

123. Frayling TM, Timpson NJ, Weedon MN, Zeggini E, Freathy RM, Lindgren CM *et al.* A common variant in the FTO gene is associated with body mass index and predisposes to childhood and adult obesity. *Science* 2007; 316(5826): 889–894.

124. Hunter GR, Brock DW, Byrne NM, Chandler-Laney PC, Del Corral P, Gower BA. Exercise training prevents regain of visceral fat for 1 year following weight loss. *Obesity (Silver Spring)* 2010; 18(4): 690–695.

125. Imbeault P, Saint-Pierre S, Almeras N, Tremblay A. Acute effects of exercise on energy intake and feeding behaviour. *British Journal of Nutrition* 1997; 77(4): 511–521.

126. Bauman A, Bellew B, Vita P, Brown W, Owen N. *Getting Australia active: towards better practice for the promotion of physical activity.* National Public Health Partnership: Melbourne, 2002.

127. Wing RR, Hill JO. Successful weight loss maintenance. *Annual Review of Nutrition* 2001; 21: 323–341.

128. Chen SY, Chen SM, Chang WH, Lai CH, Chen MC, Chou CH *et al.* Effect of 2-month detraining on body composition and insulin sensitivity in young female dancers. *International Journal of Obesity (London)* 2006; 30(1): 40–44.

129. Zeller L, Sukenik S. [The association between sports activity and knee osteoarthritis]. *Harefuah* 2008; 147(4): 315–9, 374.
130. Wing RR, Jeffery RW. Prescribed "breaks" as a means to disrupt weight control efforts. *Obesity Research* 2003; 11(2): 287–291.

Index

Also available

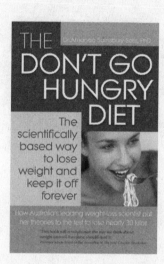

The Don't Go Hungry Diet: The scientifically based way to lose weight and keep it off forever, by Dr Amanda Sainsbury-Salis, PhD, Bantam

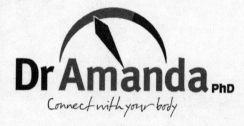

Available from bookstores or www.DrAmandaOnline.com.

Also available from www.DrAmandaOnline.com

- Speaking engagements with Dr Amanda
- Dr Amanda's newsletter
- Live workshops
- Books
- Success Diaries
- Weight loss tools
- Coaching
- Professional training

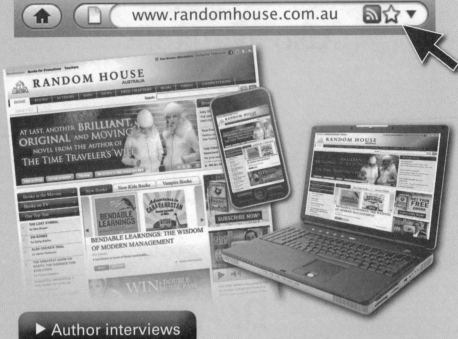